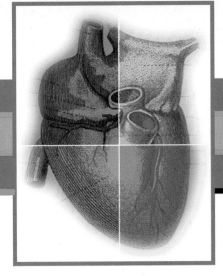

PREHOSPITAL ADVANCED CARDIAC LIFE SUPPORT

SECOND EDITION

Joseph J. Mistovich, M.Ed, NREMT-P
Chairperson and Professor, Department of Health Professions;
Youngstown State University, Youngstown, Ohio

Randall W. Benner, M.Ed, NREMT-P
Program Director, Emergency Medical Technology;
Instructor, Department of Health Professions;
Youngstown State University, Youngstown, Ohio

Gregg S. Margolis, MS, NREMT-P
Assistant Professor of Emergency Medicine,
The George Washington University, Washington, D.C.

Howard A. Werman, M.D., *Medical Editor*
Professor of Clinical Emergency Medicine,
The Ohio State University School of Medicine and Public Health, Columbus, Ohio

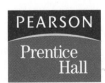

PEARSON
Prentice
Hall

Upper Saddle River, New Jersey 07458

Library of Congress Cataloging-in-Publication Data

Mistovich, Joseph J.

   Prehospital advanced cardiac life support / Joseph J. Mistovich, Randall W. Benner,
Gregg S. Margolis ; Howard A. Werman, medical editor.—2nd ed.

    p. ; cm.

   Rev. ed. of: Advanced cardiac life support. c1998.

   Includes index.

   ISBN 0-13-110143-9 (alk. paper)

   1. Cardiovascular emergencies. 2. Cardiovascular emergencies—Case studies. 3. Life
support systems (Critical Care) I. Benner, Randall W. II. Margolis, Gregg S. III. Werman,
Howard A. IV. Mistovich, Joseph J. Advanced cardiac life support. V. Title.

   [DNLM: 1. Heart Arrest—therapy. 2. Life Support Care. 3. Resuscitation. WG 205
M678p 2004]

RC675.M57 2004

616.1'025—dc22

2003065605

Publisher: Julie Levin Alexander
Publisher's assistant: Regina Bruno
Senior acquisitions editor: Tiffany Price Salter
Senior managing editor for development: Lois Berlowitz
Project manager: Sandy Breuer
Editorial assistant: Joanna Rodzen-Hickey
Senior marketing manager: Katrin Beacom
Channel marketing manager: Rachele Strober
Marketing coordinator: Janet Ryerson
Director of production and manufacturing: Bruce Johnson
Managing editor for production: Patrick Walsh
Production liaison: Julie Li
Production editor: Barbara J. Barg/Navta Associates, Inc.
Copy editor: Terse Stamos
Media editor: John Jordan
Manager of media production: Amy Peltier
New media project manager: Stephen J. Hartner
Manufacturing manager: Ilene Sanford
Manufacturing buyer: Pat Brown
Creative director: Cheryl Asherman
Senior design coordinator: Christopher Weigand
Interior designer: Lee Goldstein
Cover designer: Blair Brown
Composition: Barbara J. Barg/Navta Associates, Inc.
Printing and binding: The Banta Company
Cover printer: Coral Graphics

Notice: The authors and the publisher of this book have taken care to make certain that the equipment and schedules of treatment are correct and compatible with the standards generally accepted at the time of publication. Nevertheless, as new information becomes available, changes in treatment and in the use of equipment and procedures become necessary. The reader is advised to carefully consult the instruction and information material included in each piece of equipment or device before administration. Students are warned that the use of any techniques must be authorized by their medical adviser, where appropriate, in accord with local laws and regulations. The publisher disclaims any liability, loss, injury, or damage incurred as a consequence, directly or indirectly, of the use and application of any of the contents of this book.

Note: The rendition of the heart on the cover and chapter opener pages is an abstract image.

Studentaid.ed.gov, the U.S. Department of Education's website on college planning assistance, is a valuable tool for anyone thinking of pursuing higher education. Designed to help students at all stages of schooling, including international students, returning students, and parents, it is a guide to the financial aid process. The website presents information on applying to and attending college as well as funding your education and repaying loans. It also provides links to useful resources, such as state education agency contact information, assistance in filling out financial aid forms, and various forms of student aid.

Pearson Education LTD.
Pearson Education Australia PTY, Limited
Pearson Education Singapore, Pte. Ltd
Pearson Education North Asia Ltd
Pearson Education Canada, Ltd
Pearson Educación de Mexico, S.A. de C.V.
Pearson Education—Japan
Pearson Education Malaysia, Pte. Ltd

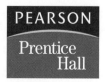

10 9 8 7 6 5 4 3 2 1
ISBN 0-13-110143-9

To my beautiful wife Andrea for her love and encouragement and for being my best friend. To my girls Katie, Kristyn, Chelsea, Morgan, and Kara for their unconditional love and the constant hugs, kisses, smiles, and laughter that make life worth living to its fullest. In memory of my father Paul, who is without any doubt my hero in life.

JJM

I'd like to simply dedicate this work in memory of my mother Rose. While Dad and we five children attempt to continue with life, we know that Mom's love will continue to span all distances—and every measure of time—to influence our thoughts and actions. We miss you, Mom.

RWB

This book is dedicated to my uncle, Gerald Margolis, and the people who cared for him. He survived two out-of-hospital cardiac arrests due to the strength of the chain of survival.

GSM

CONTENTS

◫ CHAPTER 3

AIRWAY MANAGEMENT, VENTILATION, AND OXYGEN THERAPY

35

CHAPTER 4

CHAPTER 5

CHAPTER 6

CHAPTER 7

ELECTRICAL THERAPY: DEFIBRILLATION, CARDIOVERSION, AND CARDIAC PACING   179

CHAPTER 8

PHARMACOLOGICAL THERAPY

CHAPTER 9

CHAPTER 10

CHAPTER 11

CHAPTER 12

CHAPTER 13

▦ CHAPTER 14

SPECIAL TREATMENT CONSIDERATIONS
IN THE PREHOSPITAL ENVIRONMENT   411

Management of acute cardiovascular emergencies requires rapid and decisive actions by advanced level prehospital care personnel. Standardized procedures must be established so that an effective continuum of cardiac care can be provided from the prehospital environment to the emergency department and through the more definitive care that is provided in the cardiac care unit. The approach to emergency cardiac care in the prehospital environment is quite different from that which is provided in the medical facility setting. The uncontrolled environment and limited resources make the provision of emergency cardiac care a challenge to the prehospital care provider. To accommodate the needs of this specialized group of providers, *Prehospital Advanced Cardiac Life Support* presents comprehensive information regarding emergency cardiac care procedures in a condensed format.

Prehospital Advanced Cardiac Life Support contains fourteen chapters that provide the core information necessary to prepare a candidate for the American Heart Association's ACLS Provider course or an equivalent adult advanced cardiac life support course. The information is presented in a logical manner that allows the reader to progresses from a foundation of basic core knowledge to more complex case management material. The first ten chapters are the core knowledge-building chapters. These chapters help the reader comprehend and master the algorithms, emergency cardiac care protocols, and scenarios presented in the later chapters. As the reader progress from one chapter to the next, the information, scenarios, and algorithms become more complex, requiring integration of the knowledge gained from the previous chapters. Review questions at the end of each chapter allow the reader to use the text as an ACLS review manual as well as for the purpose of self-assessment.

Key Features of the Text

Presentation   The material is presented in a logical order that is relevant to the prehospital care provider and that lends itself to continuous reinforcement of previously learned information. The reader is provided a suitable knowledge base before being asked to analyze and apply the knowledge to the understanding of algorithms or scenarios.

In this text, the algorithms are separated and introduced in different chapters. When an algorithm is presented, it is in the chapter in which the background information has prepared the reader to understand the algorithm. Each algorithm and emergency cardiac care protocol is designed to specifically meet the needs of the prehospital care provider.

Case Studies   A brief case study is presented at the beginning of each chapter (with a Case Study Follow-up at the end of the chapter) to reinforce the material presented in the chapter. While each case is specific and relevant to the information in that chapter, it also builds on information that was presented in the previous chapters. For example, the Chapter 5 "ECG Monitoring and Dysrhythmia Recognition" case study focuses on dysrhythmia recognition but also incorporates respiratory and intravenous therapy concepts from the previous two chapters. This cumulative approach to the case studies allows the reader to review previously learned material while applying it to a practical scenario. In Chapter 11, the core case scenarios are presented to help the reader integrate and apply learned knowledge.

Review Questions   Each chapter ends with a set of multiple-choice or short-answer items that can be used for self-assessment and review. The answers, with rationales, are provided in the back of the text. This feature makes the book especially useful for those who need to review when repeating an ACLS course.

Reinforcement   A key feature of this text is the inclusion of four distinct levels of information reinforcement. This systematic reinforcement should aid the reader in mastering the information and in attaining a level of comfort with the knowledge necessary to successfully complete the ACLS course. More important, it should provide efficient emergency cardiac care.

The four levels of information reinforcement include:

▶ Initial introduction of information in a logical progression

▶ Algorithms and emergency care protocols that are introduced at points of relevancy to chapter topics and geared specifically to prehospital care

▶ Case studies that address new information in each chapter while also reinforcing information from prior chapters

▶ Review questions that allow the students to assess their own understanding of the information and determine the need for remediation

The methods of teaching the concepts of emergency cardiac care in this textbook have evolved from the authors' many years of classroom instruction of hundreds of students in ACLS and advanced level emergency cardiac care courses. We have pulled together our experience as educators and clinicians and have compiled what we believe to be the most logical and comprehensive approach to emergency cardiac care in the prehospital environment. We wish you success in your educational and clinical endeavors and hope that you find this textbook a useful resource in expanding your knowledge and developing your skills in emergency cardiac care.

JJM
RWB
GSM

ACKNOWLEDGMENTS

A special thanks to our contributing writers for this edition: **Glenn Miller,** EMS Coordinator, Sharon Regional Health Center, Sharon, Pennsylvania, and **Shawn Salter,** Chief Flight Nurse, San Antonio Airlife, San Antonio, Texas.

Thanks also to **Dr. Howard A. Werman,** Professor of Clinical Emergency Medicine, The Ohio State University School of Medicine and Public Health, Columbus, Ohio. Dr. Werman carefully reviewed all the material in the text. His reviews, insights, and suggestions were greatly appreciated and contributed significantly to the development of this textbook.

We also wish to express appreciation to the following individuals:

Helen Verdream, Secretary, Department of Health Professions, Youngstown State University, for her encouragement and support on a daily basis, and for doing all the extra things that make our work a little easier.

Dr. John J. Yemma, Dean of the College of Health and Human Services, Youngstown State University, for providing Joe Mistovich and Randy Benner with the necessary encouragement to pursue scholarly activities.

Carl Leet, Photographer, Youngstown State University, for his professional photography, flexibility, and great sense of humor.

Chief Gary Borman and **Jack Martin,** firefighters, EMT-Basics, Beaver Township Fire Department, for their willingness to participate in the photography shoots for the benefit of EMS students.

Reviewers

The authors thank the following EMS professionals who reviewed material for the Second Edition of *Prehospital Advanced Cardiac Life Support*. Their insights and assistance are deeply appreciated.

Brenda M. Beasley, RN, BS, EMT-P
Department Chair, Allied Health,
EMS Program Director
Calhoun Community College
Decatur, AL

Jerry Brungardt, BS, CCNREMT-P, EMS-I
Midwest Medical Critical Care Transport Service
Grand Island, NE

S. Christopher Suprun, Jr., NREMT-P
Adjunct Instructor in Emergency Medicine,
The George Washington University
Paramedic Firefighter,
Manassas Park Fire Department
Manassas, VA

Diana Van Wormer
Century College EMS Program Director
White Bear Lake, MN

We also thank the following EMS professionals who reviewed the First Edition of this text. Their suggestions helped to make this program a successful teaching tool.

Brenda M. Beasley, RN, BS, EMT-P
Department Chair, Allied Health,
EMS Program Director
Calhoun Community College
Decatur, AL

Terry Bitterlich, NREMT-P
Safety Training, Ltd.
Albuquerque, NM

Jerry Brungardt, BS, CCNREMT-P, EMS-I
Midwest Medical Critical Care Transport Service
Grand Island, NE

Douglas K. Cline, BSW, NREMT-P
Lead EMS Instructor
Chapel Hill Fire Department
Chapel Hill, NC

Garry L. DeJong, NREMT-P
Flight Paramedic
Albuquerque Fire Department
Albuquerque, NM

Rudy Garrett
Paramedic Training Coordinator
Somerset-Pulaski Co, EMS
West Somerset, KY

Tonnie Glick, RN, MED, CCRN, CRRN
Program Director
Union County College Paramedic Program
Cranford, NJ

Paul R. Hinchey, BA, EMT-P
Paramedic Curriculum Chairperson
Westchester Community College
Valhalla, NY

Lindi Kempfer, MS, EMT-P
EMS Educator
Methodist Hospital of Indiana
Indianapolis, IN

David J. Kuchta, RN, NREMT-P, BSAS
Advance Life Support Coordinator
Division of Emergency Medical Services
Mississippi State Department of Health
Jackson, MS

Baxter Larmon
Associate Professor of Medicine
UCLA School of Medicine
Los Angeles, CA

Danny Marcum, RN, NREMT-P
Flight Nurse Health Net III
Cabell-Huntington Hospital
Huntington, WV

Lori L. Moore, MPH, EMT-P
EMS Director
International Association of Fire Fighters
Washington, DC

Judith Rafkin, RN, CEN
Peninsula Regional Medical Center
Salisbury, MD

Suzann E. Schmele, NREMT-P
Department of Emergency Medicine
School of Medicine
Oregon Health Sciences University
Portland, OR

Randy L. Smith, MS, NREMT-P
National Director EMS Education
Rural/Metro Corporation
Scottsdale, AZ

Richard G. Stump
Betsy Johnson Memorial Hospital
Carey Area EMS
Dunn, NC

Paul A. Werfel, NREMT-P
Paramedic Program Director
SUNY Health Science Center
Stony Brook, NY

Sonya Young, RN, NREMT-P
EMS Coordinator/Emergency Dept.
Good Samaritan Hospital
Cincinnati, OH

ABOUT THE AUTHORS

Joseph J. Mistovich, M.Ed, NREMT-P

Joseph Mistovich is the Chairperson of the Department of Health Professions and a Professor at Youngstown State University in Youngstown, Ohio. He has 18 years of experience as an educator in emergency medical services and multidisciplinary allied health courses, including advanced cardiac life support.

Mr. Mistovich received his Master of Education degree in Community Health Education from Kent State University in 1988. He completed a Bachelor of Science in Applied Science degree with a major in Allied Health in 1985 and an Associate in Applied Science degree in Emergency Medical Technology in 1982 from Youngstown State University. He is also certified as a Nationally Registered Emergency Medical Technician-Paramedic. Mr. Mistovich has over 22 years of experience providing advanced life support in the prehospital environment. He is an author or co-author of several EMS textbooks. He is a frequent presenter at local, state, and national conferences.

Randall W. Benner, M.Ed, NREMT-P

Randall Benner, Instructor in the Department of Health Professions at Youngstown State University, has over 16 years of experience as an educator in emergency medical services and as a field paramedic. He serves as the Director of the Emergency Medical Technology Program at Youngstown State University and is responsible for all levels of emergency medical education. In addition, he actively functions as a paramedic on an advanced life support unit.

Mr. Benner has served as a contributing author for a variety of EMS textbooks and instructor resource materials. He also serves as a medical content reviewer for emergency medical services and allied health publications. He is a contributing author to the revision of the United States Department of Transportation National Standard EMT-Intermediate and Paramedic curricula. He serves on several local, state, and national EMS committees. Mr. Benner is completing his Ph.D program in curriculum and instructional design at Kent State University.

Gregg S. Margolis, MS, NREMT-P

Gregg S. Margolis has been involved in emergency medicine and emergency medical education for over 20 years. He served as a faculty member and in leadership positions in the Departments of Emergency Medicine in two major academic institutions. In addition to his clinical, research, and educational experience, Mr. Margolis served as the Principal Investigator for the development of the Paramedic and EMT-Intermediate National Standard Curricula. He is a renowned expert and frequent lecturer on a variety of topics in emergency medicine and the author of dozens of publications. Mr. Margolis consults nationally and internationally in emergency medical services development and education.

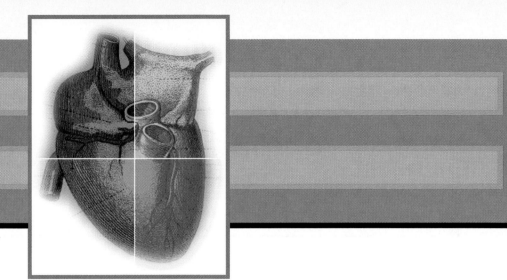

Key Concepts of Advanced Cardiac Life Support for Prehospital Care Providers

Prior to the inception of prehospital care, when an individual went into cardiac arrest and spontaneous respirations and circulation ceased, it would often mean the person would die. This grim reality, though, has slowly changed since the inception and provision of emergency medical care. Such care, when delivered in an precise and expedient fashion, can promote the return of spontaneous respirations and circulation. The overriding goal is the return of cerebral perfusion before the brain becomes permanently damaged. As such, the goal of both basic and advanced cardiac life support is to restore the cardiac rhythm and myocardial contractility as quickly as possible so that the patient can, ultimately, regain both physical health and cognitive ability. Since the success of this endeavor is so inextricably time dependent, the role of the prehospital care provider is of utmost importance.

This chapter presents an overview of key concepts of advanced cardiac life support as it applies to the prehospital environment.

Topics in this chapter are:

Key Elements of Prehospital Cardiac Resuscitation

Legal and Ethical Considerations in Prehospital Cardiac Resuscitation

 The key icon marks each key element of cardiac resuscitation.

CASE STUDY

"Medic 107—respond code 3 to 2234 West Chalmers for a 48-year-old male patient who is pulseless and apneic. YFD is on the scene. This is a confirmed nonbreather. AED has been initiated. Time out 0923 hours."

▦ INTRODUCTION

Prehospital care providers on a daily basis encounter scenarios like the one above. For many patients in the out-of-hospital environment, cardiac arrest may be the first indication that the patient has been suffering some type of coronary artery disease. Unfortunately, a large number of these patients do not survive, and therefore they never get a chance to receive medical treatment to correct the condition. However, through organized resuscitative efforts by well-educated prehospital providers, survival rates may be significantly improved.

To maximize the effectiveness of the resuscitation effort, the following knowledge areas and skills must be mastered:

- ▶ Basic and advanced airway management
- ▶ Ventilation and oxygen techniques
- ▶ Ability to recognize and manage the following cardiovascular conditions:
  - – bradycardia
  - – tachycardia
  - – acute myocardial infarction (AMI)
  - – hypotension
  - – cardiogenic shock
  - – pulmonary edema
  - – stroke
- ▶ Ability to recognize and manage lethal dysrhythmias including:
  - – ventricular fibrillation (VF, or V-fib)/pulseless ventricular tachycardia (VT, or V-tach)
  - – pulseless electrical activity (PEA)
  - – asystole/agonal rhythm
- ▶ Electrical therapy to include defibrillation, cardioversion, and transcutaneous pacing
- ▶ Intravenous therapy techniques, medication administration, and invasive monitoring
- ▶ Ability to recognize and manage the following dysrhythmias:
  - – artifact
  - – bradycardias
  - – tachycardias
  - – atrial dysrhythmias
  - – sinus rhythm
  - – pacemaker rhythms
  - – morphologic electrocardiogram (ECG) changes associated with myocardial ischemia and acute MI

▶ Ability to determine the actions, indications, dose, administration, precautions, and contraindications of the cardiovascular medications used in resuscitation of patients suffering a cardiovascular crisis

▶ Ability to recognize special considerations that necessitate specific treatment modalities in the prehospital environment for the patient suffering from:

   – stroke

   – traumatic cardiac arrest

   – drowning or submersion emergencies

   – hypothermia

   – cardiac arrest when pregnant

   – electrocution and lightning strikes

   – drug overdose

   – electrolyte imbalances

The topics listed above will all be addressed in the course of this book. However, there are several key elements that you should become acquainted with before you begin and that you should keep in mind throughout your preparation for advanced cardiac life support in the dynamic field of Emergency Medical Services—as well as throughout your career as an ACLS practitioner.

KEY ELEMENTS OF PREHOSPITAL CARDIAC RESUSCITATION

Certain elements are crucial to the efficiency of resuscitation efforts for patients suffering cardiac arrest or cardiovascular or cardiopulmonary compromise in the prehospital environment. These key elements must be considered for every patient, since the patient's survival may depend on them (Table 1-1).

TABLE 1–1 **Key Elements of Cardiac Resuscitation**

 Adapt cardiac arrest assessment and care to the prehospital environment.

 Learn how to handle the stress of prehospital resuscitation.

 Cerebral resuscitation is the fundamental goal.

 Treat the patient—not the rhythm.

 Basic-to-advanced life support is a continuum of care.

 Time to CPR and time to defibrillation are critical factors.

 Manage conditions that may lead to cardiac arrest.

 Care does not stop after successful resuscitations.

 The phase-response approach provides a standardized structure.

 Use judgment and seek medical direction regarding futile resuscitation attempts.

 Apply the chain of survival to all situations.

Cardiac Arrest in the Prehospital Environment

The application of the principles taught in advanced cardiac life support may sometimes be difficult to achieve in the prehospital environment. Many times the dynamics at the scene may leave the prehospital care provider in a situation in which "optimal" care is difficult to achieve unless you have the ability to critically (yet rapidly) determine what should be done on-scene, in the back of the EMS unit, or while en route to the hospital. You, the prehospital care provider, must realize that many aspects of a "traditional" ACLS course may not be applicable to the prehospital environment. Consider, for example, the following arrest situations: an elderly male patient collapses while at a movie theater, a middle age construction worker is trapped in an industrial accident, a young patient is shot down over a drug deal gone bad, or a female patient is found by her family in her bed in cardiac arrest. In all these situations, the patient is in need of airway management, ventilatory support, cardiac compressions, ECG monitoring, and medication administration. However, each scenario's dynamics may be impacted by the number of rescue personnel available, if there is safe access to the patient and space to provide care, extrication to the EMS unit, or even the availability of a nearby emergency departments. Any care provider with enough field experience realizes that EMS is about applying assessment and care guidelines in environments that are constantly changing.

EMS providers know that no two motor-vehicle collisions are exactly alike, no two MI patients are exactly alike, nor are two cardiac arrest scenarios exactly alike. Therefore, the prehospital provider of advanced cardiac life support must be able to adjust his assessment and treatment approach based on the patient's needs and the dynamics of the environment. This is especially true for the patient in cardiac arrest, since such a patient requires application of the most critical assessment and treatment skills taught to EMS providers. Critical thinking and decision-making skills are perhaps your most valuable allies. During your career as a prehospital provider, you will see patients and scenes that defy any of what you learned on textbook cases. However, if you are prepared with the most up-to-date knowledge as is presented in this text and then think critically and decisively about the scenarios, you will be on the right path to becoming an effective prehospital provider of advanced cardiac life support.

The Stress of Prehospital Resuscitation

EMS, obviously, can be very stressful. A cardiac arrest scenario is both a dramatic and emotionally charged event for the provider, family members, and others at the scene. You must concentrate on your critical assessment findings and apply numerous skills under the pressure of maintaining the shortest on-scene time possible. Family and friends on scene contribute to the emotional charge that surrounds a cardiac arrest. These factors, along with failed attempts at resuscitation (even when everything possible was done), can promote both emotional and physical symptoms that long outlast the original emergency. There is nothing wrong with the provider who experiences apprehension, anger, anxiety, or even grief following a cardiac arrest scenario. However, if these feelings become overwhelming and intrude into the provider's everyday life, the ramifications could be serious. Such overwhelming responses, normally referred to as "burn-out" in EMS circles, are destructive and need to be mediated.

Mental health care specialists are well aware of common reactions by providers or families who bear witness to highly charged events. These specialists recommend that the best way for providers, as well as the witnesses, to initially reduce stress is to simply talk about the event. The act of sitting down and sharing how you felt and hearing about the feelings of others allows for a certain degree of closure for all involved. Additionally, the availability of specially trained individuals in facilitating this discussion may prove beneficial, as would the initiation of a CISD team. Always remember that these feelings are normal. They simply mean that you are human, and that you care about what you do as a prehospital provider and the patients who are recipients of your care. When a patient dies despite your best efforts it is devastating, but it is an equal travesty when the stress inherent to the profession ultimately steals another excellent prehospital provider away.

Cerebral Resuscitation: The Fundamental Goal

When performing basic and advanced cardiac life support, it is important to remember the most fundamental goal of resuscitation: *Restart the heart to restore the brain.*

Resuscitating a patient to the point where he is neurologically intact, or at least is near neurologic capacity prior to cardiac arrest, is the ultimate goal of resuscitation. Restarting hearts alone is not an adequate concept of cardiac resuscitation. For this reason, Peter Safar introduced the concept of cardio-pulmonary-cerebral resuscitation (CPCR), where as much emphasis is placed on cerebral resuscitation as on cardiac resuscitation. While many of your assessment and intervention modalities may seem to be focused purely on cardiac activity, it is done so only to maintain a viable brain. Hence, starting the heart is the first step in restoring cerebral perfusion. Cerebral resuscitation involves concerns such as cerebral perfusion pressures, oxygenation, temperature control, and drug therapies, which will be discussed in Chapter 14.

Treat the Patient—Not the Rhythm

Whether in or out of the hospital, a patient in cardiac arrest is a highly charged and dramatic situation (Figure 1-1). In a circumstance like this, it is easy to lose the ability to think calmly, to see the whole picture, and to proceed in a systematic fashion.

In an emotionally charged situation, it is human nature to focus on a task which is very familiar or "safe." Subsequently, prehospital providers often develop tunnel vision and concentrate on only one skill, such as intubating the patient or starting an IV. Unfortunately, they forget to focus on other important aspects of patient care such as chest compressions, dysrhythmia recognition, and defibrillation. Remember, never treat the rhythm without considering the probable etiology (cause) of the cardiac arrest and the rhythm itself. Ask yourself, "Why is this patient in cardiac arrest?" "Why is the patient in this rhythm?" You must focus on

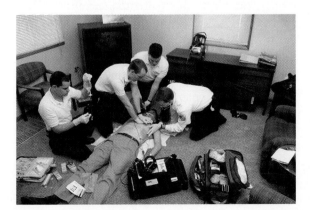

FIGURE 1–1
A cardiac arrest is a high-drama situation. Make an effort to remain calm, think clearly, and consider the big picture. "Treat the patient—not the rhythm."

treating possible causes of the problem, such as hypoxia caused by an airway obstruction. You must constantly concentrate on ensuring an adequate airway, providing effective ventilation and oxygenation, providing effective artificial circulation, administering the appropriate medications, and defibrillating the appropriate rhythms—never allowing yourself to focus on just one of these skills.

Basic-to-Advanced Life Support: A Continuum

A clear line of demarcation where basic life support stops and advanced life support begins no longer exists. Many first responders are now providing defibrillation by automated external defibrillator. Emergency Medical Technician-Basics in many states are now taught to perform tracheal intubation or use other advanced airway devices. The continuum begins with basic cardiac life support (BCLS), assuring an open airway and external cardiac compressions (or CPR), which is vital to resuscitation—and which must be performed anywhere along the continuum of care when it is needed. Advanced cardiac life support (ACLS) is at the other end of the continuum with medication administration, continued defibrillation, cardiac pacing, and other more advanced techniques. Between basic and advanced cardiac life support is intermediate cardiac life support, which is defined on a case-by-case basis.

The key is to develop a response team of trained individuals who can provide basic life support and defibrillation at the earliest possible time, followed by providers with more advanced cardiac life support techniques. Nevertheless, as an advanced life support provider, you cannot forget your BCLS skills. Administering intravenous medication is of no value if your cardiac compressions are so inadequate they do not allow for core circulation of the drug. If you cannot deliver defibrillations in an expedient fashion that does not interrupt CPR for too long a time, the patient's neurologic condition will significantly worsen, and your interventions will have only delayed the inevitable. There may come a time in your career as a prehospital provider of advanced cardiac life support when you will be the first or the only one on-scene and the only treatment modalities available will be your BCLS skills. Then the old adage "You must be a good EMT-B first" will ring true.

Remember, each cardiac arrest situation is unique. To this end, you will work with various prehospital providers with differing levels of knowledge, skills, experience, and *personalities*. It is essential that you take into consideration the differing capabilities of those working with you. Whether you are working with three other ALS providers, a new EMT-Basic, or someone you have never met, keep in mind that you are all there on the patient's behalf. Flexibility is of utmost importance. Inevitably, things will go wrong, but remember the place to discuss antagonistic differences or concerns about the arrest is not at the patient's bedside. These concerns are best handled administratively or in conjunction with your EMS system's medical director.

Time: A Critical Factor

Time is one of the most critical factors that will determine the success of resuscitation and patient outcome. With each passing minute, the chances of successfully resuscitating a *neurologically intact* patient decline.

Time to CPR is one crucial variable. Irreversible brain damage begins to occur 4 to 6 minutes following cessation of blood flow. If performed promptly, CPR will extend the time during which successful resuscitation is possible; however, CPR alone usually does not lead to successful resuscitation.

Time to defibrillation is another crucial variable. With each minute that passes by, the success rate of defibrillation declines. After 10 minutes, it is likely that the patient will have deteriorated from a rhythm that could have been defibrillated to a rhythm that cannot be defibrillated. Likewise, even if the rhythm is still one that can be defibrillated, the myocardium has become too hypoxic and acidotic and thus is no longer conducive to successful defibrillation. In addition, it is likely that the brain has suffered significant irreversible damage. The survivability of a patient in ventricular fibrillation who has not been defibrillated within 10 minutes following cardiac arrest approaches zero. This is why early defibrillation takes precedence even over chest compressions and ventilation.

Two other factors that are considered time critical are early definitive airway management by tracheal intubation to prevent potential aspiration, and early administration of epinephrine to augment cerebral and coronary perfusion. Never forget the impact of time on successful resuscitation. In fact, every action that you perform in the prehospital environment should be weighed against its contribution to patient survivability and the time in which it takes to perform the intervention.

Manage Conditions That May Lead to a Cardiac Arrest

"Treat the patient and not the monitor" is a concept that applies to a possible pre-arrest as well as to an arrest situation. Identify conditions that are likely to cause the patient to deteriorate to cardiac arrest and manage them—for example, MI or chest pain. The ability to recognize these prearrest conditions and provide rapid emergency care is critical.

Remember also that cardiac arrest is not its own diagnosis; rather it is the manifestation of the failure of some other organ or organ system in response to something. For example, pulseless electrical activity (PEA) occurs when the cardiac monitor shows an ECG rhythm that is capable of producing a pulse but does not. This is a situation where the electrical activity of the heart is present but adequate cardiac contraction or movement of blood is not. So while the manifestation (or clinical symptomatology) is cardiac arrest, the *cause* may be an undiagnosed spontaneous pneumothorax that developed into a tension pneumothorax in the elderly COPD patient. Therefore, the failure to identify and decompress the pneumothorax will doom all other efforts.

Care Does Not Stop After Successful Resuscitation

Once the pulse is regained and the patient is "resuscitated," the battle is not over. You must be prepared to handle the postarrest patient as efficiently as you managed the patient while in cardiac arrest. Without proper care, the patient can easily suffer from hypoperfusion, become hypoxic, or even deteriorate back into cardiac arrest.

The Phased-Response Approach: A Standardized Structure

In order to achieve success with the aforementioned elements of a successful resuscitation, planning is of paramount importance. The American Heart Association has developed a phased-response approach to any cardiac arrest scenario (Table 1-2). This approach provides a standardized structure that should be applied during every cardiac arrest event.

Phase 1: Anticipation
This phase, for prehospital advanced cardiac life support providers, includes the anticipation of the cardiac arrest. For EMS, this would include the presence and

TABLE 1–2	The Phased-Response Approach
Phase 1	Anticipation
Phase 2	Transfer/Reception
Phase 3	Resuscitation
Phase 4	Maintenance
Phase 5	Family Notification
Phase 6	Transfer
Phase 7	Critical Incident Stress Debriefing (or Critique Process)

proper functioning of equipment integral to arrest management (cardiac monitor, ACLS drugs, portable suction unit, etc.), identifying the team leader and the responsibilities of other providers (e.g., who intubates, who administers medications), knowing where the closest emergency department is, and so on.

Phase 2: Transfer/Reception
The transfer or reception phase occurs when the patient enters into health care. For our purposes, it is when the cardiac arrest is identified and EMS summoned, or when the patient goes into arrest in the presence of the prehospital provider. In either situation, the team leader identifies himself as the resuscitation begins, airway, breathing, circulation are assessed, and cardiac arrest management ensues.

Phase 3: Resuscitation
Resuscitation efforts should adhere to and focus on the ABCs: airway, breathing, and circulation. The team leader must be decisive and provide direction to the team; however, he must also be open to and seek suggestions from the other team members. Orders must be precise and clearly stated. The team leader's voice, inflection, and attitude can set the stage for the whole resuscitation.

Team members must seek clarification of any orders that are unclear or questionable. Team members must state aloud when procedures are completed or medications have been administered.

Phase 4: Maintenance
In this phase, the patient is stabilized and secured. Attention should be continuously directed to maintaining the airway, breathing, and circulation.

Phase 5: Family Notification
The family may be present during the resuscitation and witness the outcome. If the family is not present or choose not to be present, they should be advised that resuscitation efforts have begun and be updated as appropriate. The family is, of course, notified of the outcome of the resuscitation. The outcome that is relayed may be positive or negative. Be prepared to deliver the message with empathy, sensitivity, and honesty.

Phase 6: Transfer
The patient transfer must be as smooth a transition as possible. Patient care is assumed by a team of equal or higher qualifications and expertise, and most commonly occurs upon arrival inside the emergency department of the receiving hospital. It is essential that proper information be relayed with the patient.

Phase 7: Critical Incident Stress Debriefing (or Critique Process)

A critique of the resuscitation should be conducted regardless of the patient outcome and length of resuscitation time. This educational process provides critical feedback on the team's efforts. It also may be a time for defusing and grieving. It is always important to recognize the effects of stress on yourself as well as your partner or team. Initiation of the CISD team to help resolve any issues fosters the continued good mental health necessary to perform the job.

Use Judgment about Futile Resuscitation Attempts

There are those patients that you will encounter that have simply reached the end of their life and need to die with dignity. Resuscitation can be very demeaning and undignified to these patients and health care providers alike. Be decisive and use good judgment in determining when to start and when to stop resuscitation efforts. Be familiar with and follow your local guidelines, policies, procedures, or protocols. Seek medical direction regarding such decisions. **Out-of-hospital and hospital personnel need to have considered when to start and stop resuscitation BEFORE care is needed.**

Apply the Chain of Survival to All Situations

The basic concepts of the chain of survival, as recognized by the American Heart Association, apply to patients in out-of-hospital and hospital environments (Figure 1-2). The continuum of care must not be jeopardized as the patient is moved from the out-of-hospital to the hospital setting. It is a team effort on the part of out-of-hospital, emergency-department, and critical-care team members.

The chain of survival has four distinct but interrelated links:

▶ **Early access**—recognition of the cardiac event, activating the appropriate response and resources, and seeking the necessary equipment

▶ **Early CPR**—performance of basic life support skills as early as possible

▶ **Early defibrillation**—providing defibrillation of ventricular fibrillation and pulseless ventricular tachycardia at the earliest possible point

▶ **Early ACLS**—rapid advanced-cardiac-life-support intervention following initiation of basic life support and early defibrillation

A break in any link of the chain of survival will reduce the chances for successful resuscitation. The components of each link may vary, depending on the setting and whether the cardiac arrest occurs out of hospital or in the hospital. However, in order to reduce the number of out-of-hospital cardiac arrest deaths, phases of response must be thought out and planned for in advance.

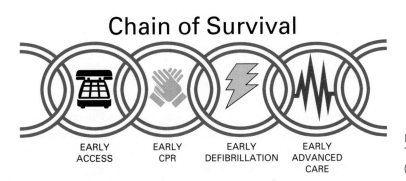

FIGURE 1–2
The chain of survival.
(American Heart Association)

Strengthening the Chain of Survival

As with any chain, the weakest link will define the strength of the chain. To this end, reduction in cardiac arrest death rates is dependent on the concerted efforts and teamwork of the community, prehospital care providers, hospitals, and long-term rehabilitation facilities. For example, the most sophisticated EMS system with the most advanced emergency departments are of little use if the community does not know how to access EMS. Efforts to strengthen the chain should be ongoing. The perception that the continuum of care is ideal can lead to complacency. Always strive for ways to improve your system.

LEGAL AND ETHICAL CONSIDERATIONS IN PREHOSPITAL CARDIAC RESUSCITATION

Cardiac resuscitation must be initiated unless an attempt to resuscitate is clearly futile according to medical direction or local guidelines and protocols or there is a binding legal directive not to proceed.

Every patient who is deemed competent and capable of making a rational decision has the legal right to refuse medical care, including basic and advanced cardiac resuscitation. For the competent patient to refuse care it is not required that the patient be suffering from a terminal illness, nor that family members agree with the decision, nor that approval be obtained from the physicians or hospital administrators.

When the patient is unable to make an informed or rational decision at the time medical intervention is needed—for example, when the patient is already in cardiac arrest and unresponsive—the provider must rely on the presence and availability of any advance directives (wishes on intents the patient had previously expressed, either orally or in writing) or decisions rendered by a legal surrogate (such as a relative who has been given a power of attorney to make health care decisions for the patient).

Living Wills and Advance Directives

In 1991, the Patient Self-Determination Act acknowledged the right of a person to make decisions regarding the medical care he may receive at any time, including at the end of life. When a person anticipates that he may, at some future time, lose the ability to make an informed or rational decision regarding his own medical care or resuscitation, he may make his wishes known in advance of such an event. Commonly, these wishes are discussed with family, friends, or health care providers. However, for obvious reasons, oral directives are considered less trustworthy than directives that are written, and unwitnessed written directives are considered less trustworthy than witnessed written directives.

Most states have passed legislation that provides some way for citizens to help ensure that their wishes will be followed, or their best interests taken into consideration, if they become unable to make such decisions themselves. Some states recognize "living wills." In a living will, *the person* states his desires regarding care in the event he becomes terminally ill and incapable of making decisions regarding his medical care. In other states, a person is permitted to designate a surrogate, or proxy—usually a close relative or friend—who holds a "durable power of attorney" to make health care decisions for the person if he becomes unable to do so for himself. In contrast to the living will, a durable power of attorney for health care applies to any medical situation, not just terminal illness.

An advance directive is not the same thing as a living will. Where the living will is the *person's* desires regarding their care in light of an unforeseen emergency, an advance directive is written by the person's *attending physician* in response to the person's current medical situation and in light of any available living will. In the absence of a living will (which is usually the case), the physician prepares the advance directive guided by his medical expertise and in consultation with available family members.

For any type of prepared advance directive to be effective, of course, the prehospital care providers must know about it. The optimal situation is when a legal document is present and can be verified before treatment begins. This is why persons who have such advance wishes and legal documents, must make an effort to discuss them with and to provide copies to their physicians, medical facilities, and prehospital services that are likely to treat them.

Very often, of course, this will not have happened when you are in a situation where care and resuscitation decisions have to be made immediately. In these circumstances, you must rely on your own judgment and common sense as well as on local protocols and, when possible, orders from the physician or the medical director in charge. Ultimately, it is your responsibility to be cognizant of the laws in your state governing these issues. If there is any doubt, initiate full advanced cardiac life support resuscitation.

Do-Not-Attempt-Resuscitation Orders

Patients with serious illnesses, whether they are in or out of the hospital, often discuss do-not-attempt-resuscitation (DNAR) orders with their physician. These orders stipulate to what extent resuscitation, if any, should be conducted if the patient deteriorates to cardiac arrest. However, such stipulations should *not* be taken to imply that other forms of patient care or management must be limited or discontinued. It is important to note that some forms of care may be limited by the patient himself. Although DNAR orders may exist, it is important to recognize that other medical treatments may be appropriate and acceptable, such as administration of antidysrhythmics or fluids. Oxygen is considered a standard comfort measure and should be administered to all patients who require it.

As of yet, the terminology regarding no-resuscitation orders has not been standardized. A variety of terms are still in use and may be confusing. The term *do not resuscitate (DNR)* implies that resuscitation would be successful if performed. Since resuscitation efforts often are not successful, the term *do not attempt resuscitation (DNAR)* may be more reflective of the chances of successfully resuscitating a patient. The term *no CPR* may be used to indicate that CPR should not be initiated or continued in the event of cardiac arrest. All three terms—*do not resuscitate (DNR), do not attempt resuscitation (DNAR),* and *no CPR*—have essentially the same meaning and are often used interchangeably.

DNR, DNAR, or no-CPR orders must not be confused with other kinds of advance wishes such as living wills. Just because a living will or other advance directive exists, it does not necessarily mean that the patient wants CPR or resuscitation withheld. For example, a living will may stipulate that the patient does not want long-term efforts such as prolonged use of a ventilator, but may not prohibit short-term resuscitation efforts such as CPR and defibrillation. Living wills and other sorts of advance directives must be interpreted by a physician and must not be automatically used as, or in place of, a DNR, DNAR, or no-CPR order.

Initiation or cessation of patient resuscitation in both the out-of-hospital and hospital setting often poses ethical dilemmas. As stated earlier, it is imperative that you follow the guidelines or protocols for resuscitation established by the prehospital medical director or hospital ethics committee, legal counsel, and medical directors.

When Not to Start Resuscitation

Death is an inevitable part of the life process. And that reality is one that health care professionals deal with on a daily basis. These professionals have developed specific criteria to use when developing protocol for those situations in which resuscitation should not be started. As always, the medical director of the EMS service should play an integral role in the adoption of these guidelines:

▶ The patient has a valid DNAR order (or such form utilized by your EMS system)

▶ The patient has obvious signs of death

– rigor mortis

– dependent lividity

– decapitation

– hemicorporectomy (severed trunk)

Termination of Resuscitative Efforts

A current trend among EMS systems is termination of resuscitative effort in the prehospital setting. This is to avoid continued investment of prehospital resources on a patient whose cardiac arrest survival is extremely improbable. Research has shown that in the absence of extenuating factors (e.g., hypothermia, cold water immersion, drug overdose), the following guidelines can be used to determine whether to terminate resuscitative efforts prehospitally:

▶ Known arrest time onset with immediate initiation of CPR

and

▶ > 30 minutes of continued BCLS

▶ Application of electrical therapy when needed (i.e., defibrillation)

▶ Successful tracheal intubation with bilateral breath sounds

▶ IV initiation

▶ Administration of appropriate pharmacology based on rhythm and arrest dynamics

▶ Absence of any positive cardiovascular response to appropriately delivered ACLS measures

▶ Consultation with the receiving emergency department physician to discuss termination of efforts

▶ The ECG rhythm upon termination is asystole

It is becoming more common practice that resuscitative efforts be terminated, and the patient be transported to the emergency department or wherever appropriate based upon local protocol for confirmation of death. Upon termination of efforts, however, the focus shifts from the deceased patient to the family and/or friends on scene. Depending on your EMS system protocols, prehospital providers must now tell the family why resuscitation has been halted and also handle the grief that accompanies such notification. EMS providers may also be called on to help the distraught family begin the next phase of funeral arrangements by placing necessary phone calls, notifying the family physician, and the like. To assist with this commonly uncomfortable situation, protocols should be clearly written to delineate how involved EMS providers should become.

▦ SUMMARY

To maximize the effectiveness of the resuscitation effort, it is essential to master the knowledge and skills relevant to basic and advanced airway management, ventilation and oxygenation, management of cardiovascular compromises, electrical therapy, IV therapy and invasive monitoring, recognition and management of lethal dysrhythmias, recognition and management of nonlethal dysrhythmias, administration of cardiovascular medications used in resuscitation, and recognition and early management for a variety of special resuscitation situations.

Certain key elements must be considered for every patient suffering cardiac arrest or cardiovascular or cardiopulmonary compromise. These include understanding the dynamic environment of prehospital arrest scenarios; inherent stress encountered on the part of the providers and others on scene; cerebral resuscitation; treating the patient, not the rhythm (keeping the big picture of patient care in mind, including airway, ventilation, oxygenation, medications, and defibrillation of appropriate rhythms); consideration of ACLS as part of a continuum of basic-to-advanced life support; consideration of time as a critical factor in successful resuscitation; management of conditions that may lead to cardiac arrest; continuation of care after successful resuscitation; applying the chain of survival to all situations; using judgment about futile resuscitations; and applying the phased-response approach to all cardiac arrest events.

It is important to be aware that patients may have given advance directives on their wishes regarding resuscitation. These advance directives may be oral or written, informal statements or legal documents. There may also be do-not-attempt-resuscitation orders that the patient has discussed with his physician or has presented as a written legal document. Use judgment and follow state and local guidelines or protocols regarding advance directives. If there is any doubt, initiate full resuscitation.

REVIEW QUESTIONS

1. One of the major goals of patient management during resuscitation is to
   a. determine the etiology of the cardiac arrest and the ECG rhythm.
   b. focus on the ECG rhythm and treat it according to the algorithm.
   c. provide medications prior to any electrical therapy or advanced airway management.
   d. administer as many medications as possible via the tracheal route to enhance absorption.

2. The most critical factor that influences successful defibrillation is the
   a. energy level at which defibrillation is performed.
   b. amount of transthoracic resistance.
   c. time delay to defibrillation.
   d. ability to administer medications prior to defibrillation.

3. Which of the following is **not** a link in the chain of survival?
   a. early access
   b. early CPR
   c. early prevention
   d. early ACLS

4. A patient has the legal right to refuse medical care only if
   a. the patient is suffering from a terminal illness.
   b. the family is in agreement with the decision.
   c. the physician agrees and acquires approval from the hospital administrator.
   d. the patient is deemed competent and capable of making a rational decision.

5. You encounter a patient in cardiac arrest. The family presents a do-not-attempt-resuscitation (DNAR) order. There is a question regarding the validity of the order. You should immediately
   a. contact the patient's family physician to verify the order.
   b. begin full advanced cardiac life support resuscitation until the order can be clarified.
   c. begin and continue basic life support until the family physician is contacted.
   d. consult the family regarding the validity of the order.

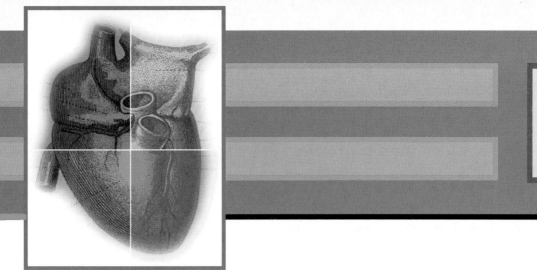

Systematic Approach to Emergency Cardiac Care: The Primary and Secondary Surveys

Emergency medical service personnel are accustomed to the familiar assessment steps often known as the ABCDs, or the primary and secondary survey. These steps have been adapted to provide a systematic approach to assessing and managing a patient who is in a prearrest state, cardiac arrest, postresuscitation state, or a patient who is suffering from a cardiopulmonary emergency.

Following the simple mnemonics of the primary and secondary survey for emergency cardiac care will ensure that the necessary basic and advanced care procedures are conducted in an organized and efficient sequence. It will counteract the tendency of some emergency medical service personnel to skip vital basic procedures and proceed directly to more advanced and dramatic skills such as placement of an tracheal tube or administration of medication. It will also provide each member of the resuscitation team with a clearer understanding of his or her role in the resuscitation effort.

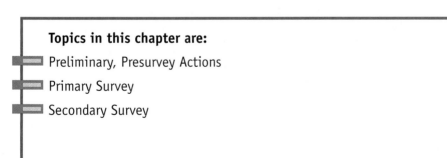

Topics in this chapter are:

Preliminary, Presurvey Actions

Primary Survey

Secondary Survey

CASE STUDY

You are summoned to an extended care facility for a patient in possible cardiac arrest. As you enter the room, you find the 58-year-old male patient lying motionless in bed. He is ashen gray. You quickly ask the wife, "How long has he been like this?" as you step to the patient's side. The wife states, "Oh, only a few minutes, I think. He looked as if he was resting so peacefully."

How would you proceed to assess and care for this patient? This chapter will describe the systematic assessment of a patient in cardiac arrest or suffering a cardiorespiratory emergency. Later, we will return to the case and apply the procedures learned.

INTRODUCTION

A systematic approach to providing care for patients suffering cardiac arrest or a cardiorespiratory emergency will assure a more organized resuscitation attempt. Also, it will lessen each emergency medical service personnel's confusion as to his or her exact responsibility and the progression of the resuscitation.

A simple approach using an "ABCD" mnemonic for both a primary and secondary survey has been developed.[1] This approach provides standard guidelines that can easily be applied to all prearrest, actual arrest, and postarrest or postresuscitation situations. In addition, if you ever reach a point where you are not sure what direction you should take next, you can step back and repeat the ABCDs to ensure that all necessary care is being provided.

Even before you conduct the primary and secondary surveys, there are some preliminary actions that must be performed. The results of these preliminary actions may determine how you will proceed in your resuscitation efforts. The preliminary actions are followed by a basic primary survey that does not involve invasive techniques, which in turn is followed by a more advanced secondary survey that requires invasive techniques of management and greater attention to determining the cause of the cardiac related problem. Both the primary and the secondary survey use the mnemonic ABCD, but the letters stand for something slightly different in each survey (Figure 2-1).

The remainder of this chapter will discuss the specifics of the preliminary actions, the primary survey, and the secondary survey for emergency cardiac care.

PRELIMINARY, PRESURVEY ACTIONS

Before providing any noninvasive or invasive care—before the "A" of the primary survey—you must take a few preliminary steps. You must assess your own safety before you approach the patient, and you must assess the patient's level of responsiveness, call for help, position the patient, and position the members of the resuscitation team as they enter the scene or resuscitation room.

Assess the Scene for Safety Hazards

Ensure your own safety before approaching any emergency scene. Keep in mind the environment that is thought to be controlled can just as easily become uncon-

[1]American Heart Association, *Textbook of Advanced Cardiac Life Support,* 1994: 1-4–1-10.

SYSTEMATIC APPROACH TO EMERGENCY CARDIAC CARE

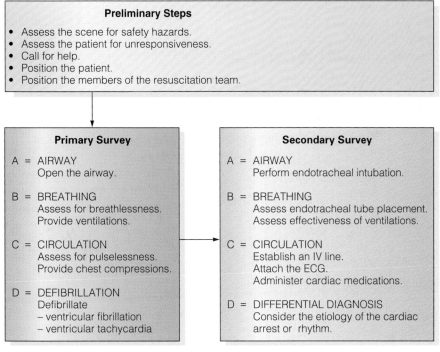

FIGURE 2–1
Systematic approach to emergency cardiac care.

trolled and hazardous. As an example, the cause of the cardiac arrest, dysrhythmia, or cardiac related emergency may be due to inhalation of a toxic substance. If you are not aware of the scene hazards, you may also fall victim to the hazardous substance. Likewise, the cardiac arrest may be the result of a traumatic incident such as a shooting or stabbing. Do not become complacent, regardless of the environment you are in.

The cardiac arrest or cardiorespiratory patient typically presents a highly charged scene; therefore it is easy for the EMT or paramedic to become totally engrossed in what care he or she is going to provide, develop tunnel vision while approaching the scene, and not use all of his or her senses to identify potential scene safety hazards. Many violent altercations have erupted, literally over patients in cardiac arrest. Emergency medical service personnel can easily walk into these scenes when they are too hasty in approaching the patient.

The out-of-hospital environment is very uncontrolled and unforgiving, with a myriad of potential hazards. The basic principle is: If the scene is not safe, either make it safe without jeopardizing your own life, or retreat until it is made safe by law enforcement, fire service, or other appropriate agencies.

Assess the scene for clues to and evidence of the nature of the emergency, such as pill bottles, unusual odors, and mechanisms of traumatic injury. Ask questions of bystanders or relatives who are at the scene who may be able to provide information regarding the events prior to the cardiac arrest or cardiac emergency. Attempt to determine the medications the patient is taking by looking on nightstands, medicine cabinets, in bathrooms, next to the sink, or in refrigerators. This information may not be recoverable or available to the emergency department personnel once you leave the scene.

Always remember the necessity of taking infection-control precautions for personal protection. Latex or vinyl gloves and eye protection must be used to reduce the risk of infectious disease transmission through contact with body fluids. The EMT or paramedic responsible for managing the airway should also use a surgical mask or a face shield that includes the mask. There is a risk of spatters and sprays from ventilation, suction, and advanced airway maneuvers that may cause contamination of the EMS provider through the nose, mouth, or eye.

Assess for Unresponsiveness

When you first come in contact with the patient, you must determine the level of responsiveness. If the patient is not obviously alert with his eyes open as you approach him, you would gently shake the person and shout, "Are you OK?" and "Open your eyes." If the patient does not respond to the verbal stimuli, quickly apply some type of painful stimuli such as a trapezius pinch, pinch to the web between the thumb and index finger, or a sternal rub. If you suspect that the patient has suffered some type of trauma that may have injured the spinal column, do not shake and shout. Obviously, shaking can further destabilize the spinal column and shouting may cause the patient to move his head or body. Instead, "touch and talk" to the possible spine-injured patient.[2]

You must keep the suspected trauma patient's cervical spine in a neutral, in-line position with the remainder of the spine as straight as possible. Ideally, bring the head and neck into a neutral in-line position and maintain manual stabilization. Do this by bringing the nose in line with the umbilicus and keeping the head and neck neutral without any extension or flexion (Figure 2-2). Keep in mind that any manipulation of the cervical spine, and certainly any shaking, may cause or aggravate a spinal cord injury.

If the non-trauma patient responds to your verbal or painful stimuli or the trauma patient responds to your touch and talk, it is obvious that he is not in cardiac arrest. Look for any other signs of a non-arrested patient such as movement, swallowing, or spontaneous breathing. If there is no response, then you must proceed to assess the airway, breathing, and circulation. Remember also that a patient may make some response to verbal or painful stimuli, or talking and touching, yet may still require airway management and ventilatory support. A patient that is able to talk without gasping for breaths in between words typically has an open airway and adequate breathing.

Call for Advanced Life Support and Backup

It is imperative to call for advanced cardiac life support (ACLS) in any potential cardiac arrest situation, either before or at the same time as basic cardiac life support (BCLS) measures are initiated. It is critical to the patient's chances for survival to get equipment and personnel to the scene for defibrillation, advanced airway management, and drug therapy as quickly as possible. Basic cardiac life support may maintain minimal perfusion of oxygenated blood until these advanced cardiac life-support measures can be initiated, but basic cardiac life support alone is unlikely to achieve a successful resuscitation. Delaying the call for advanced cardiac life support while basic cardiac life support is initiated is likely to be a fatal error. Even with CPR, the patient should optimally receive defibrillation and other advanced measures within 4 to 6 minutes and is unlikely to survive if these measures are not initiated before 10 minutes from the time of collapse.

In most systems, the EMS units are staffed with only two crew members. In the typical cardiac arrest situation, in order to perform all of the required skills and

[2]American Heart Association, *Textbook of Advanced Cardiac Life Support,* 1994: 1–5.

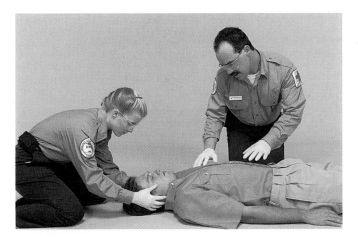

FIGURE 2–2
For the possible spine-injured patient, touch and talk to establish unresponsiveness. Maintain manual stabilization of the head and spine.

actions during the resuscitation, it is necessary to have more than two EMS crew members present. Thus, call for a backup unit as soon as you recognize cardiac arrest. In some systems, you may have a tiered or dual response of first response units followed by the EMS unit; these may provide adequate personnel at the scene to effectively carry out the resuscitation effort. In other systems, as soon as the communications officer recognizes the potential for a cardiac arrest, a second EMS unit is dispatched as a dual response.

After summoning an ALS unit or backup help, it is just as important for the EMS provider or first responder to return to the patient as quickly as possible to assess and open the airway, begin positive pressure ventilation, assess the pulse, and begin CPR if necessary. Out-of-hospital survival is directly related to decreasing the time interval from the onset of the cardiac arrest to the return of spontaneous and effective circulation. Although this is primarily achieved through defibrillation and other advanced care, don't forget that basic-life-support measures will provide the critical circulation of oxygenated blood until advanced care can begin. As soon as an automated external defibrillator or manual defibrillator is available, the patient's rhythm should be assessed and defibrillation delivered if necessary.

The layperson has been taught to "phone first," then perform the steps of CPR when dealing with an unresponsive adult and no other help is available. The trained health care provider is also generally advised to call for help first. However, health care providers may sometimes face a dilemma because of their ability to provide care beyond the basic level, which their experience and judgment tells them may be more useful to the patient than immediately getting to the phone. The trained health care provider will know that unresponsiveness may be the result of many conditions other than cardiac arrest. For example, clues in the surrounding environment may suggest a drug overdose, head injury, or a choking incident. Thus, there may be a delay in summoning EMS for these patients.

If you suspect an obstructed airway as the cause of unresponsiveness, then you must assess the airway and employ the foreign body airway obstruction maneuver immediately. You must use judgment, be decisive, and provide the most appropriate care possible given the patient situation. It may be necessary to employ invasive airway maneuvers to clear the obstruction, such as laryngoscopy and use of the Magill forceps. The key is recognition and quick intervention to clear the airway before moving on to the next management step.

Several special situations may arise when you are alone when you encounter a patient you suspect is in cardiac arrest. This situation may arise if you are off duty or acting as a first responder with limited access to equipment. One special situation may be that you have access to a defibrillator, often an automated external defibrillator. In this situation, you should not delay defibrillation to seek additional help. Instead, perform the following steps after establishing unresponsiveness:

1. Call for an advanced life support unit and backup if necessary if you have a portable radio available to you. If you are off duty, call out for help for someone to dial 911 or the emergency number to summon an advanced life support unit.

2. Manually open the airway with a head-tilt, chin-lift or jaw-thrust maneuver.

3. Deliver two breaths using a bag-valve-mask, pocket mask, or a barrier device to ensure a clear and open airway.

4. Assess the carotid pulse to confirm pulselessness.

5. Retrieve, apply, and operate the defibrillator.

Do not initiate chest compressions until after you have delivered the first set of three defibrillations unless there is a delay in retrieving the defibrillator. Only then, conduct one minute of CPR before reassessing the pulse and delivering another set of three defibrillations if the patient remains pulseless and in a shockable rhythm. The benefit of early defibrillation by far outweighs the consequent delay in initiating or continuing CPR.

Another special situation for you, as a lone responder, may be that the nearest phone is so far away it will take more than a few minutes to get to it. A delay in the initiation of CPR of 1 to 2 minutes to access EMS or obtain a defibrillator is acceptable for a patient who you suspect is in ventricular fibrillation. However, if an extended time would elapse while you activate EMS or obtain a defibrillator, you must decide whether to initiate CPR or to leave the patient to seek help.

Suppose, for example, that you are in a desolate or remote area when you witness a cardiac arrest and there is no quick way to call for help. This patient is most likely in ventricular fibrillation. In this situation, it may be most appropriate to establish an airway and positive pressure ventilation, deliver several precordial thumps, and provide CPR for approximately 10 to 15 minutes. You would realize that CPR and precordial thumps alone are very unlikely to convert the rhythm and restore circulation, but under the circumstances they are somewhat more likely to help the patient than the arrival of advanced cardiac life support after a very long delay. It is most reasonable to continue CPR for 15 minutes. If the resuscitation is unsuccessful after that period of time, and no signs of life are present, then CPR can be stopped. No signs of life would include no spontaneous pulse, no breathing or gasping respirations, no movement, body temperature that continues to decrease with mottling of the skin, dependent lividity, and fixed and dilated pupils. The traditional recommendation to continue CPR until exhausted is unrealistic, since most fit individuals may be able to perform CPR for more than one hour. The exception to this general rule is a cold-water submersion, hypothermia, and certain drug intoxications where prolonged resuscitation efforts are warranted.

Position the Patient

The patient in cardiac arrest must be placed on a firm surface. In the out-of-hospital setting, the patient is likely to be placed initially on the floor and then on a long backboard for transport. If resuscitation is to be conducted with a patient in a bed, a firm board or other support device must be placed under the posterior thorax. CPR boards, an older type wooden shortboard, or a standard longboard are typically used for this purpose.

Resuscitation cannot be attempted on a patient who is in a prone, lateral, sitting, or semi-sitting position. The prone patient or patient lying on his side must be immediately rolled as a unit to a supine position, while the patient who is in a sitting or semi-sitting position must first be placed on the floor or other hard, flat surface. If a mechanism of injury exists that is consistent with possible cervical spine injury, such as a motor-vehicle crash, diving accident, or a fall, it is necessary to take special precautions when moving the patient. The goal is to maintain the head, neck, and trunk of the body in a straight line.

If you are alone, kneel next to the patient and place one hand on the back of the head and neck. With the other hand, roll the patient over into a supine position. If two or more people are available to provide the move, position one person at the head of the patient to maintain the head and neck in a neutral in-line position. No traction or pulling force should be applied. Instead, simple manual stabilization by holding the head and neck in place is required. Other rescuers, directed by the person at the head, will roll the patient over as a unit. The patient's head, neck, and body must be maintained in a neutral in-line position throughout the resuscitation effort.

Position the Members of the Resuscitation Team

If you are working alone, your best position is at the level of the patient's shoulders. This gives you access to the chest and airway during CPR without the need to move your knees. As other members of the resuscitation team arrive, it is important to place them in key positions to facilitate the best possible care to the patient. The person controlling the airway should be placed at the head of the patient. Chest compressions should be provided by a person who is beside the patient at the level of the thorax. The person operating the monitor and defibrillator must be able to see the oscilloscope and all members of the team to avoid accidental shocks to team members. The person establishing intravenous access must be positioned at the arm and not interfering with the chest compressor or defibrillator operator. Proper positioning can identify team member responsibility and provide for optimal safety of the resuscitation team. Excuse unnecessary personnel to reduce confusion and improve safety during the resuscitation attempt.

PRIMARY SURVEY

The primary survey is a systematic approach to the patient that uses basic skills to open and maintain the airway, assess and assist ventilation, assess for pulselessness, initiate chest compressions, and provide defibrillation for ventricular fibrillation or pulseless ventricular tachycardia. It is the initial assessment performed by EMS personnel on the patient. The mnemonic ABCD is used to facilitate an organized approach to the patient and to counteract any desire to perform more invasive or advanced skills without first performing the vital basic skills of resuscitation (Table 2-1). While performing the survey, if a life-threatening condition is identified, you must stop and immediately manage the condition before moving on in the assessment. For example, if an airway obstruction is identified, you must first clear the obstruction before moving on to assess the breathing or pulse. Without an open airway, any other assessment or management is futile.

A = Airway: Open the Airway

Open and inspect inside the mouth for blood, vomitus, secretions, or other foreign materials. Immediately suction any blood, vomitus, or secretions. Remove foreign

TABLE 2-1	Primary Survey for Emergency Cardiac Care
Assessment	**Critical Actions**
A Airway	▪ Suction any vomitus, secretions, or blood from the mouth. ▪ Remove any foreign material. ▪ Open the airway with manual maneuvers.
B Breathing	▪ Assess for breathlessness. ▪ Provide positive pressure ventilation.
C Circulation	▪ Assess for pulselessness. ▪ Provide chest compressions.
D Defibrillation	▪ Assess for ventricular fibrillation or pulseless ventricular tachycardia. ▪ Defibrillate.

bodies with your gloved fingers. If you encounter heavy vomitus, turn the patient on his side and sweep the vomitus from the mouth until it is clear. Loose dentures may become completely dislodged and occlude the airway. Therefore, if the dentures are loose, remove them; if the dentures are firmly in place, leave them. If not loose, dentures provide a firm structure that enhances your ability to establish and maintain a good seal with a mask when performing bag-valve-mask or mouth-to-mask ventilation. However, dentures should be removed when intubation is attempted.

Open the airway using a manual maneuver. The head-tilt, chin-lift maneuver is the standard method of opening the airway. However, if a cervical spine injury is suspected, the head and neck must be maintained in an in-line neutral position. Use the jaw-thrust or chin-lift maneuver for the trauma patient with suspected neck or spine injury (Figure 2-3).

B = Breathing: Assess for Breathlessness and Provide Ventilation

Once the airway is opened and cleared of any foreign materials, place your ear close to the patient's nose and mouth while looking in the direction of the patient's chest. To assess for adequate breathing, you will look, listen, and feel (Figure 2-4).

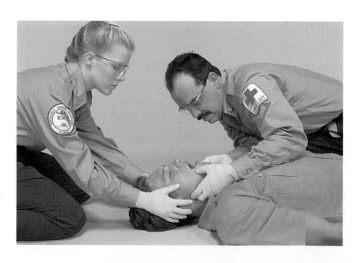

FIGURE 2-3
Use a head-tilt, chin-lift maneuver to open the airway of a medical patient, a jaw-thrust maneuver to open the airway of a trauma patient. Inspect and clear any foreign materials from inside the mouth.

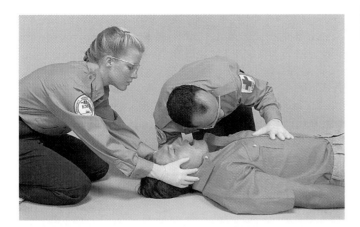

FIGURE 2–4
Look, listen, and feel to assess breathing.

▶ **Look** at the patient's chest for spontaneous rise and fall or any other respiratory movement.

▶ **Listen** for any evidence of air moving out of the patient's nose or mouth.

▶ **Feel** for any air movement out of the nose or mouth.

In order for the patient to be breathing adequately, he must have *both* an adequate respiratory rate *and* an adequate tidal volume. However, it only takes one inadequate, either an inadequate rate or an inadequate tidal volume, to have inadequate breathing. If either the respiratory rate or the tidal volume is inadequate, you must immediately begin positive pressure ventilation.

Opening the airway may be the only intervention needed to resume spontaneous ventilation in some patients. However, most patients will require some type of positive pressure ventilation with supplemental oxygen. Airway management and effective ventilation are vital to the resuscitation effort. If an airway cannot be established or adequate ventilation performed, all other resuscitation efforts will be futile.

Once you have established that the patient is not breathing, you must consider the following:

▶ Absence of air movement, which may signify an airway obstruction

▶ Whether noninvasive or invasive maneuvers are necessary to dislodge the obstruction

▶ Which ventilation device will provide the most effective positive-pressure ventilation

▶ Which ventilation device can deliver high concentrations of oxygen

▶ The rate and volume necessary to adequately ventilate the patient

▶ Methods to determine whether the ventilation is effective or not

If possible and immediately available, insert an oropharyngeal airway and begin positive pressure ventilation with a bag-valve-mask device or pocket mask. The bag-valve-mask device must have an oxygen reservoir and an oxygen inlet connection. The pocket mask should have a one-way valve to allow the patient's exhalation to be vented away from the mask and ventilator. An oxygen inlet port is also desirable.

Deliver two slow ventilations, each over a period of 2 to 4 seconds allowing for adequate exhalation between ventilations. It is important to maintain a proper airway position to allow for adequate passive exhalation. Delivering the ventilations slowly, as described, rather than quickly or abruptly, decreases the esophageal opening pressure and reduces the risk of gastric distention and subsequent regurgitation and aspiration. In addition, cricoid pressure (direct posterior pressure placed on the anterior portion of the cricoid ring) should be applied to reduce the risk of gastric distention, regurgitation, and aspiration. Cricoid pressure should not be used, however, if there is suspicion of cervical injury.

With the first two ventilations, it is necessary to determine whether the ventilations were effective or not. If resistance was met or the chest did not rise or fall with the first ventilation, reposition the head with a manual airway maneuver before attempting the second ventilation. If resistance is still met, an airway obstruction may exist. Also, suspicion of airway obstruction is based on the history of events prior to the cardiac arrest, such as eating food.

Next you must determine what methods to employ to remove the obstruction: manual foreign body airway obstruction maneuvers or more advanced techniques like laryngoscopy and the use of Magill forceps. This will be determined by your level of training, experience, and available equipment. Remember, chest compressions without effective ventilations are useless. Refer to Chapter 3 for a more detailed discussion on airway management and ventilation techniques and equipment.

C = Circulation: Assess for Pulselessness and Provide Chest Compressions

According to the primary survey's systematic approach to the patient, once the airway has been opened, breathlessness established, and two ventilations delivered, you should next check the patient's carotid pulse. Check the pulse on the side of the patient that is closer to you for 5 to 10 seconds. An unresponsive patient who is not breathing and is pulseless is in full or complete cardiac arrest and needs cardiopulmonary resuscitation immediately. However, if a defibrillator is available, immediately analyze the patient's rhythm and deliver defibrillations if necessary. Do not delay defibrillation to perform chest compressions. Only perform chest compressions and ventilation prior to defibrillation if a defibrillator is not immediately available. If a first responder crew or bystander is already performing CPR upon your arrival, after stopping the CPR and assessing the airway, breathing, and pulse, you may instruct them to continue until the defibrillator is applied and ready to be used. Again, do not wait until a cycle is completed or do not delay defibrillation in any way.

You must initiate chest compressions along with effective positive pressure ventilation (Figure 2-5). Continuously assess for effectiveness of chest compressions and ventilations. If oxygen is not connected to the ventilation device or the oxygen concentration being delivered is less than 40%, ventilate at a tidal volume of 10 ml/kg delivered over 2 seconds. If oxygen is connected to the ventilation device and is being delivered at a concentration greater than 40%, reduce the tidal volume to 6 to 7 ml/kg and deliver the ventilation over 1 to 2 seconds. The team leader will direct the initiation and cessation of compressions and ventilations.

D = Defibrillation: Defibrillate Ventricular Fibrillation and Pulseless Ventricular Tachycardia

A key concept of advanced cardiac life support is to provide defibrillation to the patient in ventricular fibrillation or pulseless ventricular tachycardia as quickly as possible (Figure 2-6). In reality, a cascade of events leads to successful resuscitation of a cardiac arrest patient, but studies show that time to defibrillation is one of the most pivotal components in determining survival. Early defibrillation takes

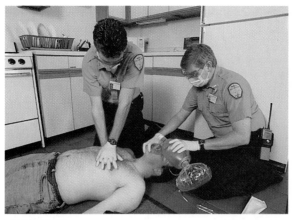

FIGURE 2–5
Initiate chest compressions and positive pressure ventilation.

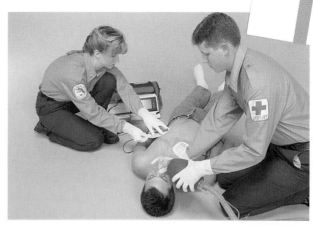

FIGURE 2–6
Provide defibrillation of ventricular fibrillation or pulseless ventricular tachycardia as soon as possible.

priority over airway management, ventilation, and chest compressions. Your goal should be to get a defibrillator to the patient as quickly as possible and provide defibrillation. As discussed earlier, that is one reason why the layperson is instructed to "phone first" after establishing unresponsiveness in the adult patient.

Two methods of external defibrillation are currently available. Many first responder units use semi-automated external defibrillators (AEDs). These devices, which automatically determine the rhythm of the patient and the need to defibrillate, are relatively easy to use and can deliver defibrillations quickly to the patient. AEDs are commonly found in locations such as airports, shopping centers, schools, and other public places. The AEDs are for public use in the case of a cardiac arrest. Thus, when responding to a cardiac arrest, it may not be a first responder from a fire department providing the defibrillation, but a layperson with no real formal training. The manual defibrillator is used by more highly trained personnel and requires the operator to determine the rhythm and need for defibrillation. Manual defibrillators are typically used by paramedics and EMT-Intermediates. Regardless of the type of defibrillator being used, it is imperative to deliver three "stacked" shocks (three shocks in quick succession, without pausing to recheck for pulselessness) in the shortest time possible prior to any basic or advanced care.

When determining the importance of defibrillation, consider the following points, which have been confirmed in a number of clinical and epidemiological studies:[3,4]

> Most adults who have been successfully resuscitated from nontraumatic cardiac arrest (greater than 90% in most studies) were in ventricular fibrillation.

> The success of defibrillation is directly related to time to defibrillation.

> The patient in ventricular fibrillation or pulseless ventricular tachycardia has an estimated probability of 70% to 80% of surviving upon succumbing to cardiac arrest at time zero. With each minute that passes, the probability of successfully defibrillating the patient to a perfusing rhythm decreases by about 2% to 10%.

> If 10 minutes have passed since the collapse of the patient and you have not been able to defibrillate him, his chance of surviving is near zero.

[3]Eisenberg, M. S., B. T. Horwood, R. O. Cummins, R. Reynolds-Haertle, T. R. Hearne, "Cardiac Arrest and Resuscitation: A Tale of 29 Cities," *Annals of Emergency Medicine*, 1990: 19:179–186.

[4]Eisenberg, M. S., R. O. Cummins, S. Damon, M. P. Larsen, T. R. Hearne, "Survival Rates from Out-of-Hospital Cardiac Arrest: Recommendations for Uniform Definitions and Data to Report," *Annals of Emergency Medicine,* 1990: 19:1249–1259.

Instruction in defibrillation has been implemented at various levels of training. This has been done to decrease the time to defibrillation of the patient. For a detailed discussion of defibrillation, see Chapter 7.

SECONDARY SURVEY

The secondary survey is conducted immediately following conclusion of the primary survey. Like the primary survey, it also uses a systematic approach and the mnemonic ABCD, however with different definitions of each component (Table 2-2). The secondary survey concentrates on more advanced and invasive care, compared to the basic care provided in the primary survey. The steps in the secondary survey should be performed almost simultaneously. The secondary survey corresponds to the rapid medical assessment and the ongoing assessment.

The resuscitation team leader is the facilitator who directs patient care. Each team member should understand his role and perform his duties without specific direction from the team leader. If not enough trained personnel are available, the team leader may need to step in and perform the most essential steps of resuscitation.

It is recommended that tracheal intubation precede intravenous access in the prehospital environment when limited personnel are available. For the first several minutes or longer after your arrival at the scene, there may be only you and your partner to perform the resuscitation. One person must perform chest compressions while the other continues with the resuscitation and performs the secondary survey. Insertion of a tracheal tube can serve two purposes. The tracheal tube can provide a secure airway and serve as a drug route for some of the initial cardiac medications which can be administered via the trachea. The effectiveness of the tracheal drug route is in question. Thus drug administration via the tracheal tube should be limited. An intravenous line should be established as quickly as possible and used as the primary drug route.

In most situations in the out-of-hospital environment, tracheal intubation takes precedence over intravenous therapy. If tracheal intubation is not successful or if you are unable to perform tracheal intubation, insert an alternative airway device. If you are able to effectively ventilate and oxygenate the patient with a bag-valve-mask device, you may delay invasive airway control to establish an

TABLE 2–2	Secondary Survey for Emergency Cardiac Care	
Assessment	**Critical Actions**
A Airway	■ Reassess basic manual maneuver effectiveness. ■ Consider advanced airway care, most likely tracheal intubation.
B Breathing	■ Assess ventilation effectiveness following tracheal intubation or other advanced airway maneuvers.
C Circulation	■ Attach the continuous ECG monitor and identify the rhythm and rate. ■ Establish an intravenous line. ■ Assess blood pressure using noninvasive technique. ■ Administer the appropriate drug therapy.
D Differential Diagnosis	■ Determine the etiology of the cardiac arrest or cardiac rhythm.

intravenous line and administer medications. However, in the uncontrolled out-of-hospital environment, the risk of regurgitation and aspiration of a patient in cardiac arrest is fairly high. Thus, invasive airway control usually is a priority.

A = Airway: Perform Invasive Airway Control by Inserting an Advanced Airway

A tracheal tube isolates the trachea and is considered a definitive method to establish and maintain an airway. With a tracheal tube in place, the airway is said to be "protected," since the distal cuff blocks any vomitus or secretions from traveling down the trachea and into the lungs (Figure 2-7). Tracheal intubation should be performed at the earliest possible point to definitively secure the airway.

Continue manual airway maneuvers while the patient and equipment are prepared for tracheal intubation. Select the appropriate laryngoscope handle and blade, proper-sized tracheal tube, a stylet, lubrication, 10 ml syringe, suction machine, and securing device. The specific equipment is dependent on the characteristics of the patient: short neck, fat neck, or anatomically challenged. Check all equipment while the patient is being hyperoxygenated. Use body substance isolation precautions, such as gloves, eye protection, and mask when performing intubation. Perform the intubation without interrupting ventilations for greater than 30 seconds. If the attempt reaches 30 seconds, remove the laryngoscope and immediately resume ventilation and hyperoxygenation for a period of 30 to 60 seconds. Reattempt the intubation following adequate ventilation and hyperoxygenation. For a detailed discussion of tracheal intubation, see Chapter 3.

Other advanced airway adjuncts exist, such as the esophageal tracheal Combitube® (ETC) and the Laryngeal Mask Airway (LMA); however, none is considered to be an equivalent substitute for a tracheal tube. The alternative airway devices are easier to use and the insertion does not require direct visualization of the glottic opening or vocal cords. The devices are very effective and can be used by those not trained or skilled in tracheal intubation.

Cricoid pressure can be used to reduce the risk of gastric distention, regurgitation, and aspiration prior to and during the attempt at tracheal intubation. Applying cricoid pressure also moves the glottic opening slightly posterior, facilitating visualization and tube placement during the intubation technique. Some studies have shown an increase of 10% in the success rate of intubation when cricoid pressure is performed.

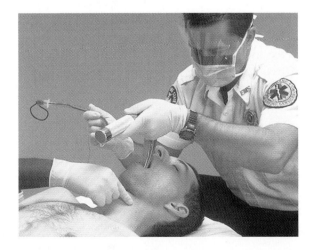

FIGURE 2–7
Protect the airway by inserting a tracheal tube.

If bag-valve-mask or pocket-mask ventilation appears to be effective in ventilating the patient, and there is no evidence of vomitus, regurgitation, or gastric distention, tracheal intubation can be delayed while other interventions are performed.

B = Breathing: Assess Tracheal Tube Placement and Effectiveness of Ventilation

The primary methods to confirm tracheal tube or advanced airway placement are through physical examination. This includes direct visualization of tracheal tube placement, inspection of the chest, and a five-point auscultation of the chest and epigastrium.

If the patient has been intubated with a tracheal tube, you must assess for proper tube placement. One of the best methods is for the intubator to ensure that he visualizes the tube passing through the glottic opening and between the vocal cords. During the first ventilation after tube placement, immediately inspect the chest for rise and auscultate over the epigastrium for sounds in the stomach (Figure 2-8). If sounds are heard over the epigastrium or the chest does not rise with the ventilation, the tube has probably been misplaced in the esophagus. Immediately remove the tube, resume ventilation and hyperoxygenation for 1 to 2 minutes, and reattempt the intubation.

If no sounds are heard over the epigastrium and the chest rises with the ventilation, the tube has been placed in the trachea. However, it is still possible that the tube may have been advanced too far into one of the mainstem bronchi, thereby directing air into only one lung. To check for this possibility, auscultate for equal bilateral breath sounds over the midaxillary line at about the fourth or fifth intercostal space and at the second intercostal space at the midclavicular line. Absent or decreased breath sounds on the left may indicate a right mainstem intubation. (Because of the lesser angle and larger diameter of the right mainstem bronchus, right mainstem intubation is far more common than left mainstem intubation.) Deflate the cuff and pull back on the tube 1 to 2 cm and reassess bilateral breath sounds. Repeat this procedure until equal breath sounds are heard bilaterally. One should also consider the unlikely possibility that a pneumothorax or fluid in the pleural cavity is the cause of inequality in breath sounds. The most reliable primary confirmation method is to visualize tube placement in the glottic opening with the laryngoscope if there is any doubt as to whether the tube is properly placed. If doubt of proper tube placement still exists, remove the tube, and continue ventilation with a bag-valve-mask or pocket mask device.

Secondary methods to confirm tube placement include an esophageal detector device (EDD) and an end-tidal CO_2 detector. The esophageal detector device may be of the bulb or syringe type. Squeeze the bulb on the device and watch for the refill time. If the bulb refills in less than 10 seconds on two separate attempts, the tracheal tube is most likely in the trachea and not the esophagus. If the bulb reexpands slowly, greater than 10 seconds, the tracheal tube is probably in the esophagus. Remove the tube immediately and resume BVM ventilation.

A qualitative or quantitative end-tidal CO_2 detector may also be used to assess for proper tube placement. A qualitative end-tidal CO_2 device is colorimetric device that changes color in response to carbon dioxide detection. A quantitative CO_2 device provides a numeric readout and a waveform. These devices are used in conjunction with physical examination. A more detailed discussion of these devices is found in Chapter 3.

Once the tube is confirmed to be properly placed, secure it with a commercial tracheal tube holder or tape. Note the centimeter marker at the level of the

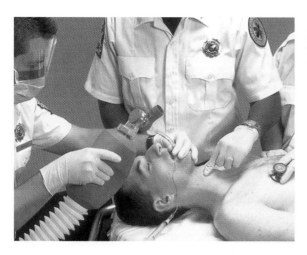

FIGURE 2–8
Ventilate the patient and assess for proper tube placement by watching for chest rise and auscultating the epigastrium and the chest.

front teeth. Insert an oropharyngeal airway to serve as a bite block to prevent occlusion of the tube if the patient would bite down.

Continue to assess effective ventilation by watching the chest rise and fall and auscultating the chest. After every move of the patient, such as from the ambulance stretcher to the emergency department gurney, tube placement must be minimally reassessed by auscultation over the epigastrium and chest. Inspect the end-tidal CO_2 detector for changes and a deterioration in the pulse oximeter reading. Also note the depth of the tube at the lip line or front teeth.

If the patient is not intubated, continue to assess for effective ventilation by watching for adequate chest rise and fall. Monitor the stomach for evidence of gastric distention which, when present, may indicate the need to reposition the head and intubate the patient quickly.

C = Circulation: Attach the ECG, Establish an IV Line, and Administer Cardiac Medications

Attach the ECG monitor to allow for continuous monitoring of the cardiac rhythm. In order to detect any changes, it is important to constantly assess the rhythm both before and following any medication administration, defibrillation, or other intervention. Any change in rhythm necessitates a pulse check. If a pulse is found, the blood pressure is measured.

An intravenous line should be initiated, using a large bore catheter in the most accessible vein available, which is usually the antecubital vein (Figure 2-9).

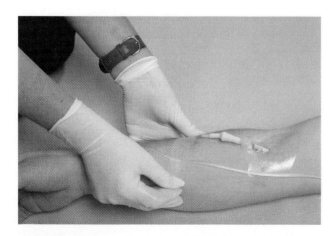

FIGURE 2–9
Initiate an intravenous line in the antecubital vein.

The solution of choice is 0.9% normal saline, which is an isotonic volume expander. The risk of causing pulmonary edema in this situation has not been found to be a significant or frequent problem. Normal saline is relatively inexpensive and has a longer shelf life than many other solutions.

The use of glucose-containing solutions, such as D_5W, has been associated with poor neurologic outcomes in postresuscitation patients and those with other types of intracranial pathology. Therefore, the use of D_5W and other glucose-containing solutions should be avoided.

When administering medication by the intravenous route, elevate the arm and deliver a 20 to 30 ml bolus of fluid following injection of the medication. This will facilitate quicker entry into the central circulation.

Use the appropriate medications for the presenting rhythm. However, be sure to treat the patient and not just the rhythm. Know the appropriate dose, indications, contraindications, actions, and side effects of each medication.

Certain medications can be administered down the tracheal tube. Lidocaine (Xylocaine), epinephrine, atropine, and naloxone (Narcan) can be given tracheally. The mnemonic LEAN provides an easy method to remember the restricted number of drugs that are acceptable for tracheal administration (Table 2-3).

To administer medication by the tracheal route, it is necessary to use a commercial tracheal drug administration device or to thread a long catheter—a 35 cm intracatheter works well—down the tracheal tube. The catheter should extend beyond the tip of the tube. Stop chest compressions, inject 2 to 2.5 times the regular dose of medication diluted to 10 ml with normal saline into the catheter and down the tube. Attach the bag-valve or other ventilation device and deliver 3 to 4 forceful ventilations to distribute the medication. A heparin lock with a 20 gauge needle pierced through the wall of the tracheal tube may be used if an intracath or commercial catheter device is not available. The medications will be aerosolized during ventilation. Drug absorption, with tracheal administration, is questionable; therefore, drugs should be administered tracheally only in situations where an intravenous line is not available and only until an IV is available.

For more detailed discussions of intravenous access and medications, see Chapters 4 and 8.

D = Differential Diagnosis: Consider the Etiology of the Cardiac Arrest or Rhythm

At this point, the team leader must consider the actual cause of the cardiac arrest or specific rhythm. Just treating rhythms and not the patient as a whole will not necessarily lead to successful resuscitation of the patient, especially if the underlying cause of the cardiac arrest or rhythm is something other than coronary artery disease. A reversible cause to the condition should be sought in an attempt to regain spontaneous circulation.

TABLE 2-3	Resuscitation Medications Administered by the Tracheal Route
L	lidocaine (Xylocaine)
E	epinephrine
A	atropine
N	naloxone (Narcan)

Examine the rhythm and explore potential etiologies of that rhythm. As an example, might the severe symptomatic bradycardia be due to organophosphate poisoning in the migrant worker brought into the emergency department? Might the pulseless tachycardia be due to a tension pneumothorax in the patient found in cardiac arrest at the bottom of the steps? Could the sinus tachycardia be due to occult gastrointestinal bleeding in the nursing home patient? or due to dehydration in the patient with the flu? These are the types of questions that must be considered when evaluating the patient.

The desire is to treat the patient as a whole, and not just the rhythm, as a part of comprehensive patient care. Decisions on patient management may be based on the questions and answers regarding cardiac arrest and rhythm etiology. Do not develop tunnel vision and treat only the rhythm when, in fact, the rhythm may have a reversible etiology. This will only lead to an unsuccessful resuscitation. Always perform a complete physical exam and patient history to identify possible reversible causes of the cardiac arrest or dysrhythmia. For more information on rhythm recognition and assessment, see Chapter 5, ECG Monitoring and Dysrhythmia Recognition, and Chapter 11, Prehospital Cardiac Emergency Scenarios: Application Exercises.

CASE STUDY FOLLOW-UP

Preliminary Presurvey Actions

You have been called to an extended care facility room for an unresponsive 58-year-old male patient. As you enter the room, there are no apparent safety hazards. You note the patient is ashen gray and motionless. You move to his side, shake him, and shout, "Mr. O'Brien, Mr. O'Brien, are you okay?" but there is no response. You call dispatch to request a backup crew to the scene *on the red*.

Primary Survey

You move to Mr. O'Brien's head and open his airway with a head-tilt, chin-lift maneuver. You note vomitus in his mouth as you open it. Two employees of the facility, Mary and John, come into the room to assist. You immediately instruct Mary to suction the vomitus from the airway. Once it is clear, you position your ear close to Mr. O'Brien's nose and mouth and look toward his chest. You inspect for chest rise and fall while listening and feeling for air movement. You do not detect any respiratory movement and indicate this to Mary.

Mary inserts an oropharyngeal airway and delivers two ventilations with a bag-valve mask over a 4-second period while you check for a carotid pulse for 5 seconds. You state, "No pulse—we need to start chest compressions." You, John, and Mary immediately move Mr. O'Brien to the floor. John finds the correct landmark on his chest, and begins compressions as you set up the monitor/defibrillator to do a "quick-look."

You move the monitor/defibrillator into position next to Mr. O'Brien. You turn on the monitor, switch the lead indicator to paddles, stop CPR, and perform a "quick-look" after applying the defibrillator pads to the chest. The oscilloscope shows coarse ventricular fibrillation. You immediately charge the paddles to 200 joules, inspect around the patient, and yell, "I'm clear, you're clear, everybody's clear," then deliver the first shock. The oscilloscope still shows ventricular fibrillation. With the paddles still on the chest, you charge to 300 joules, clear the patient a second time, and deliver the shock. Mr. O'Brien remains in ventricular fibrillation, so you charge to 360 joules, clear the patient, and deliver the third shock. You watch the oscilloscope as John checks the carotid artery for a pulse. The patient remains pulseless. You instruct John to resume chest compressions as Mary resumes ventilations.

continued on next page

Secondary Survey

Two paramedics from the back-up unit, Heather and Matt, have just arrived. Matt prepares tracheal intubation equipment as Heather spikes a 500 ml bag of normal saline and prepares equipment to gain intravenous access. Mary applies cricoid pressure as Matt performs the laryngoscopy and inserts the tracheal tube. He conducts a five-point auscultation and finds indications of proper tube placement. He quickly attaches a bulb type esophageal detection device to the tracheal tube and squeezes the bulb. It refills within two seconds. He squeezes the bulb a second time and gets a quick bulb refill of less than three seconds. Matt then attaches a colorimetric end-tidal CO_2 detector to the tracheal tube and Mary attaches the bag-valve-mask device. She ventilates six times and Matt notes a bright yellow color on the device indicating carbon dioxide. She notes the tube is at 23 cm at the level of the front teeth, inserts an oropharyngeal airway, and then secures the tube in place using a commercial tracheal tube holder. Mary resumes bag-valve ventilation with oxygen attached to the reservoir and set at 15 lpm at a tidal volume of 6 ml/kg with each breath delivered over 1 to 2 seconds.

You attach the electrodes to Mr. O'Brien's chest and set the lead selector to Lead II. Heather establishes an intravenous line with a 14-gauge angiocath catheter in the antecubital vein. Once the IV line is secure, you call for the administration of 1 mg of epinephrine intravenously. Heather calls back the order and administers the drug by IV bolus. She elevates Mr. O'Brien's arm and gives a 30 ml bolus of fluid.

Sixty seconds go by and you stop compressions to reassess the rhythm. It is still ventricular fibrillation. You clear yourself and the team, charge the defibrillator to 360 joules, and deliver the shock. John indicates "No pulse" and continues chest compressions. You continue to alternate medications with defibrillation as Mr. O'Brien remains in ventricular fibrillation.

You begin to try to determine the cause of the arrest and start looking for clues as to why the patient will not convert. Is it severe lactic acidosis? Is it profound hypoxia? How long was Mr. O'Brien in cardiac arrest?

You continue to attempt to resuscitate the patient and alter the management based on your differential diagnosis and suspected etiology.

◧ SUMMARY

Within this chapter we have covered a systematic assessment and management approach to the patient who is in cardiac arrest or suffering from a cardiorespiratory emergency. By using the mnemonic ABCD, it is easy to remember an organized, appropriate, and efficient approach to assess and manage the patient. It is imperative that the care move from the basic procedures in the primary survey to the more advanced care in the secondary survey.

Much more information will be provided in the following chapters regarding airway management and ventilation, oxygen therapy, electrical therapy, ECG interpretation, and drug therapy. Resuscitation required in specific cases and conditions will also be discussed.

It is important to apply this standard approach to every patient suffering cardiac arrest or a cardiorespiratory emergency. This will provide you and the entire resuscitation team a guideline to ensure that the best possible emergency cardiac care is afforded to the patient.

REVIEW QUESTIONS

1. Unresponsiveness should be assessed
   a. after opening the airway.
   b. after the initial pulse check.
   c. after assessing the scene for safety hazards.
   d. after delivery of the first two ventilations.

2. You are summoned by the waiter to assist a woman who suddenly becomes cyanotic while eating her dinner at a local restaurant. Upon arrival at the scene, you should immediately
   a. establish unresponsiveness, open the airway, and attempt to ventilate.
   b. immediately begin the foreign body airway obstruction removal maneuvers.
   c. apply the monitor to determine the patient rhythm.
   d. establish unresponsiveness, open the airway, and begin chest compressions.

3. A patient found at the bottom of one flight of steps is unresponsive. You should next
   a. perform a head-tilt, chin-lift maneuver to open the airway.
   b. establish manual in-line stabilization and open the airway using a jaw-thrust maneuver.
   c. take manual stabilization of the head and perform a head-tilt, chin-lift to open the airway.
   d. keep the head and neck in a neutral position and begin ventilation.

4. When conducting the primary survey, it is appropriate to
   a. perform basic airway management, ventilations, chest compressions, and initial defibrillation.
   b. establish an intravenous line, administer medications, and intubate the patient.
   c. perform chest compressions, initiate intravenous therapy, administer medications, and defibrillate.
   d. establish an airway by tracheal intubation, suction, perform hyperventilation, and initiate chest compressions.

5. The most important variable related to successful defibrillation is
   a. antidysrhythmics medication administration.
   b. successful tracheal intubation.
   c. time to defibrillation.
   d. establishing an airway.

6. The recommended order in which you should proceed during the secondary survey is
   a. perform tracheal intubation, establish an intravenous line, and administer medications.
   b. establish an intravenous line, perform tracheal intubation, and administer medications.
   c. attach the ECG monitor, administer medications, and perform tracheal intubation.
   d. determine a differential diagnosis, establish an intravenous line, and administer drugs.

7. Which of the following drugs is **not** appropriate for tracheal administration?
   a. Narcan
   b. epinephrine
   c. bretylium
   d. atropine

8. What intravenous solution is preferred for use in a cardiac arrest patient?
   a. lactated Ringer's
   b. normal saline
   c. 5% dextrose in water
   d. 45% normal saline and 5% dextrose

9. What is the appropriate dose for medications being administered tracheally?
    a. 1 to 2 times the standard IV dose
    b. the standard IV dose
    c. 2 to 2.5 times the standard IV dose
    d. half the standard IV dose

10. The differential diagnosis is conducted as part of the
    a. preliminary actions prior to patient interventions.
    b. secondary survey after medication administration has been initiated.
    c. primary survey following the initiation of chest compressions.
    d. interval between the primary and secondary survey.

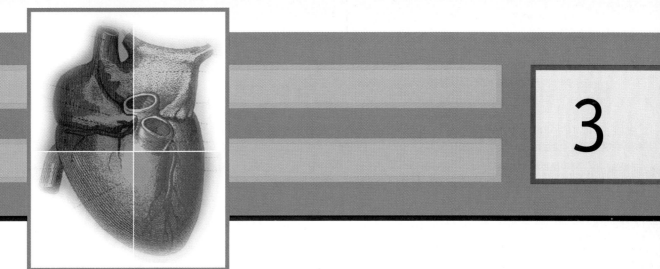

Airway Management, Ventilation, and Oxygen Therapy

The most important skills that you will perform in an acute emergency are airway management and ventilatory support, no matter what level of care is being provided to a patient. Without a patent airway and adequate ventilation and oxygenation, all other interventions will be futile. Some patients may require basic airway management, whereas others may require more advanced or surgical airway interventions. Likewise, ventilatory support may involve very basic equipment to more advanced ventilatory devices. The care you will be able to provide and equipment you can use will depend on your level of training and experience.

Topics in this chapter are:

Airway Assessment

Basic Airway Management Techniques

Advanced Airway Management Techniques

Alternative Orotracheal Intubation Techniques

Alternative Airway Adjuncts

Translaryngeal and Transtracheal Airways

Ventilation Techniques

Suction

Oxygen Therapy

CASE STUDY

You are frantically summoned by Mr. Brookley to come immediately to check on his wife. He states, "She was talking with me and suddenly fell back in bed, began gasping, and became unconscious." As you walk into the bedroom, you notice Mrs. Brookley, who is approximately 75 years of age, lying back in bed and beginning to appear ashen gray and cyanotic. Heavy vomitus is streaming from her mouth as you approach the bed. Her husband pleads, "Please do something for her," as you perform your initial assessment and ask him to leave the room.

How would you proceed to assess and manage the airway and ventilation for this patient? This chapter will describe the assessment and management of a patient with airway and ventilatory compromise. Also, oxygen therapy will be reviewed. Later we will return to the case and apply the procedures learned.

▦ INTRODUCTION

Airway management is one of the most fundamental skills you will need when caring for patients suffering from acute medical illnesses. Without a patent airway, all other interventions will be futile. Airway management may be as simple as performing a head-tilt, chin-lift maneuver or as complex as performing a surgical cricothyrotomy to relieve an airway obstruction. The key objective is to intervene rapidly to reverse any real or potential obstruction and to establish and maintain a patent airway.

Assessing the adequacy of ventilation and oxygenation is another basic skill you must master to deal with acute medical crises. Your ability to determine the severity of respiratory compromise and the need for positive pressure ventilation when spontaneous breathing is inadequate or absent will be of utmost importance. Administration of supplemental oxygen to a patient suffering from any type of cardiac or respiratory compromise is also a fundamental skill. Several methods of providing positive pressure ventilation and oxygen therapy will be discussed in this chapter.

▦ AIRWAY ASSESSMENT

In order to have adequate ventilation and oxygenation, the airway must be open. Therefore, airway assessment is the first component of the initial assessment of the patient. Upper airway obstruction may result from displacement of the tongue; from food, blood, vomitus, or foreign objects; or from edema associated with epiglottitis, burns, trauma, anaphylaxis, or other medical conditions. A patient with an altered mental status can easily suffer from an upper airway occlusion as a result of relaxation of the submandibular muscles that provide direct control of the tongue and indirect control of the epiglottis. As the muscles relax, the tongue is displaced posteriorly and occludes the airway at the level of the pharynx, while the relaxed epiglottis causes occlusion at the level of the larynx.

An alert patient who is talking or crying is assumed to have an open airway. Therefore, you can form a general impression of airway status upon your initial approach to the alert patient. If the patient has an altered mental status and is not alert, you should assume that the patient has lost his gag and cough reflex and cannot effectively control his own airway. Aggressive and rapid intervention will be necessary to reverse or prevent occlusion of the airway or aspiration of foreign material into the trachea and lungs.

In a patient with an altered mental status, you will have to open the patient's mouth to assess for airway occlusion. Use a crossed-finger technique to open the mouth (Figure 3-1). Inspect inside the mouth for any evidence of secretions, blood, vomitus, or other potential obstructions. You may need to immediately apply suction or finger sweeps to remove the material to clear a potential or actual occlusion and prevent aspiration of foreign material into the lungs. If the patient is breathing, a noisy airflow during inspiration may indicate a significant airway obstruction. When assessing the upper airway, listen for the following sounds that may indicate significant airway obstruction:

- ▶ **Sonorous sounds** or **snoring** occurs when the upper airway is partially occluded by the tongue or other tissue in the pharynx.

- ▶ **Crowing** is a sound similar to that of a cawing crow that indicates laryngeal muscular spasm and narrowing of the tracheal opening.

- ▶ **Gurgling** indicates the presence of fluids or fluidlike substances such as blood or vomitus in the upper airway. Gurgling signals the need for immediate suction to remove the substance.

- ▶ **Stridor** is a harsh, high-pitched sound. Inspiratory stridor indicates obstruction *at* or *above* the level of the vocal cords resulting from epiglottitis, foreign body, tumors, or edema. Expiratory stridor is typically associated with obstruction *below* the level of the vocal cords. Allergic reaction and croup are two conditions in which expiratory stridor may be prominent.

- ▶ **Grunting** on exhalation is a serious sign of impending respiratory failure. Patients will typically grunt at the end of exhalation. By doing so, they partially close the epiglottis over the glottic opening causing air to be trapped in the lower airway. This produces an artificial type of positive end-expiratory pressure (PEEP) that facilitates keeping the terminal airways open at the end of exhalation, making the next inhalation slightly easier due to a decreased resistance. Grunting is normally seen in lower airway diseases such as pneumonia, asthma, and bronchiolitis.

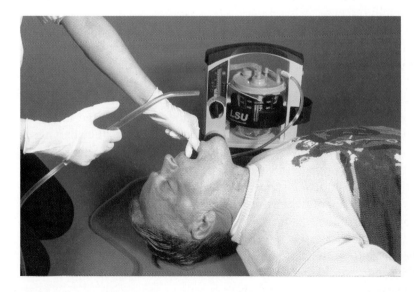

FIGURE 3–1
Use a crossed-finger technique to open the mouth.
(Carl Leet)

Other indications of an inadequate or potentially compromised airway include:

▶ Aphonia (inability to speak) or hoarseness

▶ Cyanosis—a reliable but most often a late sign of hypoxia

▶ Diaphoresis—an indication of an increased secretion of catecholamines in response to the stress

▶ Abnormal respiratory rate, either tachypnea or bradypnea

▶ Drooling—may be a sign of an obstructed airway or esophagus; indicates the patient is unable to manage his own secretions

▶ Paradoxical chest wall movement—seen as a rocking motion of the abdomen and chest as the patient makes attempts to depress the diaphragm when a partial or complete airway obstruction exists

▶ Retractions of the suprasternal notch, supraclavicular spaces, and intercostal spaces—signs of airway obstruction in the patient who appears to be breathing spontaneously; indicates use of accessory muscles to breathe. Treat patient as if a complete airway obstruction is present.

▶ Nasal flaring—early sign seen on inhalation; indicates increased work effort to breathe

▶ Tripod position—indicates increased effort to breathe; easily recognized sign and indicates impending respiratory failure

▶ Altered mental status—indicates possible airway occlusion. Hypoxia typically causes agitation; whereas hypercarbia will cause confusion. Typically these occur together and produce a patient that is agitated, sometimes aggressive, and confused.

If airway obstruction is caused by foreign material in the mouth and upper airway, you need to remove it as rapidly as possible by suction or by sweeping the substance clear from the mouth. If no spine injury is suspected, you may need to place the patient in the recovery (lateral recumbent) position to facilitate the removal of the material and prevent possible aspiration.

If the airway is obstructed by a foreign body, initially attempt to manage it with basic foreign-body-obstruction maneuvers. If unsuccessful, you may need to employ advanced techniques, such as direct laryngoscopy and removal of the foreign body by Magill forceps.

If the airway is obstructed by the tongue or epiglottis, relieve the obstruction by manually positioning the neck and head. Insert a mechanical airway if the manual maneuver is insufficient in establishing or maintaining the airway.

Tracheal intubation is a preferred method of advanced airway management. The airway is considered to be "protected" once the tracheal tube is properly placed. Alternate devices that are used to manage the airway are the laryngeal mask airway (LMA), esophageal-tracheal Combitube® (ETC), and the pharyngeo-tracheal lumen (PtL®) airway, These devices are recommended if the person managing the airway is untrained, inexperienced, or not proficient in tracheal intubation or if tracheal intubation is not available or not successful.

In the event you cannot achieve a patent airway by employing a manual maneuver or by inserting a mechanical device, you may have to proceed to a surgical airway. Transtracheal catheter ventilation (also called needle cricothyrotomy) and cricothyrotomy are the two methods to consider. These procedures are rarely performed and are used only in specific situations and after attempts at manual and mechanical airway control methods have failed.

BASIC AIRWAY MANAGEMENT TECHNIQUES

Basic airway management techniques include the use of manual maneuvers and simple airway adjuncts to establish and maintain an open airway. Use the necessary body substance isolation precautions, such as gloves and eye protection, when managing a patient's airway.

Manual Airway Maneuvers

The two manual maneuvers are the head-tilt, chin-lift and jaw-thrust technique. The head-tilt, chin-lift maneuver is most commonly used. However, if a spinal injury is suspected, the jaw-thrust maneuver is performed while the head and neck are maintained in a neutral in-line position.

Head-Tilt, Chin-Lift Maneuver

Loss of tone of the submandibular muscles in the patient with an altered mental status causes the tongue to be displaced posteriorly, partially occluding the airway at the level of the pharynx. The epiglottis indirectly loses support and creates an airway occlusion at the level of the larynx. By lifting the mandible forward, the tongue is displaced anteriorly away from the hypopharynx and the epiglottis is pulled up away from the glottic opening, relieving the obstruction at both the pharynx and larynx.

Perform the head-tilt, chin-lift maneuver by placing the palm of one hand on the patient's forehead and the tips of the fingers of the other hand under the bony part of the mandible. Avoid compression of the soft tissues under the mandible, which might obstruct the airway. Lift the mandible while tilting the head backward (Figure 3-2).

The full head-tilt, chin-lift maneuver is recommended for adults and children greater than 8 years of age. This maneuver is typically the initial management of a compromised airway. Performing the head-tilt, chin-lift may provide a stimulus to the respiratory drive in a patient with an altered mental status and a decreased respiratory effort.

Contraindications for the head-tilt, chin-lift maneuver include

▶ Cervical spine injuries due to trauma or cervical spine diseases or conditions such as ankylosing spondylitis and rheumatoid arthritis

▶ Down's syndrome patient due to a higher incidence of incomplete ossification of C1 and C2 and subluxation of the cervical vertebrae

When using the head-tilt in conjunction with the chin-lift maneuver in children, the head tilt can push the posterior pharynx toward the tongue and epiglottis due to the flexibility of the cervical spine in children less than 5 years of age. The head should remain in a neutral position as the chin is lifted forward. Excessive hyperextension of the neck in an adult can result in a compromised airway. Also, when grasping the mandible to maintain the chin-lift, be sure not to compress the soft tissue below the chin. This may displace the tongue and create or worsen an airway obstruction.

Jaw-Thrust Maneuver

The jaw-thrust maneuver, like the head-tilt, chin-lift maneuver, moves the mandible forward, causing the tongue to be pulled away from the hypopharynx. Unlike the head-tilt, chin-lift maneuver, however, the jaw-thrust maneuver does

FIGURE 3–2
The head-tilt, chin-lift maneuver.

ADULT

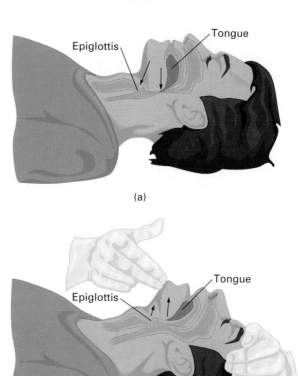

(a)

(b)

not tilt the head backward. In the spine-injured patient, the head and spine must be maintained in a neutral in-line position to prevent or reduce the chances of further injury to the spinal column and spinal cord. The jaw-thrust maneuver is the preferred method used to open the airway, since the head and neck are not flexed or extended during the maneuver. The jaw thrust should be employed if the head-tilt, chin-lift maneuver is unsuccessful in opening the airway or if a spine injury is suspected.

To perform a jaw thrust, position yourself at the head of the patient. Place one hand at each side of the patient's head. While maintaining the head in a neutral in-line position, grasp the angles of the mandible with the index, middle, and ring fingers. With the thumbs on the chin, move the mandible forward. Retract the lower lip with the thumb if necessary to open the mouth (Figure 3-3).

Either the head-tilt, chin-lift or the jaw-thrust maneuver must be performed prior to insertion of any type of airway adjunct. An airway occlusion may be relieved simply by manual positioning. However, it may be necessary to insert an airway adjunct to maintain airway control. **It is important to note that when a basic airway adjunct is used, a manual airway maneuver must be maintained**.

Basic Mechanical Airway Adjuncts

The simple airway adjuncts that require minimal skill to insert are the oropharyngeal airway and the nasopharyngeal airway. Both adjuncts extend down to the level of the hypopharynx. It must be emphasized that neither manual maneuvers nor simple airway adjuncts protect the airway or prevent aspiration of substances

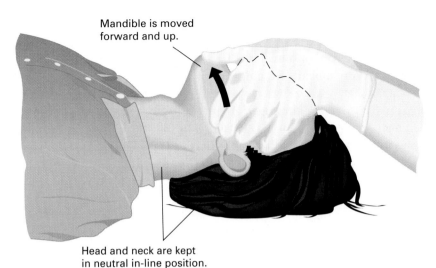

Mandible is moved forward and up.

Head and neck are kept in neutral in-line position.

FIGURE 3–3
The jaw-thrust maneuver.

into the trachea and lungs. The following general principles apply to both oropharyngeal and nasopharyngeal airway adjuncts:

▶ The adjunct can become obstructed by secretions or vomitus. For an adjunct to be effective, it must be kept clear of any foreign material.

▶ The adjunct must be properly sized to avoid potential complications from its use.

▶ The adjunct does not protect the airway. Aspiration of blood, secretions, vomitus, or other foreign substances can occur with the adjunct properly in place.

▶ Both adjuncts require the patient to have an altered mental status. The oropharyngeal airway requires that the patient have a complete loss of gag reflex. Careful and continuous monitoring of the mental status is necessary when either device is used. Recovery of the gag reflex as a result of improved mental status while an airway adjunct is in place is likely to cause vomiting and aspiration.

Oropharyngeal Airway

Also known as the oral airway, the oropharyngeal airway is semicircular, typically disposable, and made of a hard plastic. The Guedel and Berman are the two most frequently used types. The Guedel is tubular and has a hollow center. The Berman is solid and has channeled sides (Figure 3-4).

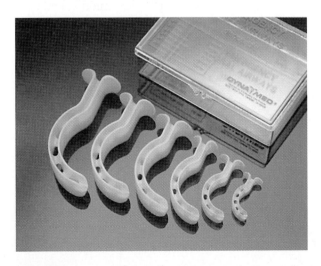

FIGURE 3–4
Oropharyngeal airways.

It is inserted into the oral cavity and displaces the tongue away from the posterior pharyngeal wall.

Even with this airway in place, it is necessary to maintain manual positioning of the airway by a head-tilt, chin-lift or jaw-thrust maneuver.

Indications for the Oropharyngeal Airway   The oropharyngeal airway is used as an adjunct for airway control. The patient must be unresponsive and must not have a gag reflex. Insertion of the device in a patient with a gag reflex may stimulate gagging, vomiting, or laryngeal spasm, further complicating the airway. If the patient regains a gag reflex, it is necessary to remove the airway. The airway may be inserted following successful tracheal intubation to serve as a bite block to prevent the patient from biting down on and possibly occluding the tracheal tube.

Contraindications for the Oropharyngeal Airway   The only absolute contraindication to insertion of the oropharyngeal airway is an intact gag reflex. A relative contraindication includes a fracture to the mandible.

Sizing the Oropharyngeal Airway   Oropharyngeal airways come in a variety of infant, child, and adult sizes. The size is a measurement of the distance from the distal tip to the proximal flange. Determine the proper size by holding the airway next to the side of the patient's face and measuring the length of the airway from the corner of the mouth to the tragus of the ear or tip of the earlobe, or from the center of the mouth to the angle of the mandible (Table 3-1).

Technique of Oropharyngeal Airway Insertion   There are various methods of insertion. In the first method, insert the airway upside down with the distal tip facing the back of the hard palate. When the tip reaches the end of the hard palate, rotate the airway to a ninety-degree position. As insertion continues, rotate the airway into the proper anatomical position until the flange of the proximal end of the airway is seated on the teeth (Figures 3-5A to 3-5D). Rotating the airway too early may actually push the tongue into the hypopharynx, worsening or causing an airway obstruction.

An alternative method is to insert the airway into the mouth at a ninety-degree angle, with the airway in a sideways position, then proceed with the insertion into the pharynx.

The preferred method of insertion, especially for infants and children, is with the use of a tongue blade (Figure 3-6). Insert the tip of the tongue blade into the mouth to the base of the tongue, then lift the tongue up and forward away from the posterior pharyngeal wall. Insert the airway in its correct anatomical position, past the tongue, into the airway. The airway is inserted properly when the tongue is displaced forward and the flange is seated on the teeth (Figure 3-7).

If the patient gags during insertion, immediately remove the airway and be prepared for vomiting. It may be necessary to see if the patient can tolerate a

TABLE 3-1 Recommended Sizes of Oropharyngeal Airways

	Length	Guedel Size
Large Adult	100 mm	5
Medium Adult	90 mm	4
Small Adult	80 mm	3

INSERTING AN OROPHARYNGEAL AIRWAY

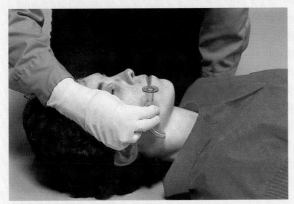

FIGURE 3–5A
Measure to assure correct size.

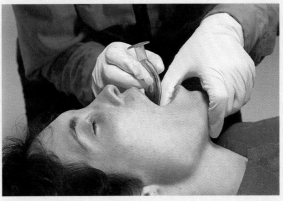

FIGURE 3–5B
Insert with top pointing up toward roof of mouth.

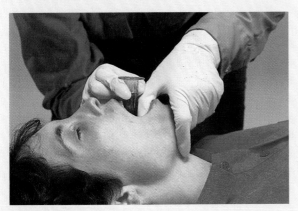

FIGURE 3–5C
Advance while rotating 180°.

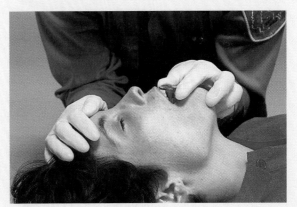

FIGURE 3–5D
Continue until flange rests on the teeth.

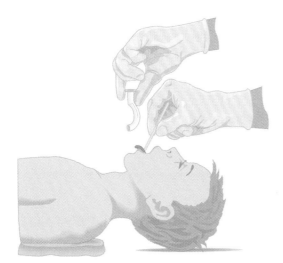

FIGURE 3–6
The preferred method of inserting the oropharyngeal airway in the infant or child is to use a tongue blade to hold the tongue forward and down toward the mandible as the airway is inserted.

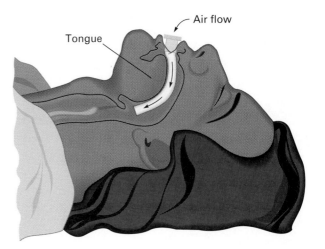

FIGURE 3–7
Oropharyngeal airway properly placed. The tongue is kept from falling back to occlude the patient's airway.

nasopharyngeal airway, if an adjunct is still desirable, or to reconsider the use of an adjunct. If the patient dislodges the airway with his tongue, remove the airway by gently pulling-it out. Be prepared for vomiting.

Complications Associated with the Oropharyngeal Airway   As already mentioned, insertion of the oropharyngeal airway in a conscious or responsive patient or one who has an intact gag reflex will likely cause severe retching and vomiting. This will further complicate the airway and may lead to aspiration of gastric contents. Also, laryngeal spasm caused by insertion of the airway may result in airway obstruction at the level of the larynx. Positive pressure ventilation may be necessary to relieve the laryngospasm.

An improperly sized airway may result in one of two complications: If it is too long, it may push the epiglottis closed over the glottic opening of the larynx, causing a complete airway obstruction. Too short an airway may be easily misplaced and the distal opening of the airway obstructed by the tongue.

Complications may also arise from insertion. An improperly inserted airway can easily push the tongue back into the pharynx, causing or aggravating an airway obstruction.

Aggressive insertion, especially if using the technique in which the airway is inserted in its reverse position, may cause trauma to the upper airway and bleeding, particularly in children. To prevent any additional trauma, be sure that the lips and tongue are not between the teeth and the airway. Never tape the airway in place since it may have to be removed quickly if the patient begins to retch or vomit. Insertion of the airway in a patient with reactive airway disease, such as asthma, may cause an acute attack to worsen.

The lumen of the tube is not large enough to allow for suctioning. Suctioning must be performed around the tube.

Nasopharyngeal Airway

The nasopharyngeal airway, also known as the nasal airway, is a curved hollow tube constructed of soft plastic or rubber with a bevel at the distal end and a flange or flare at the proximal end (Figure 3-8). This airway is less likely to stimulate gagging and vomiting because the soft, pliable tube moves and flexes as the patient swallows, lessening the gag response. Therefore, it may be used in a less responsive patient who is spontaneously breathing but needs assistance in maintaining a patent airway. If a patient does not tolerate insertion of an oropharyngeal airway but needs an airway adjunct, insert the nasopharyngeal airway.

The tube is approximately 15 cm in length. When properly sized and inserted, the distal tip sits at the posterior pharynx while the proximal flare or flange is seated on the external nare. The hollow tube facilitates air flow from the proximal end, past the tongue, and into the hypopharynx.

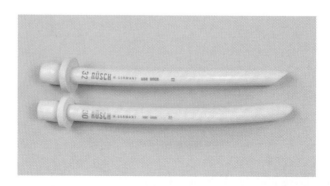

FIGURE 3–8
Nasopharyngeal airways.

The nasopharyngeal airway also requires that a manual airway maneuver, the head-tilt, chin-lift or jaw-thrust maneuver, be maintained during its use.

Indications for the Nasopharyngeal Airway   Insertion of the nasopharyngeal airway is indicated when the oropharyngeal airway is not able to be inserted due to trismus (lockjaw), mandibular trauma, mandibulo-maxillary wiring, or an intact gag reflex. This is the airway of choice for the spontaneously breathing, but less-responsive patient needing airway control.

Contraindications for the Nasopharyngeal Airway   Contraindications to the insertion of a nasopharyngeal include an occluded nasal passage, fracture of the nose, basilar skull fracture, severely deviated septum, blood clot disorders, and leakage of cerebrospinal fluid from the nose. Use caution when inserting a nasopharyngeal airway in a patient who has nasal jewelry in place. The jewelry may obstruct the nares and result in trauma if a nasopharyngeal airway is inserted. If necessary, remove the nasal jewelry prior to insertion.

Sizing the Nasopharyngeal Airway   The size of the nasopharyngeal airway indicates the internal diameter (i.d.) in millimeters (mm). As the internal diameter increases, so does the length of the tube. To size the airway, place the proximal end of the tube at the tip of the nose and the distal end at the earlobe on the side of the face. The properly sized tube should extend from the tip of the nose to the earlobe. In addition, be sure not to select a tube with an external diameter that is greater than the internal diameter of the nare (Table 3-2).

Technique of Nasopharyngeal Airway Insertion   Make sure the nasopharyngeal airway is well lubricated with a water-soluble lubricant or an anesthetic jelly such as 2% lidocaine gel. This facilitates insertion and reduces the incidence of nasopharyngeal trauma and subsequent bleeding. Be sure to select the proper-sized airway prior to insertion. Advance the nasopharyngeal airway, with the distal beveled end toward the septum, posteriorly, aiming toward the back of the head (Figures 3-9A to 3-9C).

Attempting to advance the airway cephalically (upward) will only result in resistance. Gently guide the tube along the floor of the nostril through the nasopharynx and into the posterior pharynx. In the spontaneously breathing patient, you should feel airflow at the proximal end of the tube. Immediately remove the tube if you feel no airflow in the spontaneously breathing patient.

If you meet resistance when inserting the airway, rotate the tube slightly while continuing. If you continue to meet resistance, you may have to remove the airway and insert it in the opposite nare. Significant trauma and bleeding may result if you force the airway into the nasopharynx.

Complications Associated with Use of the Nasopharyngeal Airway   Several complications associated with the nasopharyngeal airway may arise during its use. An airway that has been improperly sized and is too long may be inadvertently

TABLE 3–2	Recommended Nasopharyngeal Airway Sizes
Large Adult	8.0 to 9.0 i.d.
Medium Adult	7.0 to 8.0 i.d.
Small Adult	6.0 to 7.0 i.d.

INSERTING A NASOPHARYNGEAL AIRWAY

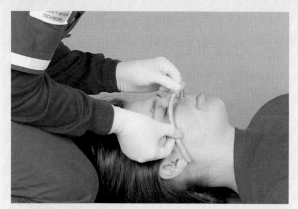

FIGURE 3–9A
Measure the airway.

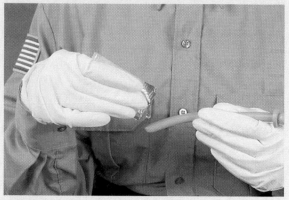

FIGURE 3–9B
Lubricate it with water-soluble lubricant.

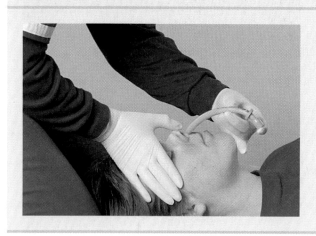

FIGURE 3–9C
Insert with the bevel toward the septum or the base of the tonsil.

inserted into the esophagus. Also, if the airway is too long it may stimulate the laryngeal or glossopharyngeal reflex producing laryngospasm, retching, or vomiting. This will result in gastric insufflation and subsequent gastric distention and hypoventilation during positive pressure ventilation. An airway that is too short may easily be occluded by the tongue in the posterior pharynx.

Insertion of the airway in the less responsive patient may cause laryngospasm. If the gag reflex is still intact and stimulated, vomiting may occur. This will further complicate airway management and may lead to aspiration of gastric contents.

Trauma to the nasal mucosa with bleeding may also result from insertion. Because the nasopharyngeal airway does not isolate the trachea, the blood may be aspirated into the trachea and lungs.

ADVANCED AIRWAY MANAGEMENT TECHNIQUES

You may have to perform advanced airway management techniques to establish, maintain, or protect the patient's airway. Also, when prolonged ventilation is necessary, you must consider advanced airway management to avoid some of the common complications associated with traditional airway management and ventilation techniques. Advanced airway management techniques are most commonly used:

▶ To protect the patient from aspiration of secretions, blood, vomitus, or other foreign substances

▶ To facilitate better oxygenation and ventilation when performed over a longer period of time

▶ When basic airway management techniques have failed or are inadequate

▶ To establish a limited drug route for the patient in cardiac arrest

▶ To create a means to perform tracheobronchial suctioning

Even though most advanced airways provide a more effective means of airway control and ventilation, you must usually initially establish an airway and ventilate the patient by using basic airway management techniques. However, there are some situations in which immediate intervention with advanced airway techniques is necessary, such as upper airway burns with laryngeal edema or massive bleeding into the upper airway.

The preferred method of advanced airway management is the insertion of a tracheal tube. Alternative devices to control the airway include the esophageal-tracheal Combitube® (ETC), the pharyngeo-tracheal lumen airway (PtL®), and the laryngeal mask airway (LMA).

Tracheal Intubation

Tracheal intubation is the preferred method of airway control in the patient with an altered mental status who lacks a gag or cough reflex, the nonbreathing unresponsive patient, or the cardiac arrest patient. A properly placed tracheal tube truly protects the airway by isolating the trachea and preventing aspiration of secretions, blood, vomitus, or other foreign material into the lungs. In addition, the tracheal tube limits the amount of dead air space during ventilation and ensures delivery of adequate tidal volumes.

When providing positive pressure ventilation to a patient who is not intubated, higher pressures must be generated to deliver the necessary tidal volume and achieve subsequent lung inflation. During the process, high pharyngeal pressure may be created, thereby opening the esophagus and causing insufflation of large amounts of air into the stomach. This results in gastric distention, which may lead to regurgitation of gastric contents and potential aspiration. Also, the gastric distention may elevate the diaphragm and impede lung expansion during ventilation. This may reduce the tidal volume delivered and lead to hypoxia. To reduce the risk of these complications, the trachea should be intubated as soon as possible during resuscitation.

Placement of a tracheal tube requires skill. A significant number of complications can occur from an improperly placed tube or poor technique of insertion by an inexperienced EMT-Basic, EMT-Intermediate, or paramedic. Therefore, only EMS personnel who are well trained and perform or practice tracheal intubation on a regular basis should be intubating the patient. Complications associated with tracheal intubation performed by inexperienced EMS personnel include:

▶ Trauma to the oropharynx and larynx

▶ Interruption of chest compression and ventilation for an unacceptable period of time while the intubation is being performed

▶ Insertion of the tracheal tube into the esophagus or bronchus

▷ Failure of the EMS crew to recognize a misplaced tracheal tube

▷ Inability to secure the tube adequately or failure to secure the tube completely

Once a tracheal tube is placed and confirmed, chest compressions and ventilations can be performed asynchronously. Ventilations should be administered at 12–15 per minute while delivering a tidal volume of 10 ml/kg. At this rate and volume, with the addition of supplemental oxygen at as close to 100% as possible, adequate oxygenation should occur.

Advantages of Tracheal Intubation

The following are advantages of intubation with an tracheal tube:

▷ It isolates the trachea and prevents aspiration of foreign material.

▷ It permits tracheobronchial suctioning.

▷ It provides more effective delivery of tidal volume and lung expansion.

▷ It enables delivery of higher concentrations of oxygen.

▷ It provides a secondary route for administration of certain drugs.

▷ It prevents gastric insufflation and resultant gastric distention.

▷ It permits asynchronous chest compressions and ventilations, allowing faster compression rates.

Indications for Tracheal Intubation

Not every patient requires tracheal intubation. The following are indications for tracheal intubation:

▷ Patient in cardiac arrest

▷ Need for prolonged positive pressure ventilation

▷ Inadequate spontaneous ventilation in the patient with no gag reflex

▷ Patient unable to protect his own airway due to altered mental status, coma, absent gag reflex

▷ Inability to effectively ventilate the patient with other basic or less invasive techniques

▷ Inability to achieve or maintain acceptable oxygenation during ventilation

▷ Airway compromise due to trauma, infection, or inflammation

Evaluate the Patient

It is necessary to take a few seconds to minutes to evaluate the patient prior to intubation. This is done to identify a potentially difficult intubation due to the patient's anatomy or situations that may impede normal intubation procedures. The evaluation may aid you in selecting the most appropriate equipment and technique.

Information collected from a patient history could provide you with valuable indicators of possible difficult intubation. History of a previous surgery with difficult intubation is typically known by the family, which can predict difficult intubation in the present situation. Other indicators of potentially difficult intubation are:

▷ Oral surgery

▷ Neck surgery

▷ Temporal mandibular joint problems

▷ Rheumatoid arthritis

▶ Degenerative joint diseases

▶ Upper airway burns

▶ Trauma to the neck

▶ Short, thick neck

▶ Cervical spine immobilization

Assess the oropharynx for potential signs of a difficult intubation. The Mallampati classification system is used to determine the potential difficulty of the intubation. This system was designed for use in the non-emergent situation and has little use in the emergent setting when an airway must be established quickly. The Mallampati and other types of guides for intubation require the patient to sit up and protrude his or her tongue. Most often, this is not feasible in the emergency situation prior to intubation. As a general rule, if you cannot see the posterior pharyngeal wall upon visualization inside the mouth, assume that the intubation will be difficult.

Measure the distance from the mandibular symphysis to the thyroid cartilage (Adam's apple). When the distance is less than three finger-widths in an adult, visualization of the glottic opening may be very difficult since the angle at which you can view the glottic opening is changed.

Another method is to measure the distance from the chin to the hyoid bone. If it is less than three fingerbreadths or 60 mm, a short, anterior larynx should be suspected. The space between the hyoid bone and the thyroid cartilage should be about two finger-widths. This is also an indication of an anterior larynx. A straight blade is considered the preferred blade, rather than a curved, in this patient. Also, using the Sellick's maneuver to displace the glottic opening posteriorly would facilitate visualization during laryngoscopy. The BURP (backwards, upwards, rightwards pressure) maneuver will provide the best glottic displacement and line of sight for intubation.

Also inspect the oropharynx for dentures, loose teeth, caps, or plates which may become dislodged and possibly aspirated. Inspect the neck for evidence of surgery, which may narrow and distort the airway anatomy and make visualization and tube insertion difficult. Thick, fat, and muscular necks typically have limited mobility, which may make alignment of the airway difficult and may lead to problems in visualization and a difficult intubation.

Patients with spine and face trauma require in-line stabilization of the head and neck. Facial trauma also poses additional problems of bleeding in the airway, loss of bony structure, and distortion of anatomy for visualization and tube insertion. Bleeding in the airway may block visualization. Suction is required to clear the airway prior to the intubation technique. It may be necessary to continuously apply suction to the hypopharynx during the laryngoscopy.

Expect a large amount of secretions when intubating a submersion patient. A pulmonary edema patient may need to be intubated while in a seated position. This technique requires more skill than the conventional intubation.

Equipment Needed for Orotracheal Intubation

Several pieces of equipment are needed for tracheal intubation. It is vital to check the equipment to ensure it is in proper working order prior to the procedure. The equipment needed for tracheal intubation includes:

▶ Body substance isolation equipment (gloves, eye protection, mask)

▶ Laryngoscope (includes handle and several blades)

▶ Tracheal tubes

▶ Malleable stylet

▶ Water-soluble lubricant

▶ 10-ml syringe

▶ Device to secure the tracheal tube

▶ Suction unit

▶ Stethoscope

▶ Magill forceps (optional)

▶ Secondary confirmation devices, such as a CO_2 monitor and esophageal detection device

Laryngoscope   The laryngoscope consists of two parts, the handle and the blade. It is inserted into the hypopharynx where it is used to lift the epiglottis and view the glottic opening and the vocal cords. The procedure is termed *laryngoscopy.* Laryngoscopes may be reusable or disposable.

The laryngoscope blade is the component that is used to manipulate the tongue and epiglottis to expose and view the glottic opening and vocal cords. It is critical to be able to see this area in order to make sure that you are guiding the tracheal tube between the vocal cords and into the trachea, and not misdirecting the tube into the esophagus. The laryngoscope handle holds batteries that provide energy for a light at the end of the blade that facilitates visualization. Fiber-optic handles contain the bulb within the handle. The light is transmitted by a fiber-optic strand to the end of the blade.

There are two basic types of laryngoscope blades: the curved blade (McIntosh) or the straight blade (Miller, Wisconsin, Flagg) (Figure 3-10). The name of each blade describes its shape. Both types of blades are designed to lift the epiglottis; however, each blade achieves this differently.

▶ **Straight Blade** The straight blade is a long, straight, hollow-channeled blade with a rounded distal end. It comes in a variety of sizes ranging from 0, the smallest, to 4, the largest. A 0 blade would be used in an infant, whereas, a 4 blade would be used to intubate a large adult. The straight blade is the preferred blade in infants and children. It is also the blade of choice in larger patients with short necks because the larynx is usually more anterior.

The straight blade is inserted into the hypopharynx and is used to directly lift the epiglottis (Figure 3-11). The blade is inserted in the right side of the mouth. With a sweeping motion to the midline, the blade moves the

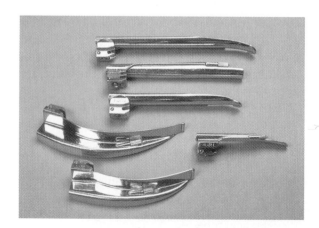

FIGURE 3-10
Straight and curved
laryngoscope blades

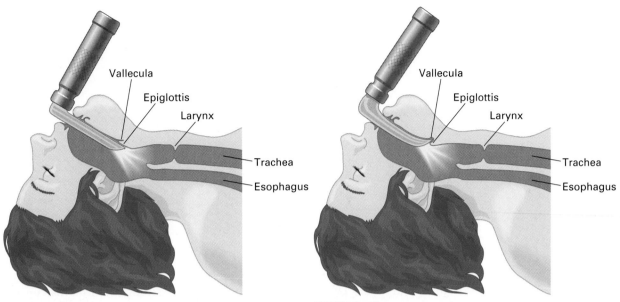

FIGURE 3–11
The straight blade is placed under the epiglottis and directly lifts the epiglottis upward to expose the vocal cords and glottic opening.

FIGURE 3–12
The curved blade is placed into the vallecula and indirectly lifts the epiglottis.

tongue to the left to provide for better visualization. The rounded distal end of the blade is inserted under the epiglottis. With an upward movement of the laryngoscope handle, the epiglottis is directly lifted upward, exposing the glottic opening and the vocal cords. The tracheal tube is advanced along the right side of the blade. The hollow channel is a sight to allow for visualization of the tube passing through the vocal cords. Note that it is *not* a conduit for the tube insertion. This is a common mistake that ends in a torn or damaged tracheal tube and the subsequent need to extubate and reintubate the patient.

▶ **Curved Blade** The curved blade has a round, beaded distal edge. The blade has a broad surface and a tall flange that is used to move and hold the tongue out of the way, allowing for better visualization of the airway anatomy during the intubation procedure. Like the straight blade, the curved blade comes in sizes ranging from 0 for infants to 4 for larger adults.

The distal, beaded end of the blade is inserted into the vallecula, the space located between the tongue and the epiglottis (Figure 3-12). With the edge of the blade resting on the glossoepiglottic ligament, upward and forward movement of the handle will put pressure on the ligament, causing the epiglottis to be indirectly lifted up off the glottic opening.

A variety of other types of blades are available. The GRANDVIEW laryngoscope blade is 80% wider than the standard McIntosh blade allowing for a better view of the glottic opening and vocal cords. Because of the improved view, less maneuvering, repositioning, and manipulation is needed during the laryngoscopy which results in less trauma to the airway. The curve of the GRANDVIEW blade is designed to be more anatomically inline with the angles encountered in the oral cavity and it also allows the blade to be used as a curved or straight blade (Figure 3-13). Disposable laryngoscope blades and handles are also available from a variety of manufacturers.

FIGURE 3–13
GRANDVIEW laryngoscope
blade.
(Hartwell Medical)

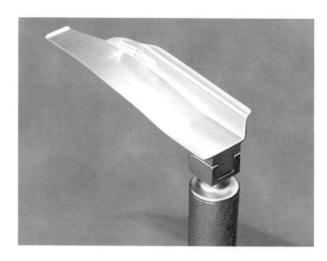

Assembly of the laryngoscope is a simple procedure. The indentation of the proximal end of the laryngoscope blade is designed to lock into the bar on the laryngoscope handle. The blade is lifted upward until at a right angle to the handle. This will lock the blade into the handle, make electrical contact, and light the bulb at the distal end of the blade (Figure 3-14).

The light at the distal end of the laryngoscope should be white and bright. If the light is not lit or is poorly lit, check that the blade is properly locked in the handle. Also, check the bulb to be sure it is tightly screwed in. A loose bulb can be dislodged while intubating and aspirated down the trachea. An absent or poor light may indicate weak or dead batteries. Spare batteries and bulbs should be available.

Fiber-optic laryngoscope handles and blades are also available. The fiber-optic light source is located in the handle. The blade contains a fiber-optic strand, rather than a bulb, to provide illumination at the distal end of the blade. The light source is brighter than with the conventional bulb system.

Tracheal Tube   The tracheal tube is a flexible, translucent tube made of polyvinyl chloride. It is open at both ends. The proximal end has a standard 15 mm connector that allows for attachment of a bag-valve or other ventilation device. The distal end has a cuff that seals and isolates the trachea. An inflation tube extends from the cuff up the tube to a pilot balloon and a one-way inflation valve. A syringe is connected to the inflation valve to fill the distal cuff with air. The pilot balloon is designed to verify cuff inflation (Figure 3-15). Uncuffed tracheal tubes are available and are used in children and infants, typically up until age eight.

The size noted on the outside of the tube is the internal diameter (i.d.). In general, an adult male will require an 8.0 to 8.5 mm i.d. tube, whereas an adult female will take a 7.0 to 8.0 mm i.d. tube. If you are uncertain as to what tube size to use, it is more prudent to use the smaller-sized tube to prevent damage to the glottic structures. In an emergency situation, both average sized males and females can usually take an 8.0 mm i.d. tube. It is a good idea to have available, when intubating, one size larger and one size smaller than the selected tube size for the patient.

A Murphy eye (a small hole) is located at the distal end of the tracheal tube opposite the side of the bevel. The eye reduces the chances of distal tube obstruction from the tracheal wall, blood clots, or secretions.

The length is measured in centimeters (cm) and is marked at several intervals along the tube. The average length of the tube for the adult is 33 cm. When properly placed, the front teeth of the patient will be at the 19–23 cm marking on the

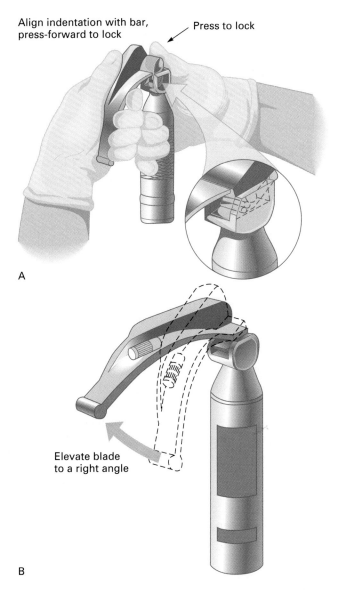

Align indentation with bar, press-forward to lock

Press to lock

A

Elevate blade to a right angle

B

FIGURE 3–14
(A) Affix the laryngoscope blade to the handle. (B) Lift the laryngoscope blade until the blade locks into place and the light at the end of the blade is lit.

tube. These measurements are available to continually monitor for tube movement or displacement. The distal tip of the tracheal tube sits midway between the carina and the vocal cords when properly placed. Once proper tube placement is confirmed, note the centimeter level marking on the tube at the front teeth. This will be used as one indicator of possible tube movement and dislodgement. The IT or Z79 markings indicate that the tube has met certain standards or tests.

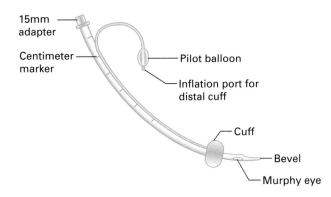

15mm adapter

Centimeter marker

Pilot balloon

Inflation port for distal cuff

Cuff

Bevel

Murphy eye

FIGURE 3–15
Tracheal tube components.

Alternative types of tracheal tubes are also available. An Endotrol tube contains a flexible stylet and trigger built into the side wall of the tube. When the trigger is pulled the stylet redirects the distal end of the tube upward. This facilitates placement of the tube in the patient with an anterior larynx. Also available is a tube with a built-in medication injection port and catheter for tracheal medication administration.

Stylet   The malleable stylet is a piece of pliable metal wire, typically coated in plastic, that is inserted into the tracheal tube prior to insertion to alter its shape and provide stiffness (Figure 3-16). The stylet should be lubricated with a water-soluble jelly to facilitate easy removal. The stylet should never project beyond the level of the Murphy eye and should always be recessed at least 1/2 inch from the distal end of the tube. Trauma to or perforation of the trachea may result from a stylet that is inserted beyond the distal end of the tube. Hold the tube securely while removing the stylet, so you do not accidentally dislodge the tube.

Other Equipment   If time permits, water-soluble lubricant is applied to the distal end of the tracheal tube to facilitate insertion into the trachea. In addition, the lubricant is applied to the stylet to allow for easier removal. Do not use petroleum-based products, since they can damage the tracheal tube and irritate and inflame the mucosal lining of the airway.

A 10 ml syringe is used to inflate the distal cuff of the tracheal tube. Test the cuff integrity with the syringe when checking the equipment prior to intubation. Once the air is inserted in the cuff, remove the syringe. If the syringe is left attached to the inflation port, the cuff may deflate.

Magill forceps are used to remove foreign material from the upper airway. Also, the forceps may be used to direct the tip of the tracheal tube into the glottic opening.

A commercially available securing device or tape must be used to hold the tube in place once proper placement has been confirmed. Some systems use IV tubing as a securing device.

A suction unit must be available during tracheal intubation to remove any fluid, vomitus, blood, or other material from the upper airway to prevent aspiration. A rigid catheter is used to suction the oropharynx, whereas, a soft suction catheter should be available to perform tracheobronchial suctioning.

A stethoscope must be at hand to listen for breath sounds at the lungs and epigastrium to help confirm correct placement of the tracheal tube, or to help detect incorrect placement. In addition, an end-tidal carbon dioxide ($ETCO_2$) detector and an esophageal detection device should be used to provide secondary confirmation of tracheal tube placement.

Sellick's Maneuver (Cricoid Pressure)

As explained earlier, a major complication associated with both basic and advanced airway management is the regurgitation and aspiration of gastric con-

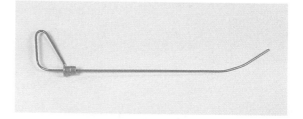

FIGURE 3–16
The stylet may be inserted to
stiffen and shape the tracheal tube.

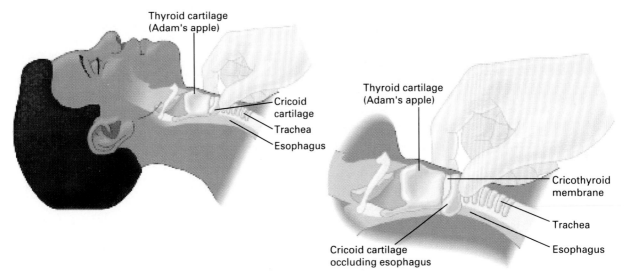

FIGURE 3–17
To perform Sellick's maneuver, locate the cricoid cartilage inferior to the thyroid cartilage. Apply firm posterior pressure with the thumb and index finger.

tents. When an tracheal tube is not in place, high pharyngeal pressure is generated during positive pressure ventilation. This opens the esophagus and causes gastric insufflation. The resultant gastric distention may impede effective artificial ventilation or may lead to regurgitation of gastric contents with subsequent aspiration.

To protect the airway, posterior pressure (Figure 3-17) is applied to the cricoid cartilage to seal off the esophagus when unprotected positive pressure ventilation is performed. This reduces the amount of air traveling down the esophagus to the stomach and blocks vomitus from moving up the esophagus.

In addition, cricoid pressure is used to better visualize the glottic opening. By applying pressure on the anterior cricoid ring, displacing the larynx posteriorly, the glottis will be less anterior and the visual field used for tracheal tube insertion is improved. Remember the BURP technique during cricoid pressure which provides better visualization of the glottic opening. Be careful not to apply too much backward pressure to the cricoid cartilage during Sellick's maneuver since it may occlude the airway and impair tracheal intubation.

Technique of Orotracheal Intubation
When properly placed in the trachea, the tracheal tube is the ultimate airway. However, if the tube is misplaced in the esophagus, it will lead to rapid deterioration of the patient. If this mistake is not detected and corrected immediately, it can be fatal or result in irreversible brain damage from hypoxia.

The steps for tracheal intubation (Figures 3-18A to 3-18H) are as follows:

1. *Take the necessary universal precautions against contact with body fluids.* In addition to gloves and eye protection, consider a surgical mask because of the potential for spattering of secretions during intubation.

2. *Clear the airway of any potential obstructions.* Establish manual positioning of the airway, and insert an oropharyngeal or nasopharyngeal airway.

3. *Begin positive pressure ventilation to hyperoxygenate the patient while the equipment is being prepared.* A spontaneously breathing patient may continue to receive close to 100% oxygen via a nonrebreather mask. Place the patient on an ECG monitor and apply a pulse oximeter.

OROTRACHEAL INTUBATION

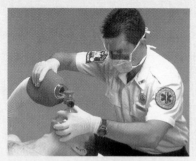

FIGURE 3–18A
Hyperoxygenate the patient.

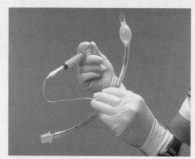

FIGURE 3–18B
Prepare the equipment.

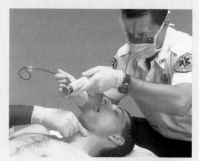

FIGURE 3–18C
Apply Sellick's maneuver and insert laryngoscope.

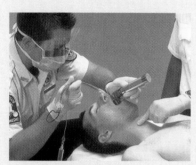

FIGURE 3–18D
Visualize the larynx and insert the ETT.

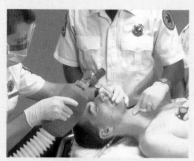

FIGURE 3–18E
Inflate the cuff, ventilate, and auscultate.

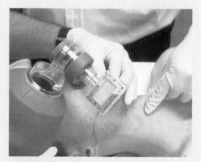

FIGURE 3–18F
Confirm placement with an $ETCO_2$ detector.

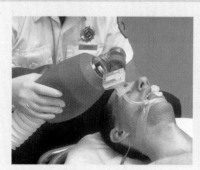

FIGURE 3–18G
Secure the tube.

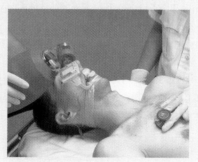

FIGURE 3–18H
Reconfirm tracheal tube placement.

4. *Assemble and check the equipment.* Select the proper laryngoscope blade according to patient size and personal preference. Assemble the laryngoscope blade and handle. If a conventional laryngoscope is used, check the light at the distal end of the blade. The light should be bright and secure. If the light is dim, you will have difficulty in visualizing the glottic opening and will be more likely to misplace the tracheal tube in the esophagus. Orotracheal intubation is a completely "visual" technique, and it is imperative that you visualize the tube as you pass it through the vocal cords and into the larynx. Orotracheal intubation should not be performed blindly. Therefore, the light emitted from the blade must be very white and bright. Obtain another handle or change the batteries if necessary.

Select the proper size tracheal tube. Women usually require a 7.0 mm to 8.0 mm i.d. tube, whereas men usually take an 8.0 mm to 8.5 mm i.d. tube. In an emergency situation, an 8.0 mm i.d. tube is acceptable for use in both average sized men and women.

Lubricate the stylet and insert it into the tracheal tube. Be sure the stylet is recessed at least 1/2 inch (1.27 cm) from the distal end of the tube. The use of a stylet is based on your personal preference, the patient's anatomy, and any difficulty in passing the tube. The stylet merely conforms the tube to a desired configuration and facilitates insertion into the glottic opening and trachea. Shaping the tube and stylet into an open J, or "hockey-stick," configuration can facilitate the tube insertion.

Attach a 10 ml syringe to the inflation port, inject 10 ml of air, and check the distal cuff for leaks. The cuff and pilot balloon should remain inflated. Replace any defective tubes prior to intubation. Insertion of a tube with a defective cuff will not isolate the trachea, therefore leaving the airway unprotected and allowing for air leakage and potential subsequent aspiration.

Have a suction unit available. Check the suction unit to ensure it is working properly. Have both a rigid and soft suction catheter available.

If time permits, lubricate the tracheal tube with a water-soluble lubricant to ease insertion.

5. *Open the patient's mouth and inspect for any potential obstructions. Suction any secretions, blood, or other substances from the oropharynx. Remove any loose dental appliances.*

6. *Position the patient's head to align the three axes of the mouth, pharynx, and trachea to achieve better visualization* (Figure 3-19). Place the head in a "sniffing" position. Accomplish this by extending the head and flexing the neck (extension at C1 and C2, flexion at C5 and C6). You can aid flexion of the neck by placing folded towels under the occiput. The neck is extended by the person performing the intubation. Do not allow the patient's head to hang over the end of the bed or table.

If a cervical spine injury is suspected, you must place the patient's head and neck in a neutral in-line position. In this position, the nose is aligned with the umbilicus on a sagittal (vertical, midbody) plane, and the head and neck are maintained in a neutral position without any flexion or extension. To

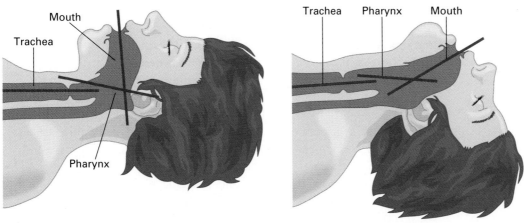

FIGURE 3–19
The three axes of the mouth, pharynx, and trachea should be aligned to achieve optimal visualization for tracheal intubation.

protect the patient's spine, open the airway with a jaw-thrust maneuver and perform laryngoscopy with a second person maintaining in-line stabilization. Apply cricoid pressure any time you are intubating a patient with a suspected cervical spine injury.

7. *Hyperoxygenate the patient by providing positive pressure ventilation with a ventilation device delivering as close to 100% oxygen as possible for a 30-second period.* This will raise the PaO$_2$ and reduce the effects of hypoxia associated with the absence of ventilation during the intubation procedure.

    At any time the intubation process reaches 30 seconds, stop the procedure and resume ventilation of the patient for at least 30 to 60 seconds before attempting intubation again.

8. *Open the mouth using the fingers of the right hand. If any secretions or other substance are again found inside the mouth, suction it out immediately.* Apply cricoid pressure until the tracheal tube is successfully placed and the distal cuff is inflated.

9. *Insert the laryngoscope and visualize the vocal cords.* Hold the laryngoscope handle in your left hand. Insert the blade into the right side of mouth. Move the blade to the midline while advancing it to the base of the tongue. With the tip of the blade at the base of the tongue, lift the blade up and forward toward the patient's feet—in the direction that the handle is pointing. This should be a nice, fluid motion without prying or digging. Do not pull back on the handle or use the teeth as a fulcrum. This will potentially cause trauma to the lips, gums, or teeth. To avoid trauma to the lower lip, you can retract it with your right index finger during the laryngoscopy. In the patient without suspected spinal injury, point and direct the end of the handle at a 30- to 45-degree angle toward and above the patient's feet. This will place the patient's head and neck in the "sniffing position," which will allow for better visualization of the glottic opening and vocal cords.

    To visualize the vocal cords for tube insertion, you must use the laryngoscope blade to lift the epiglottis off the glottic opening. If you are using a straight blade, insert the tip under the epiglottis. With upward and forward movement on the laryngoscope handle, directly lift the epiglottis to expose the glottic opening. If you are using a curved blade, insert it into the vallecula, the space between the base of the tongue and the base of the epiglottis. Lift the handle to place pressure on the glossoepiglottic ligament, which will indirectly cause the epiglottis to be lifted away from the glottic opening.

    To aid in visualization, you may slightly elevate the patient's head. Also, cricoid pressure may be applied to slightly displace the laryngeal structures posteriorly, facilitating visualization. These measures should not be used, however, if a cervical spine injury is suspected.

    The identifiable structures that you should view during laryngoscopy are the epiglottis, the cuneiform, corniculate, and aretynoid cartilages, the glottic opening, and the vocal cords. If the straight laryngoscope blade is inserted too far, it may enter the esophagus, and no identifiable structures will be seen. Remember that the opening of the esophagus is more oval in shape and lacks cartilaginous structures, whereas the opening of the glottis is surrounded by cartilage and is round in shape. Pull back on the blade to remove it from the esophagus while watching for the glottic opening and vocal cords to come into view.

    If you do not see any identifiable structures, remove the blade and resume ventilation of the patient. Never exceed 30 seconds from the time artificial ventilation is stopped until it is resumed. Hyperoxygenate the patient for at least 30 to 60 seconds prior to any further attempt at intubation.

10. *With the vocal cords visualized, insert the tracheal tube.* Insert the tube through the right side of the mouth. Watch the tube as it passes through the vocal cords. The proximal end of the cuff should be advanced 1/2 to 1 inch (1 to 2.5 cm) beyond the level of the vocal cords. This should place the tip of the tracheal tube midway between the vocal cords and the carina. The tube marking in an average-sized adult will be between 19 and 23 cm at the level of the front teeth.

    Hold the tube firmly in place and remove the stylet if you used it.

11. *Inflate the distal cuff with 8–10 ml of air.* Inject enough air to assure cuff inflation that is adequate to isolate the trachea. This may require 10–20 ml of air. Check the pilot balloon to ensure the cuff is still inflated. If the pilot balloon does not remain inflated, remove the tracheal tube, ventilate the patient, and repeat the procedure using a new tracheal tube. The cuff is used to isolate the trachea and prevent aspiration of foreign materials. It does not secure the tube in place. Be sure to hold the tube firmly until it is properly secured.

12. *Assess tube placement with primary confirmation techniques.* While simultaneously delivering the first ventilation, auscultate over the epigastrium while watching for chest rise and fall. If gurgling sounds are heard over the epigastrium, or the chest does not rise with the ventilation, assume the esophagus has been inadvertently intubated and immediately remove the tube. Immediately resume ventilation and hyperoxygenation for approximately 30 to 60 seconds prior to another attempt. Be prepared to suction vomitus.

    If the chest wall rises and no sounds are heard over the epigastrium, auscultate over the right and left lung fields at the second intercostal space midclavicular line on the anterior chest. Then auscultate over the left and right lateral chest at the fourth intercostal space at the midaxillary line with subsequent ventilation. If equal breath sounds are heard bilaterally, secure the device.

    Right mainstem intubation may occur from insertion of the tube too far into the trachea. If diminished or no breath sounds are heard on the left but good breath sounds are heard on the right, deflate the cuff and pull back on the tube about 1 to 2 cm. Recheck breath sounds. Repeat this procedure until equal breath sounds are heard bilaterally. (A left mainstem intubation may also occur; however, because of the anatomy and angles of the right and left mainstem bronchi, it is much more likely that the right mainstem bronchus will be inadvertently intubated. The same procedure would be used to correct a left mainstem intubation.)

    Confirm the tube placement using secondary confirmation techniques. An end-tidal carbon-dioxide ($ETCO_2$) detector may also be used to confirm tube placement (Figures 3-20, 3-21A, and 3-21B). Lack of CO_2 typically indicates an esophageal intubation in patients with spontaneous circulation. However, in pulseless patients or those with low pulmonary blood flow or large dead space, the amount of carbon dioxide may be negligible and not detected. Both electronic and less-expensive colorimetric CO_2 detectors are available. Be familiar with the limitations of both devices.

    A minimum of six ventilations must be provided prior to determining the CO_2 level. If any CO_2 is present in the stomach as a result of BVM ventilation, it will be washed out within the six ventilations. Thus, if CO_2 is present after six ventilations, it is a reliable indicator that the tracheal tube is in

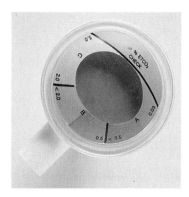

FIGURE 3–20
Colorimetric end-tidal CO_2 detector.

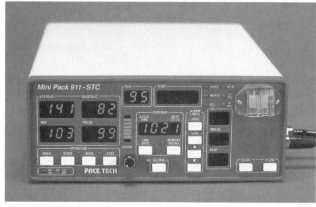

FIGURE 3–21A
Combined devices check pulse oximetry, end-tidal CO_2, blood pressure, pulse, respiratory rate, and temperature.

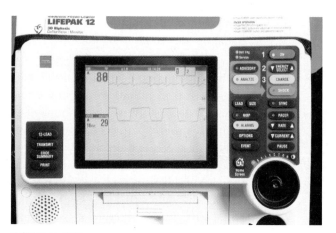

FIGURE 3–21B
LifePak 12 with end-tidal CO_2 monitoring capability.
(Carl Leet)

the trachea. If after six breaths there is no CO_2 being exhaled, the tube is most likely in the esophagus. Be cautious when the patient is in cardiac arrest due to poor pulmonary blood flow. In cardiac arrest, a carbon dioxide level reading of 2% or greater is an indication of correct tracheal tube placement.

The colorimetric CO_2 detection device is disposable, reliable, inexpensive, and easy to read. When CO_2 is present, the device changes color. Around the edges of the detection indicator window, a scale is provided and color coded to match the color in the patient exhaled CO_2 level window. Due to the low metabolic state and poor perfusion, the electronic device may be more reliable in determining tube placement.

Pulse oximetry is a reliable tool to detect oxygen desaturation in a patient. The pulse oximeter will show a decline in the oxygen saturation levels if a patient is intubated in the esophagus; however, the desaturation may not occur for several minutes. Thus, pulse oximetry is not a good tool to quickly determine esophageal intubation.

Esophageal detector devices are also available to assess for esophageal intubation (Figures 3-22 and 3-23A to 3-23C). If the tracheal tube is in the esophagus, when suction is applied to the device either by squeezing the bulb or pulling back on the syringe, the suction will cause the esophageal mucosa to be pulled up against the distal end of the tube. This will not allow the bulb

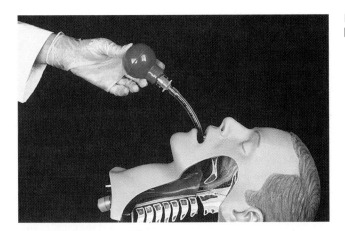

FIGURE 3–22
Esophageal detector device.

FIGURE 3–23
An esophageal intubation detector—bulb style. (A) Squeeze the device and then attach it to the tracheal tube. (B) If the bulb refills easily and within 10 seconds upon release, it indicates correct placement. (C) If the bulb does not refill, or refills in greater than 10 seconds, the tube is improperly placed.

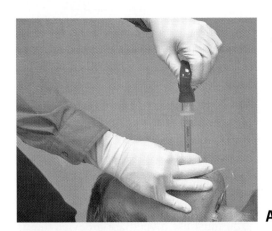

A

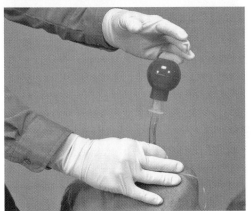

B

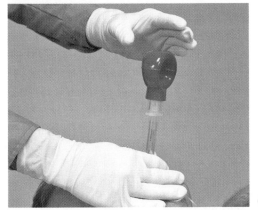

C

to refill quickly or it will prevent the operator from pulling back on the syringe. This is an indication that the tube is in the esophagus. The esophageal detection devices may not be very reliable in patients that are morbidly obese, in late pregnancy, in status asthmaticus, or those with copious amounts of tracheobronchial secretions. In these patients, the trachea may have a tendency to collapse or the airways may be small and obstructed by secretions providing a false reading when the tube is properly placed in the trachea.

These devices are only adjuncts to proper assessment of tube placement. A chest x-ray, if it is feasible to obtain one, can also be used to confirm tube placement. However, the best method to ensure proper tube placement is direct visualization. If in doubt, reconfirm the tube placement by performing a laryngoscopy and visualizing the tube between the vocal cords. If you are in doubt that the tube is properly positioned, remove it and resume ventilation with a bag-valve mask or other acceptable ventilation device.

13. *Secure the tube with tape or a commercially available securing device.* IV tubing can be used as a temporary securing device, especially when sweat or vomit make taping impossible. Note the cm marker at the level of the front teeth. You may insert an oropharyngeal airway after the tube is secured to prevent the patient with spontaneous circulation and breathing from biting down and occluding the tube. Following any patient movement, you must reassess tube placement. Even when the tube is secured, it can become dislodged when the patient moves or is moved.

14. *Ventilate the patient with a tidal volume of 10 ml/kg.* You can adjust the volume up for larger patients and down for smaller patients. During respiratory or cardiac arrest, provide ventilation at a rate of 12 to 15 ventilations per minute (one every 4 to 5 seconds). You must use a ventilation device that is capable of being connected to an oxygen source and is able to deliver as close to 100% oxygen as possible with each ventilation. In a patient who suffers from severe obstructive pulmonary disease, lower the respiratory rate to 6 to 8 per minute to avoid air trapping and an auto-PEEP effect. Air trapping may lead to a drop in cardiac output and a decrease in perfusion. It is necessary to reduce the respiratory rate to allow for more adequate time for exhalation.

Complications Associated with Tracheal Intubation

Numerous complications are associated with the procedure of tracheal intubation. These include the following:

▶ Trauma to the lips and tongue from compression between the teeth and the blade, causing lacerations

▶ Trauma to the teeth from the laryngoscope blade

▶ Bleeding, hematoma, or abscess formation associated with laceration of the pharyngeal or tracheal mucosa caused by the tip of the tube or an improperly placed stylet

▶ Rupture of the trachea

▶ Injury to the vocal cords and avulsion of an arytenoid cartilage

▶ Pharyngeal-esophageal perforation

▶ Intubation of the pyriform sinus or glottic opening

▶ Stimulation of the gag reflex with subsequent vomiting and aspiration

▶ Hypertension, tachycardia, and dysrhythmias from stimulation of the sympathetic nervous system in the patient with spontaneous circulation

▶ Right mainstem intubation—the most frequent complication, which can lead to hypoxia from underinflation of a lung

▶ Esophageal intubation, resulting in no ventilation or oxygenation

▶ Hypoxia resulting from prolonged interruptions in ventilation during attempts at intubation

▶ Airway obstruction associated with laryngospasm from stimulation of the epiglottis or larynx

▶ Accidental displacement of the tube during movement of the patient due to failure to properly secure the tube

▶ Excessive delay in performing chest compressions during the intubation attempt

To reduce the possibility of complications associated with tracheal intubation, the following precautions must be observed:

▶ Only properly trained personnel should perform tracheal intubation.

▶ Cardiac arrest patients should be intubated as quickly as possible to reduce the risk of gastric insufflation and aspiration of gastric contents.

▶ The intubation procedure must not exceed 30 seconds. (The 30-second time period is from cessation of ventilation to resumption of ventilation.) If the procedure is unsuccessful, the patient must be hyperoxygenated with a ventilation device connected to 100% supplemental oxygen for 30 to 60 seconds before intubation is reattempted.

▶ Apply cricoid pressure to reduce the incidence of gastric distention and aspiration of gastric contents into the lower airway. Once the patient is successfully intubated, there is no need to continue with cricoid pressure.

▶ A high-volume, low-pressure cuff is recommended for use during cardiac arrest management. The intracuff pressure should be adjusted to 25–35 cmH_2O. An intracuff pressure of 25 cmH_2O is the minimum required to isolate the trachea and prevent aspiration. An intracuff pressure greater than 40 cmH_2O will reduce capillary blood flow to the mucosa and result in tissue ischemia or necrosis.

▶ Continually reassess and confirm tracheal tube placement.

Special Considerations in the Patient with Severe Trauma

Patients who present with trauma to the face, neck, or head, or those with multiple injuries require special airway consideration due to the possibility of spinal cord or vertebral injury. If the mechanism of injury is consistent with a pattern that may cause spinal injury, take the necessary precautions against excessive manipulation of the head and neck while establishing an airway. During both manual and mechanical maneuvers to establish and maintain an airway, the head and neck must be maintained in a neutral in-line position until spinal injury can be ruled out.

When manually establishing an airway in the patient with suspected spinal injury, perform a jaw-thrust or a chin-lift maneuver without the head tilt. If the jaw thrust or chin lift alone does not clear the airway, slowly and carefully perform the head tilt until the airway is unobstructed. The goal is to keep the head in an in-line neutral position, with the nose in-line with the umbilicus and the head and neck not flexed or hyperextended. This position must be maintained until spinal injury is properly ruled out.

Blind nasal intubation may be performed in patients with suspected spinal injury since, unlike orotracheal intubation, nasal intubation does not require manipulation of the head and neck. Nasal intubation must be performed only by trained and experienced health care providers in spontaneously breathing patients. Spinal immobilization must be continuously maintained, since the technique may cause the patient to move his neck. This technique of intubation is relatively contraindicated in patients with suspected midfacial fractures and basilar skull fracture. In this case, orotracheal intubation should be performed while a second care provider maintains manual in-line stabilization of the head and neck. This procedure requires special training and skill.

If a tracheal tube cannot be successfully placed, and if ventilation cannot be adequately achieved by other methods such as bag-valve-mask ventilation, a cricothyrotomy or tracheostomy may be necessary. Paralytic agents may aid in successful intubation when the patient presents with trismus and clenched jaws. Frequent suctioning may be necessary, as bleeding is associated with facial or airway trauma.

ALTERNATIVE OROTRACHEAL INTUBATION TECHNIQUES

There are several alternative techniques that can be used to insert a tracheal tube orally. These methods do not use the conventional technique of insertion or the standard equipment. These techniques are not recommended in every situation nor for all patients needing tracheal intubation.

Digital Intubation

In digital intubation you insert your fingers into the patient's hypopharynx and use them to lift the epiglottis and guide the tracheal tube through the glottic opening. This is referred to as a "blind" technique because you do not use a laryngoscope and do not actually visualize the tracheal tube passing through the vocal cords. (The word *digits* is another word for fingers or toes. The term *digital* means "with the fingers.") Digital intubation may be used in a patient who is in cardiac arrest or is unresponsive and has no gag reflex.

The standard technique of using a laryngoscope is preferred because it allows you to visualize the tracheal tube passing through the vocal cords. However, you may encounter situations where the patient's position or condition precludes effective use of a laryngoscope, for example in situations where visualization of the glottic opening is difficult because of bleeding in the airway.

Digital intubation may also be recommended in the patient with a possible cervical spine injury. Since this patient is immobilized and the head and neck cannot be manipulated, it is very difficult to achieve an axis that allows for proper visualization with a laryngoscope. Digital intubation can be performed without visualizing the vocal cords, so it eliminates the need to manipulate the head or neck.

Also, consider the patient who is entrapped in a vehicle and needs to be intubated. Extrication time may be lengthy and the airway problem may be severe. Proper positioning for intubation with a laryngoscope is virtually impossible to achieve, but digital intubation may be possible.

In addition, in the case of failure of the laryngoscope batteries or bulb when no spares are available or working properly, you may be able to insert a tracheal tube using the digital technique.

Equipment Needed for Digital Intubation

The equipment needed to perform digital intubation includes:

- Appropriate size tracheal tube
- Malleable stylet
- Water-soluble lubricant
- 10 cc syringe
- Bite block
- Device to secure the tracheal tube

Digital Intubation Procedure

The procedure for digital intubation is listed below:

1. *Take the necessary body substance isolation precautions.* Gloves, eye wear, and a mask are recommended.
2. *Ventilate and hyperoxygenate the patient for approximately 30 seconds prior to initiating the insertion technique.*
3. *Check and lubricate the tracheal tube as you normally would.* Lubricate the tube with a water-soluble lubricant. Lubricate the stylet and insert it to form the tube into a J-shape.
4. *Assure correct positioning.* If spinal injury is suspected, have a trained rescuer or health care provider manually stabilize the patient's head and neck. Face the patient and kneel at his left shoulder.
5. *Instruct the person ventilating the patient to stop.* Quickly place a bite block between the patient's molars to prevent the patient from biting down on your fingers during the procedure.
6. *Insert the middle and index fingers of your left hand into the patient's mouth.* Advance your fingers down the midline while simultaneously lifting the tongue up and out of the way.
7. *Palpate the epiglottis with your middle finger. Press upward and move the epiglottis forward* (Figure 3-24A).
8. *Insert the tracheal tube into the mouth with your opposite hand.* Advance the tube using your index finger to maintain the tip of the tube against the middle finger. The tip will be directed upward toward the epiglottis. Guide the tip of the tube into the glottic opening with the index and middle fingers (Figure 3-24B).
9. *Remove your fingers, hold the tube in place, and remove the stylet carefully.*
10. *Ventilate.* Inflate the cuff with 8 to 10 cc of air. Attach a bag-valve device to the tube and ventilate. Artificial ventilation must not be interrupted for greater than 30 seconds during the insertion.
11. *Confirm placement.* Auscultate over the epigastrium and watch for chest rise and fall while a ventilation is delivered. If no gurgling sounds are heard, auscultate over the right and left chest at the apex and midaxillary area of the lungs. If primary confirmation indicates proper tube placement, perform secondary confirmation by using an end-tidal CO_2 detector or an esophageal detection device.
12. *If correct placement is not confirmed, remove or reposition the tube.* If gurgling sounds are heard over the epigastrium, cease ventilation through the tube and immediately remove it. Ventilate the patient with a bag-valve-mask

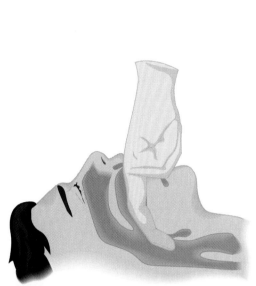

FIGURE 3-24A
Insert your index and middle fingers into the patient's mouth. Elevate the epiglottis with your middle finger.

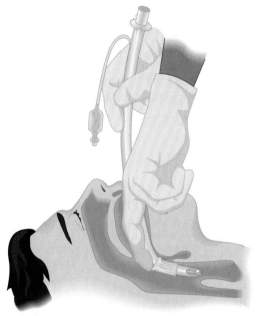

FIGURE 3-24B
Guide the tube forward and into the glottic opening with your index and middle fingers.

device. If breath sounds are absent or diminished on the left but are good on the right, suspect a right mainstem intubation. Deflate the cuff and pull back on the tube until equal breath sounds are heard bilaterally and then re-inflate the cuff.

13. *If correct placement is confirmed, secure the tube.* If no sounds are heard over the epigastrium, breath sounds are heard equally bilaterally, and the chest rises and falls equally with each ventilation, secure the tube in place. Use tape or a commercial securing device.

14. *Resume ventilation of the patient.*

15. *Reassess tube position with each movement of the patient.*

Transillumination (Lighted Stylet) Intubation

Another alternative method of orotracheal intubation is transillumination, or the "lighted stylet" technique. In this technique, a special lighted stylet is inserted into the tracheal tube which is then inserted through the mouth and hypopharynx and down into the trachea. If correctly placed in the trachea, the bright light can be seen through the soft tissues of the neck. If incorrectly placed in the esophagus, the light will be very dim or hard to see.

With the transillumination method, the intubator can confirm passage of the tracheal tube through the glottic opening into the trachea without having to use a laryngoscope to directly visualize the glottic structures. This eliminates the need to manipulate the head or neck during intubation. For this reason, the transillumination technique can be an effective means of intubation in the trauma patient.

The transillumination stylet has a high intensity bulb at the distal end. Power for the device is supplied by a small battery housed at the proximal end and is controlled by an on-off switch. A major complication with this technique is the inability to effectively see the stylet light because of the ambient light. For this reason, transillumination is best performed in a darkened environment. In sunlight or a brightly lit room, shield the neck to be sure whether the stylet light is or is not shining through the neck.

Equipment Needed for Transillumination Intubation
The equipment needed to perform transillumination tracheal intubation includes:

▶ Appropriate size tracheal tube
▶ Lighted stylet
▶ Water-soluble lubricant
▶ 10 cc syringe
▶ Scissors (to trim the tube)
▶ Securing device for the tracheal tube

Procedure for Transillumination (Lighted Stylet) Intubation
The procedure for transillumination intubation is:

1. *Take the necessary body substance isolation precautions* including gloves, eye wear, and a mask.
2. *While maintaining ventilatory support, ventilate and hyperoxygenate the patient for approximately 30 to 60 seconds prior to the attempt.*
3. *Assemble and check the equipment.* The tracheal tube should be between 7.5 and 8.5 mm i.d., and will need to be cut to 25–27 cm in order to accommodate the stylet. Place the stylet into the tube and bend it just proximal to the cuff.
4. *Kneel on either side of the patient, facing the head.*
5. *Turn on the stylet light.*
6. *Insert the tube/stylet.* With your index and middle fingers inserted deeply into the patient's mouth and your thumb on the chin, lift the patient's tongue and jaw forward. Insert the tube/stylet combination into the mouth and advance it through the oropharynx and into the hypopharynx. Using a "hooking" motion, lift the epiglottis out of the way and advance the tube/stylet through the glottic opening into the larynx (Figure 3-25A).
7. *Confirm that the light is visible.* When you see a circle of light at the level of the larynx on the anterior neck, hold the stylet stationary (Figure 3-25B). Advance the tube off the stylet into the larynx approximately one-half to one inch. A diffuse, dim, or hard-to-see light indicates that the tube/stylet combination is in the esophagus. The tube should be immediately withdrawn and hyperventilation resumed. A bright light that appears laterally to the upper aspect of the thyroid cartilage (Adam's apple) indicates that it is placed into the right or left pyriform fossa. Immediately withdraw the tube and resume ventilation. A second attempt can be tried after a few minutes. Artificial ventilation must not be interrupted for greater than 30 seconds when performing this technique.
8. *Hold the tube in place with one hand and remove the stylet.*
9. *Ventilate.* Inflate the cuff with 8–10 cc of air and attach the bag-valve device to the end of the tube.
10. *Confirm placement.* Auscultate for sounds over the epigastrium while inspecting for chest rise with the first ventilation. If gurgling is heard, immediately remove the tube and begin positive pressure ventilation with

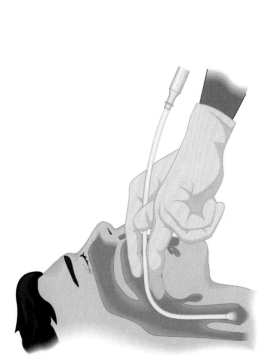

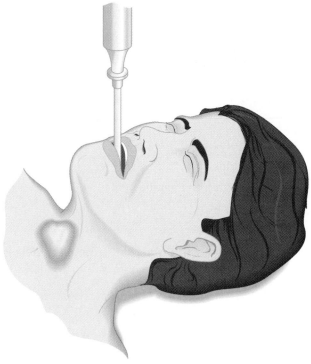

FIGURE 3–25A
Lighted stylet (transillumination) tracheal tube in position.

FIGURE 3–25B
The properly positioned stylet should be visible at the front of the patient's neck.

the bag-valve-mask device. If no sounds are heard, auscultate breath sound on both sides of the chest in the apical and midaxillary areas of the lung. Breath sounds should be equal on each side. If breath sounds are diminished or absent on the left, suspect a right mainstem intubation. Deflate the cuff of the tube and pull back until breath sounds are heard equally bilaterally. Re-inflate the cuff. Observe for equal rise and fall of the patient's chest. Confirm tube placement using secondary confirmation techniques.

11. *Secure the tube* with tape or a commercial securing device that has been approved by medical direction.

12. *Reassess tube placement often, especially after each patient move.*

ALTERNATIVE AIRWAY ADJUNCTS

A variety of alternative adjuncts for airway management are available. These alternative devices are designed to be inserted blindly; therefore, less skill is required for their use. These devices are effective in managing the patient's airway and delivering ventilation. Three of the more common devices are the esophageal-tracheal Combitube® (ETC), the pharyngeo-tracheal lumen (PtL®) airway, and the laryngeal mask airway (LMA).

Esophageal-Tracheal Combitube® (ETC)

The esophageal-tracheal Combitube® (ETC) airway is a double-lumen airway. The ETC lumens are not placed one inside the other. Instead, the lumens are situated side by side and separated by a partition wall within a larger tube (Figure 3-26).

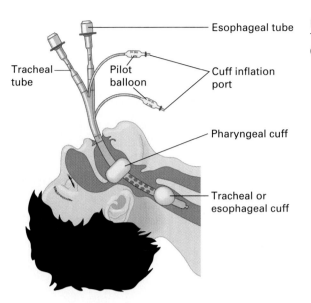

FIGURE 3–26
The esophageal-tracheal Combitube® (ETC).

Esophageal tube

Tracheal tube

Pilot balloon

Cuff inflation port

Pharyngeal cuff

Tracheal or esophageal cuff

The distal end of the ETC has a cuff that is used to seal either the esophagus or the trachea, depending on the placement. A proximal pharyngeal cuff, which is self-positioning and self-adjusting, is used to seal the pharynx, eliminating the need for a mask device. The #1 tube is slightly longer and delivers the ventilation through a series of holes located between the distal cuff and the pharyngeal cuff. The holes are located just proximal to the glottic opening when the tube is placed in the esophagus. The #2 tube is slightly shorter than the #1 tube and provides ventilation from the end of the tube below the distal cuff, similar to a tracheal tube. The #2 tube is used to ventilate when the tube has been placed in the trachea. Based on the tube design and operator use, it is more likely that the tube will be placed in the esophagus (Figures 3-27A and 3-27B).

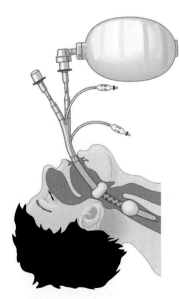

FIGURE 3–27A
Esophageal placement of the Combitube® airway.

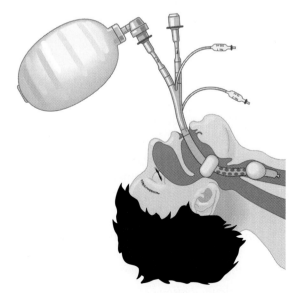

FIGURE 3–27B
Tracheal placement of the Combitube® airway.

Advantages

The following are advantages of the ETC:

- ▶ The pharynx is sealed by the large balloon cuff located in the pharynx; therefore, a mask is not necessary for performing ventilation. This eliminates the complication of a poor mask seal during ventilation.
- ▶ The risk of inadvertent tracheal intubation is not considered a true complication since the tube is designed to be placed in either the trachea or esophagus.
- ▶ There is no obturator in the distal lumen; therefore, immediate suctioning of gastric contents may be performed.
- ▶ A spontaneously breathing patient may breathe through the series of small holes in the opposite lumen.
- ▶ The pharyngeal cuff is self-positioning and self-adjusting, allowing for a better pharyngeal seal.

Contraindications

The Combitube should not be used in patients that are under 5 feet tall and less than 16 years of age. A Combitube SA is used for patients who are 4 to 5 feet tall. There is no pediatric device available. The Combitube should not be used in a patient with a known esophageal disease or one who has ingested a caustic substance. Also, never attempt to insert the device in a patient with a gag reflex or if the patient is not unresponsive.

Equipment

Equipment needed for ETC insertion includes:

- ▶ Oxygen source
- ▶ Bag-valve-mask device
- ▶ ETC device
- ▶ Water-soluble lubricant
- ▶ 10 or 20 ml and 100 ml syringe
- ▶ Suction equipment
- ▶ Stethoscope
- ▶ Secondary confirmation equipment ($ETCO_2$ or esophageal detector device)

Technique

The ETC is inserted using the following procedure:

1. *Hyperoxygenate the patient by performing positive pressure ventilation and a 100 percent oxygen source for one to two minutes.*
2. *Lubricate the ETC using water soluble lubricant.*
3. *Place the patient's head in a neutral position. Pull the tongue and mandible forward.* Insert the ETC through the mouth along the natural curvature of the pharynx. Continue to insert the tube until the black rings on the tube are at the level of the patient's teeth.
4. *Inflate the balloon cuff on the large tube with 100 ml of air. Inflate the smaller cuff with 10–15 ml of air.*
5. *Ventilate through the shorter tube port marked #1 (blue tube).* Auscultate over the epigastrium and assess for chest rise and fall. If no air is heard in

the epigastrium, auscultate over the chest at the second intercostal space at the midclavicular line and at the fourth intercostal space at the midaxillary line. If breath sounds are heard, continue to ventilate through this port and confirm using a secondary confirmation device.

6. *If air is heard over the epigastrium when ventilating through tube #1, remove the BVM or ventilation device and connect it to the other port (clear tube). Auscultate over the epigastrium and chest while ventilating through this port. Confirm tube placement using a secondary confirmation device.*

7. *Secure the tube in place.*

The complication rate with the use of the ETC has been low. Studies have shown that ventilation and oxygenation have been comparable to the tracheal tube. The ETC requires the operator to make a proper assessment of the tube's placement, which requires some skill.

Pharyngeo-tracheal Lumen Airway (PtL®)

The pharyngeo-tracheal lumen (PtL®) airway is a dual-lumen device that is blindly inserted into the airway without the need for direct visualization. The PtL® is actually a tube within a tube, thus the dual lumen reference. (Figure 3-28). A long, clear tracheal-type tube with a cuff at the distal end is located inside a shorter, wider tube that is designed to fit just proximal to the glottic opening. The shorter tube has a large balloon cuff that is used to seal the pharynx. The longer tube, which is designed to be inserted in either the trachea or esophagus, also has a distal cuff that is used to occlude the esophagus or isolate the trachea. An obturator is located within the long tube for cases of esophageal placement.

When the long, clear tube has been inserted into the trachea, the plastic obturator is removed and ventilation is performed through that tube. However, if the long tube is placed in the esophagus, the plastic obturator is left in place and the ventilation is performed through the shorter (green) tube (Figure 3-29). The

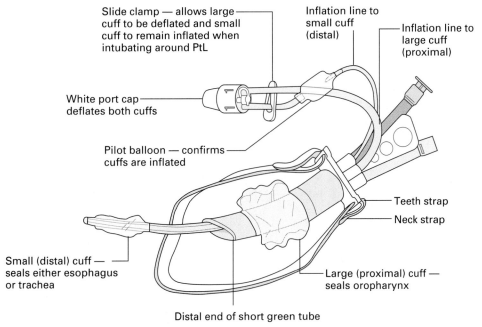

Slide clamp — allows large cuff to be deflated and small cuff to remain inflated when intubating around PtL

Inflation line to small cuff (distal)

Inflation line to large cuff (proximal)

White port cap deflates both cuffs

Pilot balloon — confirms cuffs are inflated

Teeth strap

Neck strap

Small (distal) cuff — seals either esophagus or trachea

Large (proximal) cuff — seals oropharynx

Distal end of short green tube

FIGURE 3–28
The pharyngeo-tracheal lumen (PtL®) airway.

FIGURE 3–29
The PtL® airway in place. The longer tube is shown placed in the esophagus while ventilations delivered through the shorter tube are directed into the trachea.

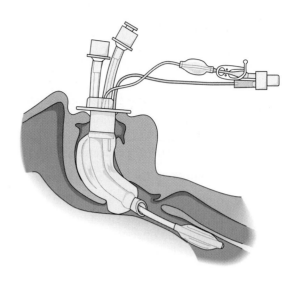

pharyngeal cuff seals the pharynx and allows for effective ventilation. The airway is secured in place with a strap that is fastened around the neck.

Advantages

Two major advantages of the PtL® airway design are:

▶ The pharynx is sealed by the large balloon cuff located in the pharynx; therefore, a mask is not necessary for performing ventilation. This eliminates the complication of a poor mask seal during ventilation.

▶ The risk of inadvertent tracheal intubation is not considered a true complication since the tube is designed to be placed in either the trachea or esophagus.

Disadvantages

The greatest limitation with the PtL airway is the need for the emergency care provider to assess the patient to determine whether the longer tube has been placed in the esophagus or the trachea. This requires skill and good assessment techniques. The PtL is not used in patients younger than 16 years of age or those patients who are shorter than 5 feet tall. It should not be used in patients with known esophageal disease or patients who may have ingested a caustic substance.

Equipment

Equipment needed for PtL insertion includes:

▶ Oxygen source

▶ Bag-valve-mask device

▶ PtL® device

▶ Water-soluble lubricant

▶ Suction equipment

▶ Stethoscope

▶ Secondary confirmation equipment (ETCO$_2$ or esophageal detector device)

Technique

The PtL is inserted using the following procedure:

1. *Hyperoxygenate the patient by performing positive pressure ventilation and a 100 percent oxygen source for one to two minutes.*

2. *Lubricate the PtL using water soluble lubricant.*

3. *Place the patient's head in a hyperextended position. Pull the tongue and mandible forward.* Insert the PtL through the mouth along the natural curvature of the pharynx. Continue to insert the tube until the teeth flange and strap are at the level of the patient's teeth.

4. *Fasten the strap around the patient.* Inflate both balloon cuffs by ventilating into the common balloon port.

5. *Ventilate through the shorter and wider (green) tube.* Auscultate over the epigastrium and assess for chest rise and fall. If no air is heard in the epigastrium, auscultate over the chest at the second intercostal space at the midclavicular line and at the fourth intercostal space at the midaxillary line. If breath sounds are heard, continue to ventilate through this port and confirm using a secondary confirmation device. This is an indication that the longer tube is occluding the esophagus.

6. *If air is heard over the epigastrium when ventilating through the shorter (green) tube, remove the stylet from the other tube and attach the BVM or ventilation device.* Begin ventilation. Auscultate over the epigastrium and chest while ventilating through this port. Confirm tube placement using a secondary confirmation device. This indicates the long tube is placed in the trachea.

7. *Ensure the tube is secured in place.*

Laryngeal Mask Airway (LMA)

The laryngeal mask airway (LMA) is an alternative airway device that can be used in all age groups (Figures 3-30). The LMA provides for ventilation through the proximal 15/22 mm port that forces air directly into the glottic opening at the distal opening of the tube. The tube consists of an airway tube, laryngeal mask, and inflation line that connects to the mask. When properly seated, the laryngeal mask sits above the laryngeal inlet just above the glottic opening. When inflated, the mask fills the hypopharynx and covers the laryngeal opening. The tip of the device rests in the esophagus. Two bars in the mask prevent the epiglottis from falling

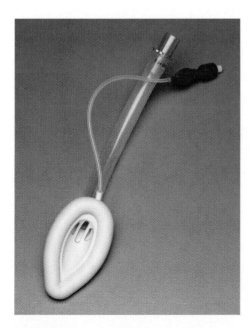

FIGURE 3-30
The standard laryngeal mask airway (LMA).
(LMA North America, Inc.)

TABLE 3–3 Maximum LMA Cuff Inflation Volumes

LMA Size	Cuff Volume (air)	LMA Size	Cuff Volume (air)
1	up to 4 ml	3	up to 20 ml
1-1/2	up to 7 ml	4	up to 30 ml
2	up to 10 ml	5	up to 40 ml
2-1/2	up to 14 ml	6	up to 50 ml

Source: LMA Instruction Manual, Table 5, p. 28

down and occluding the opening into the glottis. The distal mask of the LMA is too large to be inserted into the esophagus.

The LMA is a reusable device. It comes in several sizes. Size 1 is used in infants who weigh less than 6.5 kg. Size 2 is used in patients who weigh between 6.5 to 25 kg. Size 3 is used for patient who weighs greater than 25 kg to a small adult patient. Size 4 is used for a normal sized adult and size 5 is used for a larger sized adult (Table 3-3).

Limited training is needed for insertion of a LMA. Insertion of a LMA does not require a laryngoscope or direct visualization. It uses a blind insertion technique. Since no laryngoscope is used, trauma to the airway is not an issue during the insertion. Insertion of the LMA may cause some stimulation with changes in the heart rate and the blood pressure.

Complications

Aspiration is a major complication of the LMA. The device does not fully protect the glottic opening. Other complications may include laryngospasm and unsuccessful placement, which are rare complications. The trauma patient, obese patient, a patient who has recently eaten, and the patient who has ingested a large quantity of alcohol are not good candidates for LMA insertion due to the risk of aspiration.

Equipment

Equipment needed to insert the LMA include:

▶ Oxygen source

▶ Bag-valve-mask device

▶ LMA device

▶ Water-soluble lubricant

▶ Suction equipment

▶ Stethoscope

▶ Secondary confirmation equipment (ETCO$_2$ or esophageal detector device)

Technique

Insertion of the LMA should be performed as follows (Figures 3-31A to 3-31F):

1. *Hyperoxygenate the patient by performing positive pressure ventilation and using a 100 percent oxygen source for one to two minutes.*

2. *Place the patient in a "sniffing" position.*

3. *Lubricate the dorsal (back) portion of the tube.* Do not lubricate the ventral surface due to the risk of aspiration. Completely deflate the cuff.

STANDARD LMA INSERTION

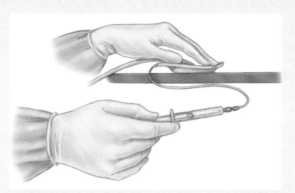

FIGURE 3–31A
Tightly deflate the cuff so that it forms a smooth "spoon shape." Lubricate the posterior surface of the mask with water-soluble lubricant.

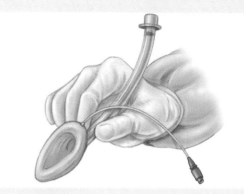

FIGURE 3–31B
Hold the LMA like a pen, with the index finger at the junction of the cuff and the tube.

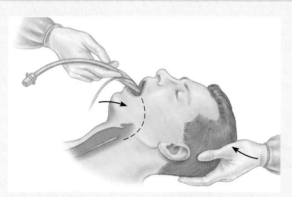

FIGURE 3–31C
With the patient's head extended and the neck flexed, carefully flatten the LMA tip against the hard palate.

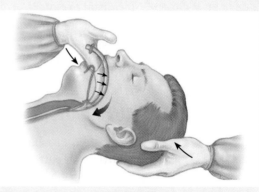

FIGURE 3–31D
Use the index finger to push cranially, maintaining a pressure on the tube with the finger. Advance the mask until definite resistance is felt at the base of the hypopharynx.

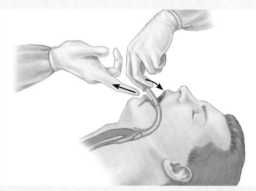

FIGURE 3–31E
Gently maintain cranial pressure with the one hand while removing the index finger.

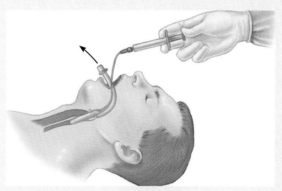

FIGURE 3–31F
Without holding the tube, inflate the cuff with just enough air to obtain a seal (to a pressure of approximately 60 cm H_2O).

(LMA Instruction Manual, p. 28)

4. *Pull the mandible and tongue forward.* While holding the LMA like a pen, insert the device with the tip firmly against the hard palate and facing toward the patient's feet and away from the emergency care provider. Continue to insert the tube until resistance is met. The black line on the tube should be located on the posterior side. If the black line is anterior or lateral, the tube is not properly positioned. A laryngoscope can be used to verify the proper position of the LMA.

5. *Inflate the cuff with approximately 30 ml of air for a #4 mask and 40 ml of air for a #5 mask.*

6. *Attach the BVM or ventilation device.* If possible, monitor peak airway pressure an do not exceed 20 cmH$_2$O pressure while ventilating. This will reduce the amount of gastric insufflation. Ventilate the patient and assess for tube placement using both primary and secondary confirmation techniques.

A modified LMA is available that allows for the passage of a tracheal tube through the lumen of the LMA. This device is referred to as an intubating LMA (Figure 3-32). A tracheal tube is inserted through the lumen of the LMA and out of the distal opening. A rigid steel shaft and handle lies over the ventilation tube. The mask has a V-shaped ramp that directs the tracheal tube upwards and toward the glottic opening. An epiglottic elevating bar is found in the distal mask to keep the epiglottis up and away from the mask opening. Use of this device requires more skill than the standard LMA.

Cuffed Oropharyngeal Airway (COPA)

The cuffed oropharyngeal airway (COPA) is basically a standard Guedel airway with a distal cuff. The inflatable distal cuff is designed to form a seal in the proximal laryngopharynx. The pointed end of the anterior cuff elevates the epiglottis and provides a clear glottic opening (Figure 3-33).

The COPA comes in a variety of sizes ranging from an 8 to an 11. The standard Guedel airway is approximately 1 cm shorter than the COPA airway. The COPA also has a lip tooth guard and securing posts for an elastic securing strap. The proximal end of the tube has a standard 15/22 mm connector. The proper size is determined by placing the distal tip of the COPA at the angle of the jaw with the tooth lip guard extending 1 cm beyond the level of the lips.

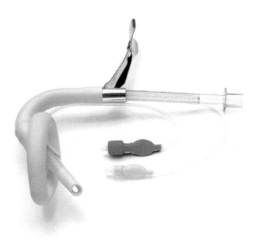

FIGURE 3–32
The intubating LMA.
(LMA North America, Inc.)

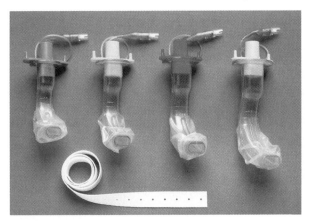

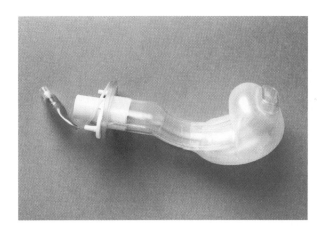

FIGURE 3–33
Cuffed oropharyngeal airway (COPA).
(Carl Leet)

To insert the airway, place the patient's head in a "sniffing" position and proceed as you would with a standard Guedel airway. It may be necessary to manipulate the airway several times to achieve an adequate seal for positive pressure ventilation. The COPA carries the same complications as the LMA; however, the LMA has been shown to perform better in some patients.

Esophageal Obturator Airway (EOA) and Esophageal Gastric Tube Airway (EGTA)

The esophageal obturator airway (EOA) and esophageal gastric tube airway (EGTA) are both obsolete airway adjuncts and are mentioned here for historical purposes only (Figure 3-34). Both devices employed an esophageal tube-mask system. The esophageal tube had a cuff at the distal end. The esophageal tube was designed to be inserted directly into the esophagus. Once the distal cuff was inflated, the tube occluded the esophagus. Thus, vomitus could be regurgitated and the risk of aspiration was eliminated. Also, since the esophagus was occluded, there was no risk of gastric insufflation and subsequent gastric distention. The emergency care provider was responsible for maintaining a good mask seal with the device properly in place. The primary reason for failure of the EOA and EGTA was inadequate mask seal. With the development of better airway devices, the EOA and EGTA have been phased out by emergency medical services.

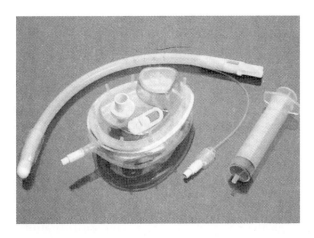

FIGURE 3–34
The esophageal obturator airway
(EOA).

TRANSLARYNGEAL AND TRANSTRACHEAL AIRWAYS

In the event of an airway obstruction when it is not possible to establish an airway by using conventional manual or mechanical techniques, it may be necessary to puncture or incise the larynx or trachea to provide ventilation and oxygenation. These techniques are performed in the acute setting only after failure to gain control of the airway by tracheal intubation and inability to ventilate using less invasive measures.

Transtracheal Catheter Ventilation

Transtracheal catheter ventilation, also known as needle cricothyrotomy or needle jet insufflation, is an emergency procedure for gaining rapid access to the airway in an acute obstruction that cannot be relieved by other methods. An over-the-needle catheter is inserted through the cricothyroid membrane in the lower larynx and angled downward into the trachea. Intermittent jet ventilation is provided through a valve system connected to a 100% oxygen source.

Equipment
Since this is performed only as an emergency procedure, it is important to have all the necessary equipment readily available. Unless a commercially made device is available, the following equipment is needed:

- A 12- to 14-gauge over-the-needle catheter (angiocath)
- A 5- or 10-ml syringe
- Pressure regulating valve and a pressure gauge
- High-pressure oxygen source (30–60 psi)
- High-pressure tubing to connect the pressure regulating valve to a hand-operated release valve
- Relief valve connected by tubing to the catheter

Technique
The cricothyroid membrane forms the soft depression located just inferior to the thyroid cartilage (Adam's apple) and superior to the cricoid cartilage, the large bulky circumferential ring that is the most inferior part of the larynx (Figure 3-35). A 5–10-ml syringe is attached to the back of the flashback chamber of the angiocath. Insert the angiocath at a 45-degree angle caudally (toward the feet) through the cricothyroid membrane (Figures 3-36A and 3-36B). Pull back on the syringe, creating a negative pressure during insertion. When air freely moves into the syringe, the angiocath is in the trachea. Stop the insertion to prevent inadvertent puncture and placement of the angiocath into the esophagus. Advance the catheter off of the stylet and into the trachea until the hub rests on the skin. The tubing is connected to the hub of the catheter while it is held in place. Open the release valve, allowing the oxygen under high pressure to flow through the catheter and inflate the lungs. Adjust the pressure so that the chest rises adequately with each insufflation. As soon as the chest rises during ventilation, stop the insufflation of oxygen. Exhalation occurs passively. This device and technique actually provides for more oxygenation than true ventilation since exhalation is minimal.

Generally, even with acute blockage of the airway, there is enough opening to permit passive exhalation through the pharynx. However, you must carefully

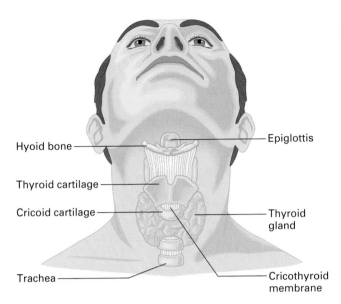

FIGURE 3–35
The cricothyroid membrane is inferior to the thyroid cartilage and superior to the cricoid cartilage (lower border of the larynx).

Hyoid bone

Epiglottis

Thyroid cartilage

Cricoid cartilage

Thyroid gland

Trachea

Cricothyroid membrane

monitor the chest during inhalation and exhalation. If the chest remains inflated after the exhalation period, a complete airway obstruction may be present proximal to the cricothyroid membrane, thus blocking passive exhalation. In this situation, a second catheter will need to be inserted next to the first to allow for adequate exhalation. If this procedure does not correct the exhalation problem, cricothyrotomy should be considered.

Complications

Several complications of transtracheal catheter ventilation may occur both from the insertion and from the technique of ventilation itself. A major disadvantage of using this device and technique is carbon dioxide retention and buildup from inadequate ventilation. Although transtracheal catheter ventilation provides oxygenation, adequate ventilation is not possible. The following are potential complications associated with the device:

▶ Barotrauma resulting in a pneumothorax from the high pressure and air entrapment

▶ Hemorrhage at the site of needle insertion

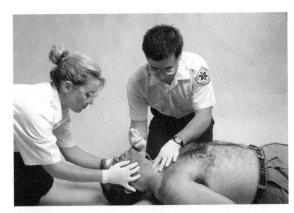

FIGURE 3–36A
To perform a transtracheal catheter ventilation, insert the angiocath at a 45-degree angle caudally through the cricothyroid membrane.

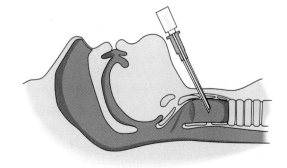

FIGURE 3–36B
The angiocath properly placed through the cricothyroid membrane into the trachea.

▶ Laceration of the thyroid gland

▶ Perforation of the esophagus

▶ Inability to suction secretions

▶ Subcutaneous or mediastinal emphysema

Employing this technique when other more suitable and less complicated methods of establishing and maintaining an airway are available is a major error. Transtracheal catheter ventilation should only be performed when all other conventional methods of airway control are not possible or not effective. This technique is used when an obstruction prevents successful intubation of the trachea. It is not intended to be employed as an alternative because of lack of skill of the health care provider to intubate the trachea successfully.

Cricothyrotomy

The cricothyrotomy is another technique that is used to establish an emergency airway in a patient when other methods are not possible or effective. An incision or puncture is made through the cricothyroid membrane and a tracheal tube or other similar device is inserted into the trachea. Like transtracheal catheter ventilation, a cricothyrotomy provides a temporary avenue for ventilation and oxygenation. However, this technique provides a much better airway, ventilation, and oxygenation than the transtracheal catheter ventilation technique.

Indications
Indications for a cricothyrotomy include:

▶ Inability to intubate the trachea because of a complete airway obstruction that is not relieved by manual foreign body obstruction techniques or laryngoscopy

▶ Trauma to the face or upper airway, hemorrhage, or swelling that prevents tracheal intubation or other airway techniques

Surgical Technique
The surgical technique uses conventional equipment that is readily available. There are commercially prepared devices specifically designed for cricothyrotomy that differ slightly from the surgical technique as described below:

1. Locate the cricothyroid membrane between the thyroid and cricoid cartilage.
2. Cleanse the site with alcohol or another antiseptic solution.
3. While stabilizing the larynx with your nondominant hand, make a horizontal incision with a scalpel into the cricothyroid membrane (Figure 3-37).
4. Insert the handle of the scalpel into the incision and rotate it 90 degrees.
5. Insert the largest possible tracheal tube, usually a pediatric size (5.0 or 5.5 mm), into the opening. The tube only needs to be inserted a few centimeters until the cuff is completely in the trachea. The tip of the tube must be above the carina.
6. Inflate the cuff with 8–10 ml of air.
7. Attach a bag-valve-mask device to the 15/22 mm adapter on the tube and ventilate with the highest concentration of oxygen that can be provided.

Another suggested method requires the scalpel to be left in place. A curved hemostat is inserted in the opening in a closed position, rotated, and then opened

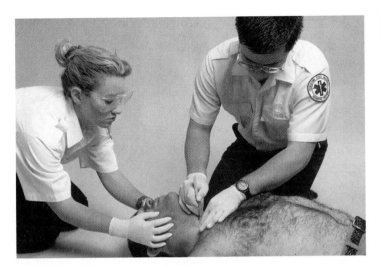

FIGURE 3-37
In the cricothyrotomy, a surgical incision or puncture is made into the cricothyroid membrane.

widely to create a larger opening. Then the scalpel is removed. This provides a much larger opening that facilitates easier insertion of an tracheal tube.

Complications

The following are complications associated with the cricothyrotomy technique:

▶ Damage to blood vessels, causing significant hemorrhage

▶ False passage

▶ Perforation of the esophagus

▶ Subcutaneous or mediastinal emphysema

▶ Tracheal stenosis

A contraindication to performing a cricothyrotomy is the ability to establish and maintain an airway using other possible techniques and devices. The risks of the procedure outweigh the potential benefits when other means are available.

Tracheostomy

Tracheostomy, which is a surgical opening directly into the trachea, is not a technique that should be performed in an emergency setting. It is better performed by a skilled care provider in the operating room under a controlled setting. The airway should first be secured by tracheal intubation, transtracheal catheter ventilation, or cricothyrotomy prior to consideration of performing a tracheostomy.

▦ VENTILATION TECHNIQUES

Several techniques and devices are available to perform positive pressure ventilation when ventilatory support is necessary. These include mouth-to-mouth; mouth-to-nose; bag-valve-mask devices; flow restricted, oxygen-powered ventilation devices; and automatic transport ventilators.

Mouth-to-Mouth and Mouth-to-Nose Ventilation

This basic technique of ventilation uses the expired air of the care provider to provide positive pressure ventilation to the patient. Adequate tidal volumes of air can be delivered by this method. An average of 10 ml/kg of tidal volume is necessary to adequately inflate a person's lungs. The vital capacity of the average person is several liters more than that required to provide adequate lung inflation; therefore, this method provides sufficient tidal volumes during positive pressure ventilation.

Exhaled air contains approximately 17% oxygen. This is a limitation to effective oxygenation. The rescuer can breathe oxygen from a simple face mask, nasal cannula, or other simple oxygen-delivery device to increase the percentage of delivered oxygen to the patient. This method may increase oxygen content delivered by almost 5%.

Cross contamination of infectious disease is also a concern. These techniques should be performed with a barrier device.

Mouth-to-Mask Ventilation

A mask, commonly referred to as a pocket mask, can be used to increase the effectiveness of ventilation by the emergency care provider (Figure 3-38). The mask should:

▶ Be constructed of a transparent material to allow for detection of vomitus, secretions, or other substances in the mouth

▶ Be capable of fitting tightly to the face to provide a good mask seal

▶ Contain an oxygen inlet to increase the delivered oxygen to the patient

▶ Contain a one-way valve to reduce the risk of contamination by infectious secretions

▶ Be available in sizes for the adult, child, and infant

Advantages

Mouth-to-mask ventilation has the same advantage as mouth-to-mouth ventilation of providing more-than-adequate tidal volumes. This technique has actually been shown to be more effective in delivering adequate tidal volumes on mannikins than bag-valve-mask ventilation.

The other major advantages of mouth-to-mask ventilation are:

▶ Supplemental oxygen administration is possible.

▶ There is no direct contact with the patient's mouth or nose.

▶ Exhaled gases are diverted through a one-way valve.

▶ It provides effective tidal volumes.

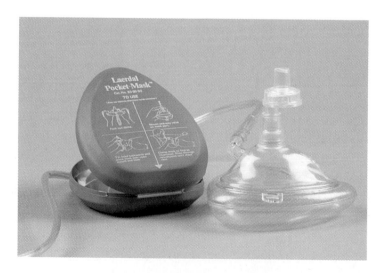

FIGURE 3–38
The pocket mask.

Technique

Connect a one-way valve to the ventilation port to eliminate exposure to the patient's exhaled gas. Connect oxygen tubing to the oxygen inlet valve and set it at 10–15 lpm. (At 10 lpm a concentration of inspired oxygen of approximately 50% will be achieved, whereas 15 lpm will deliver approximately an 80% inspired oxygen concentration.) To assure an open airway, you can use an oropharyngeal airway in conjunction with the appropriate manual airway maneuver, either a head-tilt, chin-lift or jaw-thrust maneuver. Fit the mask over the bridge of the nose and the cleft immediately above the chin. Place both hands over the mask with the thumb-sides of the hands placing pressure to the sides of the mask, creating an airtight seal. Use the fingers to bring the mandible upward toward the mask while maintaining the head tilt or jaw thrust. Use what is known as the E-C clamp technique. Form a "C" with the thumb and index finger over the mask and an "E" with the middle, ring, and little finger under the mandible.

Blow into the ventilation port while watching for chest rise (Figure 3-39). If oxygen is not connected to the mask or is not flowing at a liter flow of at least 10 lpm, ventilate the patient with a tidal volume of 10 ml/kg (approximately 700 to 1,000 ml in an adult) with each ventilation delivered over a 2-second period. The chest must rise clearly and fully with each individual ventilation. Once oxygen is connected to the mask and flowing at a rate of at least 10 lpm, reduce the tidal volume of each ventilation to 6 to 7 ml/kg (400 to 600 ml) delivered over a 1- to 2-second period. When oxygen is provided during the positive pressure ventilation at a concentration of 40% or greater, a reduced tidal is recommended to reduce the incidence of gastric inflation and subsequent regurgitation and aspiration. The lower tidal volumes with oxygen supplement can provide adequate arterial oxygen saturation but will not maintain normocarbia. You can also apply cricoid pressure to reduce the incidence of gastric insufflation and distention during pocket-mask ventilation.

Bag-Valve Devices

A bag-valve device can be used to provide positive pressure ventilation in conjunction with a tracheal tube, with an alternative airway adjunct such as an ETC®, LMA, or PtL®, or with a mask. The bag-valve device is comprised of a self-inflating bag, a nonrebreathing valve to vent all exhaled gases away from the bag, and a

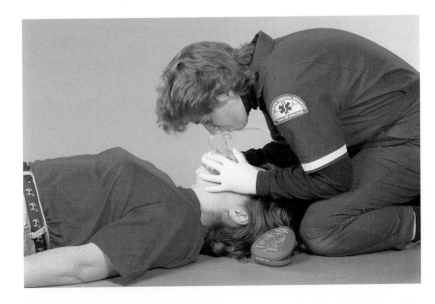

FIGURE 3-39
Mouth-to-mask ventilation.

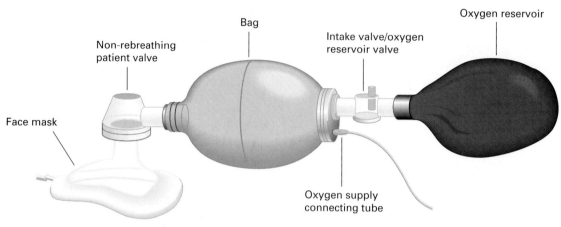

FIGURE 3-40
Bag-valve-mask device.

mask (Figure 3-40). Most bag-valve-mask devices have a volume of approximately 1600 ml. When used in conjunction with a tracheal tube, the bag-valve device can usually deliver an adequate tidal volume of 10–15 ml/kg.

When performing ventilation with a bag-valve device connected to a mask, it is imperative that you establish and maintain a proper manual airway maneuver (head-tilt, chin-lift or jaw thrust). You can use an oropharyngeal airway to facilitate better airway control. If oxygen is not connected to the bag-valve-mask device or is not flowing at a liter flow of 8 to 12 lpm, ventilate the patient with a tidal volume of 10 ml/kg (approximately 700 to 1,000 ml in an adult) with each ventilation delivered over a 2-second period. The chest must rise clearly and fully with each individual ventilation. Once oxygen is connected to the bag-valve-mask device and flowing at a rate of at least 8 to 12 lpm, reduce the tidal volume of each ventilation to 6 to 7 ml/kg (400 to 600 ml) delivered over a 1- to 2-second period. Cricoid pressure can also be used to reduce these complications. Oxygen should be attached to the bag-valve device and a reservoir used to maximize the concentration of delivered oxygen.

Desired Features
A bag-valve device that is acceptable for patient use should have the following standard features:

- A self-refilling bag that is either disposable or can be easily cleaned and sterilized
- A nonjam valve system that can accommodate at least 15 lpm oxygen inlet flow
- Standard 15/22 mm fittings to allow for connection with a tracheal tube and other airway adjuncts
- Oxygen connection and a reservoir bag or tubing that facilitates the delivery of high concentrations of oxygen
- A nonrebreathing valve that does not allow any of the patient's exhaled gases to escape into the bag
- Manufactured of material that allows for proper function under all environmental conditions and temperature extremes
- Available in adult, child, and infant sizes

▶ A pressure relief valve is not desirable; however, if one is present it must have an occlusion switch. Many pediatric and adult BVMs come with a pressure relief valve.

Advantages

Advantages to performing ventilation with a bag-valve device are as follows:

▶ It eliminates direct contact with the patient during ventilation.

▶ High concentrations of oxygen, up toward 98%, may be delivered to the patient during ventilations while using a reservoir tube or bag with high-flow oxygen.

▶ The patient's exhaled gas is vented out of the bag so no rebreathing of oxygen-poor gas occurs.

▶ It can provide adequate ventilation when used with a tracheal tube.

▶ The device is readily available and does not require an oxygen source to power it.

▶ It permits assessment of lung compliance during ventilation.

Disadvantages

The following are disadvantages of the bag-valve device ventilation:

▶ In adults, the bag-valve device may provide less tidal volume than mouth-to-mouth or mouth-to-mask ventilation.

▶ When used with a mask, one operator has difficulty in maintaining a tight mask seal and an adequate airway with one hand while squeezing the bag hard enough with the other hand to deliver an adequate tidal volume.

▶ The device is more effective when used with two experienced and well-trained care providers, one to hold the mask seal with two hands while the other squeezes the bag with two hands.

▶ Improperly over-squeezing the bag-valve device, or delivering the ventilations at too fast a rate, will increase the risk of gastric insufflation.

Indications of a Difficult Patient for Bag-Valve-Mask Ventilation

There are observable indicators that a patient may be potentially difficult to ventilate using a bag-valve-mask device due to poor mask seal, airway positioning, or airway resistance. These indicators are:

▶ Patient who has no teeth (edentulous)

▶ Obstructive airway disease such as acute asthma

▶ Obesity

▶ Structural abnormality of the face

▶ Trauma to the neck or face

▶ Facial hair

▶ Third trimester pregnancy

Technique

Position yourself at the top of the patient's head and establish an airway using the appropriate manual technique. If no cervical spinal injury is suspected, you can tilt the head back and place it on a towel or pillow to achieve a sniffing position. Insert an oropharyngeal airway if the patient has no gag reflex. Consider a

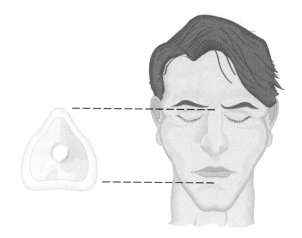

FIGURE 3–41
Always use the proper mask size. The mask should fit over the bridge of the nose and in the cleft of the chin.

nasopharyngeal airway in the patient who is not completely unresponsive but needs positive pressure ventilation. Fit the mask over the bridge of the nose and in the cleft immediately above the chin (Figure 3-41). Hold the mask tightly against the face to form an airtight seal using the E-C clamp technique.

With the head in the proper position, squeeze the bag slowly to deliver an adequate tidal volume based on the oxygen flow to the bag-valve-mask device. If only one care provider is ventilating, he will squeeze the bag with one hand while holding a mask seal with the other (Figure 3-42A). This can be better accomplished by squeezing the bag slowly against his body to deliver a greater volume. One-person ventilation with a bag-valve-mask device often leads to early fatigue and inadequate ventilation. If two care providers are available, one will squeeze the bag with two hands to deliver an adequate tidal volume while the other holds the mask seal (Figure 3-42B). Observe the chest rise to determine if adequate volume is being delivered. A third care provider may apply cricoid pressure to reduce the incidence of gastric distention and aspiration.

If spinal injury is suspected, manual in-line stabilization of the patient's head must be established and maintained during ventilation, and cricoid pressure must be avoided (Figures 3-43A to 3-43C).

Complications

A major complication associated with bag-valve devices is the inability to provide adequate tidal volumes to patients who are not intubated. Operator fatigue occurs early in one-person bag-valve-mask ventilation, which may lead to inadequate

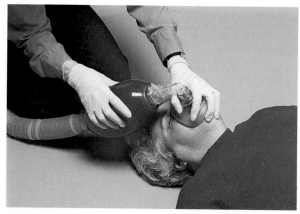

FIGURE 3–42A
One-person bag-valve-mask method.

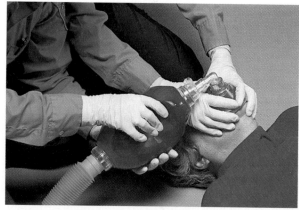

FIGURE 3–42B
Two-person bag-valve-mask method.

IN-LINE STABILIZATION DURING BAG-VALVE VENTILATION

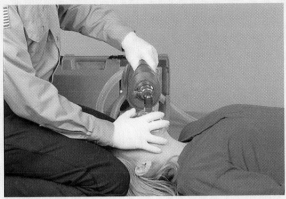

FIGURE 3-43A
Technique for one-person in-line stabilization during bag-valve ventilation.

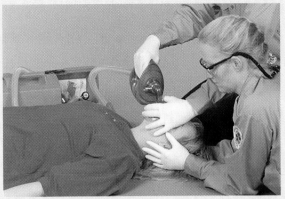

FIGURE 3-43B
Technique for two-person in-line stabilization during bag-valve ventilation.

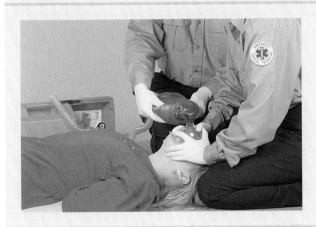

FIGURE 3-43C
Alternative technique for two-person in-line stabilization during bag-valve ventilation.

mask seal and insufficient delivered volume. This leads to ventilatory insufficiency. The proper technique requires training, practice, and demonstrated proficiency.

Flow-Restricted, Oxygen-Powered, Manually Triggered Ventilation Device (FROPVD)

Another method of providing positive pressure ventilation—to an adult patient only—is through the use of a flow-restricted, oxygen-powered ventilation device (Figure 3-44). This device is manually triggered by the practitioner to deliver the desired tidal volume. Since it is powered by an oxygen source, 100% oxygen is delivered with each ventilation. In the spontaneously breathing patient, the negative pressure generated with inspiration will automatically open the valve and allow the patient to breathe 100% oxygen. Oxygen flow ceases once inhalation ends. The device can be used in conjunction with a tracheal tube, ETC®, LMA, PtL® mask, or other acceptable airway adjunct. When used with a mask alone, the high flow and pressure from the device can easily cause gastric inflation and associated complications. When used in conjunction with airway adjuncts, the high pressure and flow can cause barotrauma. Although the FROPVD has been in use by emergency medical services personnel for many years, the device requires further investigation and is not recommended for use in the *AHA Guidelines 2000 for CPR and ECC*.

FIGURE 3–44
A flow-restricted, oxygen-powered ventilation device.

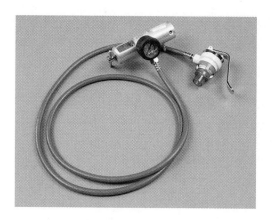

Features

The flow-restricted, oxygen-powered ventilation device should have the following features:

- ▶ A peak flow rate of less than 40 lpm of 100% oxygen
- ▶ An inspiratory-pressure-relief valve that opens at approximately 60 centimeters of water pressure and vents any remaining volume to the atmosphere or ceases gas flow
- ▶ An audible alarm that sounds whenever the relief-valve pressure is exceeded
- ▶ Adaptability to a variety of environmental conditions and extremes of temperature
- ▶ An activating trigger or on/off button positioned so the operator can keep both hands on the mask to hold a seal
- ▶ A standard 15/22 mm coupling to fit an tracheal tube, mask, and other alternative airways

Technique

If your medical director approves the use of the flow-restricted, oxygen-powered ventilation device, follow these steps:

1. Check the unit to ensure that it is functioning properly.
2. Open the airway using a manual maneuver.
3. Attach an adult mask to the ventilator port.
4. Position your hands over the mask and fit it to the patient's face, holding a tight seal with both hands.
5. Depress the button to activate the device and deliver ventilation. As soon as the chest rises, release the button to deactivate the device and stop the airflow.
6. Exhalation occurs through the one-way valve and out to the atmosphere.

Complications

The flow-restricted, oxygen-powered ventilation device is designed to be used on adults only. Because of the high pressure and flow rates, it is not acceptable for infants or children. Also because of the high pressure and flow rates, gastric distention may easily occur. In addition, overinflation can lead to barotrauma, potentially resulting in a pneumothorax. High flow rates in intubated patients may lead to intrapulmonary shunting and maldistribution of ventilation.

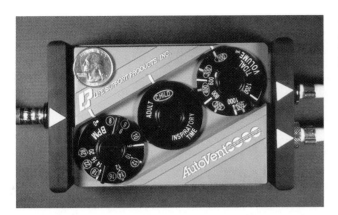

FIGURE 3–45
Automatic transport
ventilator. (The coin shows
relative size.)

Automatic Transport Ventilator (ATV)

Another device used for positive pressure ventilation is the automatic transport ventilator, or ATV (Figure 3-45). Several different devices are currently available. They have been shown to be excellent at providing and maintaining a constant rate and tidal volume during ventilation and maintaining adequate oxygenation of arterial blood. In addition, most ATVs use oxygen as their power source, thereby providing 100% oxygen during ventilation. The ATV can be used to ventilate a patient who is intubated or unintubated.

Advantages

The ATV can deliver oxygen at lower inspiratory flow rates and for longer inspiratory times. Therefore, the device is less likely to cause gastric distention in unintubated patients compared with other methods of positive pressure ventilation, including mouth-to-mask, bag-valve-mask, and flow-restricted, oxygen-powered ventilation devices. However, as with any other ventilation device, gastric distention can occur if the patient's head and neck are improperly positioned.

Advantages of the ATV are:

▶ Oxygen can be delivered at lower inspiratory flow rates and for longer inspiratory times, thereby lessening the likelihood of gastric distention.

▶ The operator is free to use both hands to hold a mask seal or perform other responsibilities if the patient is intubated.

▶ The device can be set to deliver a specific tidal volume, respiratory rate, and minute volume.

▶ Alarms indicate low pressure in the oxygen tank as well as accidental disconnection from the ventilator.

▶ Cricoid pressure can be performed with one hand while the other holds the mask seal.

Disadvantages

There are a few disadvantages associated with the ATV:

▶ Because most ATVs are oxygen powered, a constant oxygen supply is needed to power the device. A bag-valve-mask device should always be readily available when using the ATV.

▶ The ATV cannot be used in children less than 5 years of age.

▶ When using the ATV, it is not possible to feel an increase in airway resistance or a decrease in lung compliance.

Features

The minimum desirable features of the ATV are as follows:

- Time or volume cycled device
- A standard 15/22 mm adapter to fit a tracheal tube, mask, or other airway adjunct
- A rugged design that is also lightweight (2–5 kg)
- Capable of operating under temperature extremes and under all environmental conditions
- A peak-inspiratory-pressure-limiting valve that is set at 60 cmH_2O but can be increased to 80 cmH_2O or lowered to 20 cmH_2O
- An audible alarm that indicates high airway pressure or poor lung compliance when peak inspiratory limiting pressure is generated
- Minimal gas consumption so that the device can operate for a minimum of 45 minutes on an E cylinder
- Ability to deliver 100% oxygen with each ventilation
- Ability to deliver each ventilation over a 2-second period at a maximum flow rate of approximately 30 L/minute in the adult and 1-second duration in children with a maximum flow rate of 15 L/minute
- Ability to provide a rate of 10 ventilations/minute for an adult and 20 ventilations/minute for a child
- If it has a demand-valve feature, it should deliver an inspiratory flow rate of at least 100 L/minute and triggered at −2 cmH_2O inspiratory pressure to reduce the work of breathing.
- Will deliver a ventilation rate of 10 ventilations per minute in the adult and 20 ventilations per minute in the child with the ability to adjust the rate

Technique

Check that the ATV is working properly and is attached to the tracheal tube, mask, or airway adjunct. (These ventilators are most commonly used in intubated patients.) Set the tidal volume and ventilation rate if not already set on the unit. Turn the unit on and watch for adequate chest rise. Adjust the tidal-volume control to provide adequate ventilation. Continuously monitor the device to ensure adequate ventilation volumes and rate.

When using the ATV during cardiac arrest, it is best to select a ventilation rate of 10/minute in the adult and 20/minute in the child. Be cautious when using higher rates. Faster rates may cause air to be trapped in the alveoli creating an auto-PEEP or intrinsic PEEP (iPEEP) effect. This will have a tendency to lower the cardiac output and perfusion. The pulmonary vessels have a very low pulmonary pressure and are affected very easily by increases in alveolar pressure, especially in hypovolemic and cardiac arrest states. When the alveolar pressure is increased, it has a tendency to compress the pulmonary capillaries, impeding blood flow. The reduction in pulmonary blood flow will decrease left ventricular end-diastolic filling volume and will result in a decrease in cardiac output. A reduction in cardiac output will result in a decrease in organ perfusion. Maintain an inhalation to exhalation time ratio (I:E) of 1:2.

The SUREVENT (Figure 3-46) is a single-patient-use lightweight pressure-cycled automatic transport ventilator that is available to and used by emergency medical services. The disposable ATV operates by sensing airway pressures and ventilates until a set pressure is achieved. The pressure is set at 25 cmH_2O which

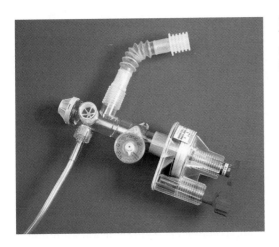

FIGURE 3–46
The SUREVENT is a single patient use ATV_2.
(Carl Leet)

is typically adequate to ventilate most patients. The SUREVENT operates using a continuous gas flow source of 50 psi at 15 lpm to 40 lpm. The pressure is adjusted to chest rise, and the rate is set accordingly. PEEP can be administered with the device. The ventilator can be used with a tracheal tube, other adjunct airway devices, or a mask. It is not recommended for patients under 40 kg and should not be used in pediatric patients.

Noninvasive Ventilatory Support

Two methods of providing noninvasive ventilatory support are through the use of continuous positive airway pressure (CPAP) and bilevel positive airway pressure (Bi-PAP or BL-PAP).

Continuous Positive Airway Pressure (CPAP)

CPAP refers to the application of continuous positive pressure after the patient has exhaled. Positive end-expiratory pressure (PEEP) is very similar to CPAP. PEEP, however, is applied during mechanical ventilation, and CPAP is used to support a patient who is spontaneously breathing. Mask CPAP is an effective way to provide noninvasive positive pressure ventilation in the emergency setting, especially for pulmonary edema. Mask CPAP has also been found to be beneficial to a patient suffering an acute asthma attack since it reduces the work of breathing, airway pressure, and air trapping.

Bilevel Positive Airway Pressure (Bi-PAP or BL-PAP)

Bilevel positive airway pressure is a combination of pressure-cycled ventilation and CPAP. Pressure-cycled ventilation (PSV) is a mode in which the spontaneously breathing patient's ventilations are supported with the ventilation device. The patient controls the ventilation and the PSV device controls the peak pressures. BL-PAP or Bi-PAP is used in spontaneously breathing patients; it provides support of inspiration through inspiratory positive airway pressure (IPAP) and support of expiration through expiratory positive airway pressure (EPAP). The IPAP setting must always be set at a higher pressure than the EPAP. When the patient begins to inspire, the IPAP is triggered and the positive pressure ventilation is delivered. This increases the tidal volume and decreases the patient's work of breathing. The IPAP continues for up to 3 seconds or discontinues when the patient stops the inspiration or begins to exhale. The EPAP is then triggered maintaining a preset positive expiratory pressure. EPAP will also decrease the patient's work of breathing.

BL-PAP or Bi-PAP has been effective in managing spontaneously breathing patients in respiratory failure. It has been used as a noninvasive positive pressure ventilatory (NPPV) device for patients with pulmonary edema, pneumonia, status asthmaticus, and COPD. Patients that typically meet the requirements for NPPV are those with reversible respiratory conditions in which the airway is patent and the respiratory drive is still intact and functioning but ineffectively. Portable devices are now available for use in the prehospital setting.

◫ SUCTION

Oropharyngeal Suctioning

Two different types of suction catheters are available. A rigid catheter, commonly referred to as a Yankauer or tonsil tip catheter, is used to suction blood, secretions, or other foreign material from the mouth and oropharynx. A soft suction catheter is used to perform suctioning through a tracheal tube to remove secretions from the tracheobronchial tree. The soft suction catheter is also used to clear secretions from the nasopharynx.

When suctioning the mouth or pharynx, high negative pressure is necessary. A suction pressure of greater than −120 mmHg should be used.

Tracheobronchial Suctioning

The soft suction catheter should have the following design features:

- ▶ Molded end and soft side holes to reduce mucosal trauma
- ▶ Available in various lengths to allow it to pass through the tip of the tracheal tube
- ▶ Made of material that produces a minimal amount of friction during insertion through the tracheal tube
- ▶ Sterile, disposable, and designed for one-time use

Technique
Follow these steps (Figures 3-47A to 3-47F) when performing tracheobronchial suctioning:

1. Check the equipment and make sure it is in proper working order. Place the patient on an ECG monitor if not already done.
2. Set the suction pressure at between −80 and −120 mmHg.
3. Preoxygenate via positive pressure ventilation for 1 minute or preoxygenate the spontaneously breathing patient for 5 minutes.
4. Insert the catheter without suction pressure applied. This is accomplished by keeping your finger or thumb off of the suction port located proximally and on the side of the catheter.
5. Advance the catheter to the level of the carina.
6. Close the suction port and apply intermittent suction while spiraling and withdrawing the catheter.
7. Never suction for longer than 15 seconds and continuously monitor the cardiac rhythm for indication of dysrhythmias. If bradycardia or other dysrhythmias are present, immediately stop the procedure and hyperventilate the patient.
8. Prior to repeating the procedure, preoxygenate the patient for approximately 30 seconds.

OROTRACHEAL SUCTIONING

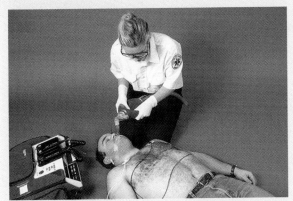

FIGURE 3-47A
Hyperventilate the patient prior to suctioning.

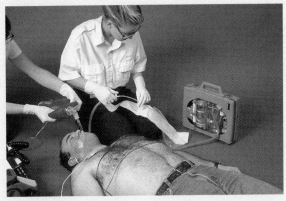

FIGURE 3-47B
Meanwhile, check the suction equipment. Orotracheal suctioning is a sterile procedure, so be careful not to contaminate the suction catheter.

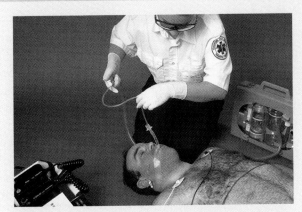

FIGURE 3-47C
Insert the catheter without suction applied.

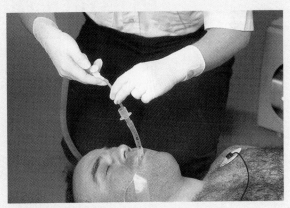

FIGURE 3-47D
Advance the catheter.

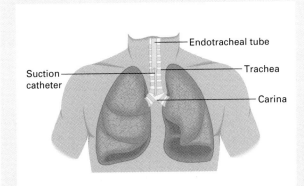

FIGURE 3-47E
Continue to advance the catheter to the level of the carina.

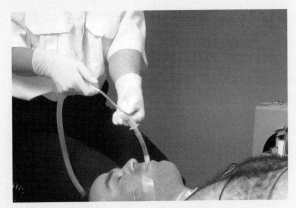

FIGURE 3-47F
Apply suction by closing the suction port (covering the open part of the catheter). Apply intermittent suction while withdrawing the catheter.

Complications

The following are complications associated with tracheobronchial suctioning:

▶ Hypoxemia may occur secondary to a decrease in functional residual volume due to interruption of ventilation and the negative pressure of the suction itself. This is the most serious complication, and may lead to cardiac arrest.

▶ Stimulation of the airway may cause an increase in arterial pressure and tachycardia or increases in intracranial pressure.

▶ Cardiac dysrhythmias, particularly bradycardia, may occur due to a decrease in myocardial oxygen supply from hypoxemia or due to an increased myocardial demand from hypertension or tachycardia.

▶ Vagal stimulation may produce bradycardia and hypotension.

▶ An increase in intracranial pressure and decrease in cerebral blood flow may result from stimulation of coughing during suctioning.

▶ Mucosal damage may result in edema, ulceration, and tracheal infection from loss of integrity.

▦ OXYGEN THERAPY

Any patient with an acute cardiac condition should receive supplemental oxygen, even in the absence of respiratory distress. A nasal cannula can be applied at 2 lpm for comfort. If the patient is exhibiting mild respiratory distress, the oxygen flow should be increased to 5–6 lpm. A high concentration of oxygen, preferably as close to 100% as possible with a nonrebreather mask, should be delivered to the patient with severe respiratory compromise or evidence of hypoxia. If positive pressure ventilation is being performed, supplemental oxygen should be attached to the ventilation device to deliver as high a concentration of oxygen as possible. Administration of 100% oxygen to any nonbreathing patient is advisable, likewise to any serious respiratory- or cardiac-compromised patient. Oxygen can then be titrated according to PaO_2, or oxygen saturation, values.

Equipment

Oxygen delivery equipment (Figure 3-48) normally consists of the following:

▶ An oxygen supply derived from a cylinder or wall unit

▶ Valve with a handle to open the cylinder

▶ Pressure gauge and flowmeter to regulate the oxygen flow

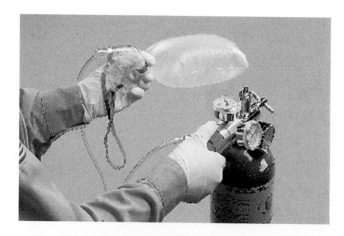

FIGURE 3–48
Oxygen delivery equipment.

▶ Tubing to connect the delivery device to the regulator

▶ Humidifier to humidify the oxygen

Four common devices are used to deliver oxygen to a patient: nasal cannula, face mask, face mask with an oxygen reservoir, and Venturi mask. Each has advantages, disadvantages, and specific uses.

Nasal Cannula

The nasal cannula is considered a low-flow oxygen system (Figures 3-49A and 3-49B). The gas flow emitted from the nasal cannula is not enough to provide an adequate tidal volume; therefore, the gas is mixed with ambient air during inspiration. The amount of oxygen inspired is dependent on the liter flow as well as the tidal volume of the patient. As a general rule, for every increase of 1 liter per minute, the inspired oxygen concentration will increase by 4%. Thus, at 1 lpm, the FiO_2 (concentration of inspired oxygen) will be approximately 25%, whereas at 6 lpm, the approximate FiO_2 will be 45%. However, the actual oxygen concentration range is said to be between 24% and 44%.

The patient must be breathing in an adequate tidal volume in order to use this device. The liter flow is restricted to no less than 1 lpm and no greater than 6 lpm. This device is best used in patients with minimal distress, when the desired FiO_2 to be delivered is low, or when the patient is unable to tolerate an oxygen face mask.

Face Mask

The simple face mask (Figure 3-50) is usually well tolerated by an adult patient. This device can deliver oxygen concentrations of between 40% and 60% at a recommended liter flow of 8–10 lpm. Like the nasal cannula, the simple face mask allows the patient to inspire ambient air, diluting the oxygen concentration. It is imperative that a minimum liter flow of 6 lpm be used to avoid accumulation of exhaled gas in the mask with subsequent rebreathing of that gas.

Face Mask with a Reservoir

This device, which consists of a face mask, nonrebreather valve, and oxygen reservoir, is commonly referred to as a nonrebreather mask (Figures 3-51A and 3-51B). A nonrebreather valve located between the mask and the reservoir bag prevents the patient's exhaled gas from entering the reservoir bag and diluting the oxygen concentration. Instead, the exhaled gas is diverted out of the mask through two side

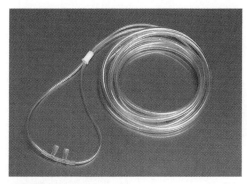

FIGURE 3–49A
Nasal cannula.

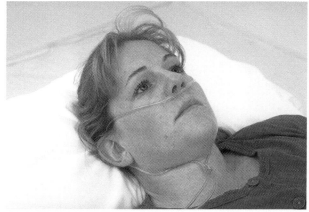

FIGURE 3–49B
Nasal cannula applied to patient.

FIGURE 3–50
Simple face mask.

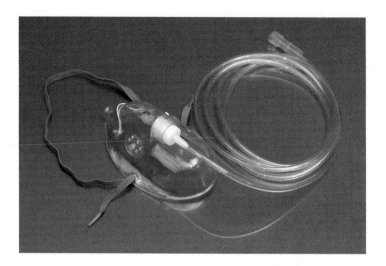

ports while the reservoir is filling with 100% oxygen. On the patient's next inspiration, the 100% oxygen that has collected in the reservoir is drawn up into the mask and breathed in. The side ports have rubber gaskets that occlude at least one port to reduce the amount of inspired ambient air. This provides the greatest concentration of oxygen.

A constant flow of oxygen is required to keep the reservoir bag inflated. An oxygen flow of 6 lpm will provide an FiO_2 concentration of approximately 60%. With each liter/minute increase, a parallel increase of approximately 10% FiO_2 will occur. Thus, at 10 lpm the device may deliver up toward 100% oxygen.

This device is used on patients who are spontaneously breathing with an adequate tidal volume but who require high concentrations of oxygen. Carbon monoxide poisoning, head injuries, and near-drowning are just a few situations that may require high concentrations of oxygen delivered by a nonrebreather. It is important to monitor these patients closely for deterioration, respiratory insufficiency, vomiting, and airway occlusion.

Venturi Mask

The Venturi mask (Figure 3-52) is capable of delivering fixed concentrations of oxygen. This is accomplished by forcing the oxygen through an entrainment valve. The oxygen concentration is adjusted by changing the entrainment valve size and oxygen liter flow. Typical concentrations of 24%, 28%, 35%, and 40% are used.

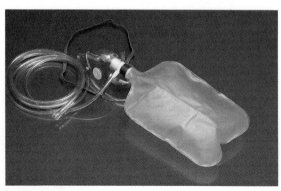

FIGURE 3–51A
Nonrebreather mask.

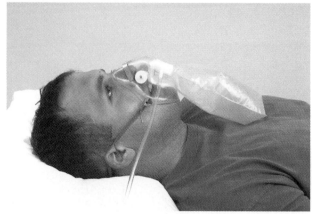

FIGURE 3–51B
Nonrebreather mask applied to patient.

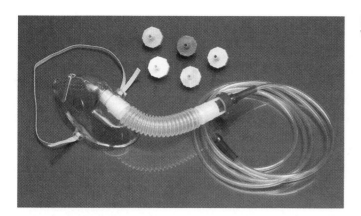

FIGURE 3–52
Venturi mask.

A Venturi mask is commonly used in chronic obstructive pulmonary disease (COPD) patients who require low or restricted oxygen concentrations. In the acute setting, however, if the COPD patient appears to be hypoxic, never withhold oxygen from him. The patient's oxygen saturation and ventilation efforts are monitored and the inspired oxygen concentration adjusted accordingly.

CASE STUDY FOLLOW-UP

Assessment

You are called to a residence for Mrs. Brookley, a 75-year-old female patient complaining of severe dyspnea. Upon your arrival, you are led back to the bedroom. Your general impression upon entering the room is a female patient in her mid-70's who is ashen gray and cyanotic, has gasping respirations, and visible vomitus coming from her mouth. You and your partner immediately turn the patient on her side to clear the vomitus in the oropharynx. Your initial assessment reveals a respiratory rate of approximately 6 per minute with minimal chest rise and fall indicating a poor tidal volume. A carotid pulse is present, strong but irregular at a rate of 78/minute. As you begin to manage the airway, your partner attaches the ECG monitor. It shows atrial fibrillation. You instruct your partner to call for a backup crew.

Treatment

You immediately attach a tonsil tip catheter to the suction tubing and set the wall suction at greater than −120 mmHg. You do a crossed-finger technique to open Mrs. Brookley's mouth and suction the vomitus from her oral cavity. Once the vomitus is clear, you perform a head-tilt, chin-lift maneuver to manually open her airway. You assess her chest for rise and fall and feel for air movement from her nose and mouth. Your patient has one gasping-type respiration. You immediately measure an oropharyngeal airway and begin to insert it into her oropharynx. She gags, so you immediately remove the airway. You quickly lubricate a nasopharyngeal airway and insert it into her right nare. She accepts the airway without incident.

With the head-tilt, chin-lift maintained, you place the mask of the bag-valve-mask device over Mrs. Brookley's face and form a tight seal. Your backup crew arrives at the scene. You instruct them to perform two-person bag-valve-mask ventilation. As they attempt ventilation, Mrs. Brookley begins to vomit copious amounts of emesis. You turn her on her side and scoop out the vomitus with a finger sweep with a gloved hand. You then apply suction to remove the remainder of the vomitus from her airway, which now appears to be clear. Your coworkers resume ventilation and provide a tidal volume of 6 ml/kg over a 1-second period with the BVM with an oxygen reservoir connected to oxygen flowing at 15 lpm.

Because of the significant decrease in her mental status and the potential for a compromised airway, you elect to intubate Mrs. Brookley's trachea with a tracheal tube to protect her airway. You select a 7.5 mm tube

continued on next page

based on the patient's size. You also choose a #3 straight blade and prepare your equipment. You lubricate a stylet, insert it into the tracheal tube, and form the tube into a "hockey stick" shape. You lightly lubricate the tube with lidocaine jelly. You also assess the proper functioning of the laryngoscope.

You instruct your coworkers to stop ventilation. You insert the straight blade into the right side of Mrs. Brookley's mouth, sweeping her tongue to the left. You insert the blade to the base of the tongue, carefully noting the lack of a gag reflex, and then into the hypopharynx. As you lift the laryngoscope handle up and forward, you expose the glottic opening. You insert the tracheal tube into the right side of her mouth and watch it disappear into the trachea past the cords. Once the proximal end of the cuff is about 1.5 cm beyond the level of the vocal cords, you stop the insertion and remove the laryngoscope handle and blade. You firmly hold the tube in place and remove the stylet while noting that the tube is at 23 cm at the level of her teeth. You inject 10 ml of air into the inflation port to inflate the distal cuff. The pilot balloon inflates, indicating that the cuff is inflated.

While holding the tube, your coworker attaches the bag-valve device to the tube and delivers a ventilation. You inspect Mrs. Brookley's chest for rise while auscultating over her epigastrium. Her chest wall rises with the ventilation, and you hear no gurgling sounds over her epigastrium.

Having confirmed that the tube is not misplaced into the esophagus, you instruct your coworker to continue to ventilate while you auscultate at the second intercostal space midclavicular and fourth intercostal space midaxillary, comparing the breath sounds on the right and left. You hear good breath sounds on the right, but diminished sounds on the left. You suspect a right mainstem intubation, so you deflate the cuff and pull back on the tube about one centimeter to 22 cm at the level of the teeth. You reinflate the cuff and auscultate with each ventilation. The breath sounds are now equal and clear bilaterally.

You reassess tube placement by watching for chest rise and fall, auscultating over the epigastrium for gurgling sounds, and listening for equal breath sounds. The chest continues to rise and fall, no gurgling sounds are heard, and equal breath sounds are heard with each ventilation. You again note the tube is at 22 cm at the level of the teeth. You place a colorimetric end-tidal CO_2 detector on the end of the tracheal tube and deliver six more ventilations. You note the color of the colorimetric device is yellow indicating exhalation of CO_2. You secure the tube with a commercial tracheal tube holder.

You continue with your assessment and management of the patient, apply a pulse oximeter, initiate an intravenous line, and prepare her for transport. Based on your history and assessment findings, you notify the emergency department that you are en route with a possible stroke patient and to alert the stroke team. The patient's condition does not change while en route. Since you are solely managing the airway and ventilation, you continue to monitor the tracheal tube placement, pulse oximeter, and ventilatory status of the patient.

■ SUMMARY

Within this chapter we have reviewed techniques and equipment necessary to secure a patent airway, provide effective ventilatory support, and administer supplemental oxygen. It is imperative that the right techniques and equipment be used to ensure effective ventilation and oxygenation of the patient.

Dependent on the patient's condition, you may initially need to manage the airway with basic manual maneuvers and basic airway adjuncts, then move to more advanced techniques and equipment if necessary. In general, the tracheal tube is the preferred advanced airway. As a last resort when tracheal intubation cannot be performed, translaryngeal or transtracheal ventilation may need to be performed.

Select the appropriate device to ventilate the patient. The device must be capable of delivering an adequate tidal volume to ensure effective ventilatory volumes. In some cases, mouth-to-mask ventilation may be more effective in delivering a sufficient tidal volume than bag-valve-mask ventilation. An automatic transport ventilator has many advantages and should be considered in certain situations.

Supplemental oxygen administration is vital when providing positive pressure ventilation. In addition, you should administer oxygen to any patient suffering from respiratory or cardiovascular compromise.

Without a patent airway, and without adequate ventilation and oxygenation, all other therapies become futile. You must carefully assess the patient and approach airway and ventilatory support and oxygen therapy aggressively.

REVIEW QUESTIONS

1. Sonorous sounds heard upon inspiration indicate
   a. an increase in airway resistance in the bronchioles.
   b. a partial occlusion at the level of the pharynx.
   c. secretions or vomitus in the hypopharynx.
   d. laryngeal occlusion due to edema.

2. With the oropharyngeal airway in place
   a. it is not necessary to maintain a manual airway maneuver.
   b. tracheobronchial suctioning may be performed.
   c. a head-tilt, chin-lift or jaw-thrust maneuver must be maintained.
   d. stimulation of the gag reflex will not occur.

3. Which of the following is **not** an advantage of tracheal intubation?
   a. It isolates the trachea, preventing aspiration of foreign material.
   b. It provides a route for administration of certain drugs.
   c. It permits asynchronous chest compressions and ventilation to be performed.
   d. It stimulates a sympathetic nervous system response.

4. The curved laryngoscope blade is designed to fit
   a. in the vallecula to indirectly lift the epiglottis.
   b. under the epiglottis to directly lift it up.
   c. in the glottic opening to expose the vocal cords.
   d. in the aryepiglottic fold to indirectly lift the epiglottis.

5. Which of the following tracheal tube sizes would be most appropriate for both adult males and females in an emergency situation where immediate tracheal intubation is necessary?
   a. 6.0 mm i.d.
   b. 7.0 mm i.d.
   c. 8.0 mm i.d.
   d. 8.5 mm i.d.

6. Insertion of the tracheal tube in the glottic opening should be stopped when
   a. the proximal end of the cuff has passed 1 to 2.5 cm beyond the level of the vocal cords.
   b. resistance is met and the tip of the tube is suspected to be at the level of the carina.
   c. the 23 cm marker on the tube is at the level of the front teeth.
   d. the distal end of the cuff is at the level of the vocal cords.

7. Which of the following should be initially performed with the first ventilation following intubation to confirm tracheal tube placement?
   a. Auscultate bilateral breath sounds.
   b. Assess chest rise and auscultate for epigastric sounds.
   c. Inspect for condensation in the tracheal tube.
   d. Inspect the centimeter marker at the level of the teeth.

8. Which of the following should be done when performing orotracheal intubation in a patient with blunt trauma to the face?
   a. Only 5 ml of air should be used to inflate the cuff to reduce the cuff pressure.
   b. The patient should not be preoxygenated because of suspected intracranial hypertension.
   c. The head and neck must be maintained in a neutral in-line position.
   d. The distal end of the cuff should only be inserted to the level of the cords.

9. Secondary confirmation of tracheal tube placement is best achieved through the use of
   a. an end-tidal carbon dioxide detector and esophageal detector device.
   b. a pulse oximeter and an end-tidal CO_2 monitor.
   c. visualization of the chest rise and fall and bilateral breath sounds.
   d. condensation in the tracheal tube and absence of epigastric sounds.

10. The cricothyroid membrane is located
    a. inferior to the cricoid cartilage and superior to the thyroid cartilage.
    b. superior to the thyroid cartilage and inferior to the hyoid bone.
    c. inferior to the thyroid cartilage and superior to the cricoid cartilage.
    d. inferior to the cricoid and superior to the suprasternal notch.

11. The tidal volume that should be delivered to an adult patient when performing positive pressure ventilation without any oxygen source is
    a. 7 ml/kg.
    b. 10 ml/kg.
    c. 15 ml/kg.
    d. 20 ml/kg.

12. Which of the following is a major complication associated with ventilation with a flow-restricted, oxygen-powered ventilation device?
    a. inability to deliver high concentrations of oxygen during ventilation
    b. delivery of inadequate tidal volume
    c. induction of barotrauma and a pneumothorax
    d. the device is restricted to use on pediatric patients only

13. Which of the following should **not** be done while performing tracheobronchial suctioning?
    a. Set the suction to greater than -120 mmHg.
    b. Ventilate the patient for one minute prior to applying suction.
    c. Insert the catheter without suction applied.
    d. Suction for less than 15 seconds at a time.

14. The most serious complication associated with tracheobronchial suctioning is
    a. stimulation of the cough and gag reflex.
    b. stimulation of the sympathetic nervous system with resultant tachycardia.
    c. mucosal damage and subsequent infection.
    d. hypoxemia secondary to a decrease in functional residual volume.

15. Which of the following is true regarding the simple face mask?
    a. An FiO_2 of 100% is possible with the mask.
    b. The liter flow should not be set at less then 6 lpm.
    c. Oxygen is collected in a reservoir bag prior to inhalation.
    d. The mask is well tolerated by pediatric patients.

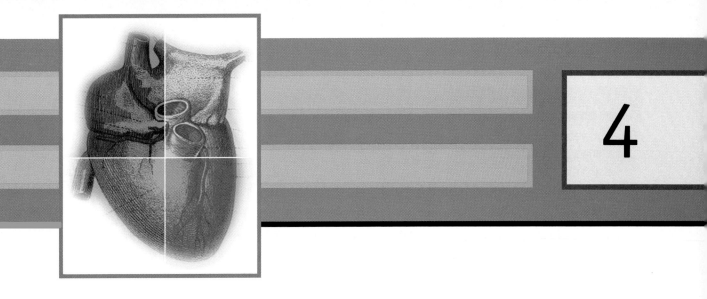

Gaining Intravenous Access

In an emergency situation with a patient experiencing severe cardiovascular instability, drug therapy is often used to help convert the abnormality. To obtain the desired effects, the drugs must reach the target cell or organ rapidly. To facilitate the quickest absorption, you will often deliver medications directly into the patient's venous circulation. You may also need to obtain samples of the patient's venous blood for analysis.

Both of these objectives—rapid delivery of medications and obtaining samples of venous blood—are accomplished by gaining intravenous (IV) access with a cannula, which may be a needle or a catheter. IV cannulation is generally a safe procedure, but there are risks, which can be reduced by following proper procedures.

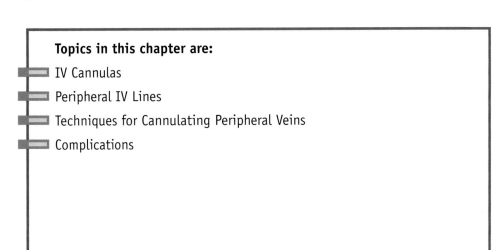

Topics in this chapter are:

IV Cannulas

Peripheral IV Lines

Techniques for Cannulating Peripheral Veins

Complications

CASE STUDY

Bill, a 56-year-old male, begins having severe chest pain just after dinner. When the pain hasn't diminished after 20 minutes, his wife dials 911. You and your partner are dispatched to Bill's home. You quickly perform an initial assessment on Bill, start him on oxygen, and place him on a cardiac monitor. You will be careful with injections and venipuncture, because you suspect that Bill might be a candidate for fibrinolytic therapy.

How should your team proceed to assess and manage this patient? What medications would be administered intravenously in this situation? This chapter will discuss the purposes of IV access in the emergency setting and describe the techniques of gaining IV access. Later we will return to the case to see how IV therapy is applied.

▓ INTRODUCTION

In non-emergency situations, most medications are given orally, intramuscularly (IM), or subcutaneously (SQ). In emergencies, you must deliver medications so that they can enter the central circulation quickly. The most reliable way to administer medications in emergency situations and cardiac arrest is by injecting them directly into the venous circulation. This is accomplished by placing a catheter or needle directly into a vein.

Intravenous (IV) cannulation is performed for two main reasons:

1. To administer medications and fluids
2. To obtain venous blood samples

There are two general categories of IVs: central and peripheral. Peripheral IVs are relatively easy to locate, and can be accessed quickly, easily, and safely, even during CPR. Central veins, however, are more difficult to cannulate because they are deeper within the body. To become efficient in central line placement, a significant amount of practice and experience is necessary.

In this chapter we will take a very practical view of IV cannulation. You should review and understand the advantages and disadvantages of peripheral and central IVs (Tables 4-1 and 4-2). You should also be familiar with the technique of cannulating peripheral IVs and how to maximize the delivery of medication in cardiac arrest.

TABLE 4–1   Advantages and Disadvantages of Peripheral IVs

Peripheral Sites	Advantages	Disadvantages
Arm	Relatively easy to master the technique	Collapse during shock or cardiac arrest
Leg	Easy to locate	Prolonged time for medication to reach the central circulation in cardiac arrest
External jugular vein	Fast to cannulate	
	Safe to perform	
	Multiple practitioners can try at once	
	Easily compressible to reduce bleeding from unsuccessful attempts	
	Can usually be accomplished during CPR	
	Low complication rate compared to central IVs	

TABLE 4-2 Advantages and Disadvantages of Central IVs

Central Sites	Advantages	Disadvantages
Femoral vein	Do not collapse in shock	Relatively difficult to master the technique
Internal jugular vein	Do not collapse during cardiac arrest	Increased incidence of:
	Can be used to monitor central venous pressure	Arterial puncture
Subclavian vein		Pneumothorax
		Air embolism
	Can be used for transvenous pacing	Catheter embolism
	The central veins accommodate large-bore catheters	Can usually not be accomplished during CPR
	More rapid delivery of medication to the central circulation during cardiac arrest	Relatively contraindicated in patients who may receive thrombolytic agents

This chapter will not discuss the techniques of central vein cannulation. If you routinely perform central IV cannulation, it is unlikely that we could add to your knowledge about the skill in this chapter. It is not the intent of this chapter to teach the technique of central cannulation. Please read other texts available that cover intravenous techniques in greater detail and for an extensive review of central vein cannulation.

In some situations, either peripheral or central IV access will have been established in the patient before the cardiac emergency. In these cases, you should obviously use this access during the emergency care or resuscitation of the patient after confirming patency of the catheter.

In non-emergency situations, you usually can spend additional time to assure that you are paying strict attention to aseptic (sterile) technique. In an emergency you must gain IV access as quickly as possible. Use the best aseptic practice that is possible during emergency IV cannulation.

Glucose-containing solutions, such as 5% dextrose in water, should be avoided. Some studies have shown worsened neurological outcomes following the use of dextrose in patients with intracranial pathology. The IV fluid of choice to keep the vein open in cardiac arrest is 0.9% sodium chloride (normal saline). The fluid should be adjusted to administer 10–20 cc/hr. Alternatively, you can also attach a saline lock to the IV cannula and eliminate the need for tubing and IV fluid.

IV CANNULAS

There are different types of IV cannulas:

1. *Hollow needles.* These are commonly called butterfly needles and are occasionally used in pediatric patients. The problem with hollow needles is that the sharp, metal needle, when inserted in the vein, often damages the vessel.

2. *Catheters inserted through a needle.* These are used occasionally for central vein access, but are quite uncommon for peripheral access (Figure 4-1A).

3. *Catheters inserted over a needle.* These are by far the most common IV catheters used for peripheral vein cannulation (Figure 4-1B).

Recently, increased emphasis on preventing needle-stick injuries, in order to decrease the risk of the transmission of blood-borne diseases such as hepatitis and HIV, has prompted development of several new types of IV cannulation devices.

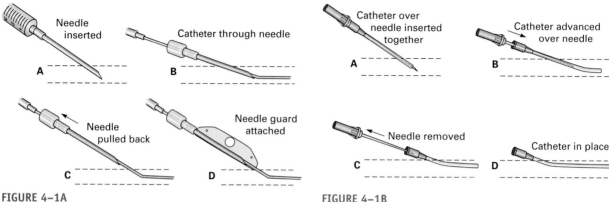

FIGURE 4–1A
Insertion of catheter through needle.

FIGURE 4–1B
Insertion of catheter over needle.

These new devices incorporate engineering controls designed to protect the rescuer from inadvertently sticking himself with the steel stylet after it is removed from the patient. A few of these devices are shown in Figure 4-2. It is important that you are familiar with the specific operational features of the IV cannula you are using prior to attempts at IV initiation.

PERIPHERAL IV LINES

If the emergency patient (or patient in cardiac arrest) has no venous access, you should consider peripheral IV cannulation as one of the first priorities of management. Peripheral veins used for venous access include the veins in the arm, the leg, and the external jugular vein (Figures 4-3, 4-4, and 4-5). These veins lie superficially and are easy to see and palpate. Although a relatively easy skill, cannulating peripheral veins requires practice.

In cardiac arrest, venous blood flow is severely compromised. As a result, medications administered peripherally have significant delays in reaching the central circulation. To increase the, effectiveness in cardiac arrest, you should administer IV drugs rapidly by IV bolus injection, followed with a 20 cc bolus of IV fluid, and elevation of the extremity for 10–20 seconds. When selecting a site for cannulation, the closer to the central circulation you can cannulate a vein the better. Try to use the large antecubital or external jugular veins in cardiac arrest (Figures 4-6 and 4-7).

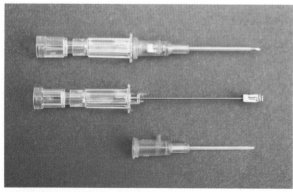
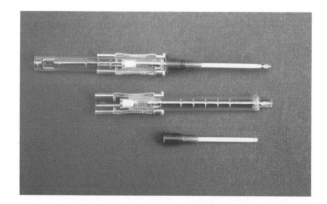

FIGURE 4–2
IV cannulation devices designed to prevent needlestick.
(Carl Leet)

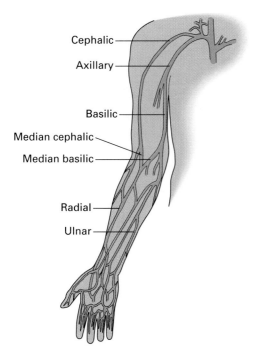

FIGURE 4–3
Veins of the hand and arm.

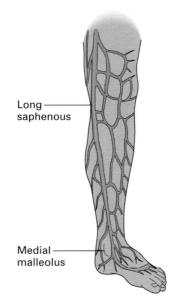

FIGURE 4–4
Long saphenous vein of the leg.

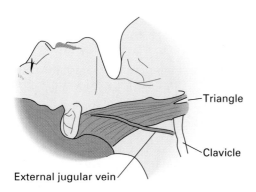

FIGURE 4–5
External jugular vein.

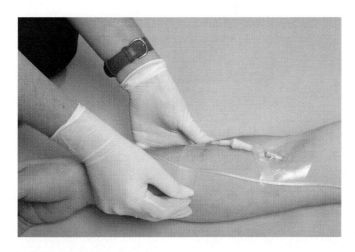

FIGURE 4–6
Antecubital venipuncture.

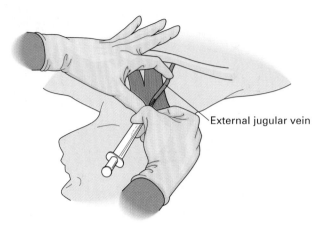

FIGURE 4–7
External jugular venipuncture.

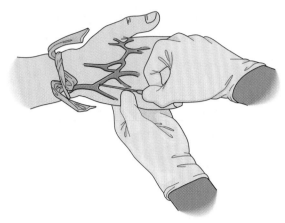

FIGURE 4–8
Dorsal hand venipuncture.

In non-arrest situations, the veins in the dorsum of the hand, the wrist, and the forearm are the preferred IV sites (Figure 4-8). As a last resort, you can use the long saphenous vein in the leg, but a higher rate of thrombophlebitis and other complications is associated with IVs started in the lower extremities.

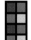 # TECHNIQUES FOR CANNULATING PERIPHERAL VEINS

Cannulating an Arm or Leg Vein

The vast majority of IVs are started in the upper extremities. The veins are superficial and easily located on the back of the hand, the forearm, and the antecubital fossa. In cardiac arrest, the preferred sites are the antecubital and external jugular vein. Below are the steps for cannulating a superficial arm or leg vein.

1. Apply a venous tourniquet proximally to the site of the attempt. The purposes of the constricting band are to impede venous return and to engorge the veins. Engorgement makes the distal veins easier to locate.

2. Locate the vein and cleanse the skin with alcohol or a similar antiseptic.

3. Hold the skin taut.

4. With the needle bevel-up, puncture the skin.

5. Enter the vein either from the side or from above. You will feel a "pop" as you enter the vein, and you will see a flash of blood returning through the flash-back chamber.

6. Advance the needle slightly to be sure that the catheter is completely within the lumen (interior) of the vein.

7. Advance the catheter over the needle and into the vein. Remove the tourniquet.

8. Completely remove the needle stylet, attach the tubing to the catheter, and slowly start the flow of fluids.

9. Cover the injection site with sterile dressing material and tape the catheter in place.

10. Watch for complications. (See "Complications" below.)

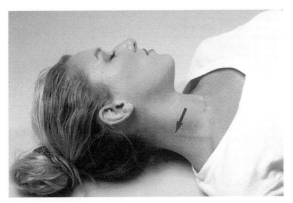

FIGURE 4–9A
Location of the external jugular vein.

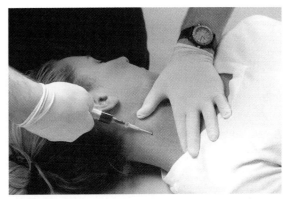

FIGURE 4–9B
Cannulation of the external jugular vein.

Cannulating an External Jugular Vein

The external jugular vein is considered a peripheral vein because it lies superficially in the neck (Figure 4-9A). However, it is very close to the central circulation and has significant advantages over other peripheral IVs. Below is the technique for cannulating the external jugular vein (Figure 4-9B).

1. Place the patient in a Trendelenburg position (supine, feet slightly elevated) and turn the patient's head to the side.
2. Cleanse the injection site.
3. Attach a 10 cc syringe filled with a few cc's of saline to the IV cannulation device.
4. Occlude the venous return by placing one finger on the external jugular vein just above the clavicle.
5. Puncture the vein midway between the angle of the jaw and your finger.
6. Enter the vein while withdrawing the plunger of the syringe. Stop when blood flows briskly into the syringe.
7. Advance the catheter into the vein and remove the needle stylet.
8. Attach the tubing to the catheter, start the flow of fluid, and secure the catheter.
9. Watch for complications.

⊞ COMPLICATIONS

IV cannulation is not without some risks. The complications can be divided into local and systemic complications. Local complications of IV cannulation include hematoma formation, cellulitis, thrombosis, and phlebitis. Systemic complications are sepsis, pulmonary embolism, and air or catheter emboli. The probability of any of these complications can be reduced by following proper technique, as described above.

For patients who are potential candidates for fibrinolysis, special care must be taken to avoid unnecessary bleeding. Sites of IM injections, blood draw, IV cannulation, and unsuccessful IV attempts can result in bleeding or significant hematomas after fibrinolytics are administered, since fibrinolytics act to dissolve clots that lead to myocardial infarction and will therefore increase the risk of or

CASE STUDY FOLLOW-UP

Assessment

You and your partner continue your treatment and conduct a focused history and physical exam on Bill, a 56-year-old male who is suffering from chest pain. You quickly insert an intravenous catheter into a vein in his right forearm. You take blood samples from the IV site and then attach the IV line to the catheter hub. You infuse normal saline at 20 cc/hr. Then, as you are preparing to do a 12-lead ECG, Bill suddenly slumps over, unresponsive. The monitor shows ventricular fibrillation.

Treatment

You and your partner immediately defibrillate Bill at 200, 300, and then 360 joules, but are unsuccessful in converting the rhythm. You administer a 1 mg bolus of 1:10,000 epinephrine intravenously. Since the IV is in Bill's antecubital fossa, you raise his arm and open the line to let about 20 cc of fluid flush the medication into the vein. You deliver a fourth defibrillation without success. Your partner continues chest compressions and ventilations as you administer a 300 mg bolus of amiodarone. You deliver a fifth defibrillation and convert the rhythm to a sinus tachycardia. You assess pulses and the breathing status. Your partner continues to ventilate Bill at 12 times per minute. You assess the blood pressure and reassess the pulses. You then set up an amiodarone infusion 360 mg and set the drip rate at 1 mg/minute. You closely monitor Bill as you transport him to the medical facility.

He leaves the hospital four days later, starts a cardiac rehabilitation program, and recovers fully.

aggravate bleeding or hematomas. In this situation be especially diligent in attempting to establish a patent IV on the first attempt. Candidates for fibrinolytic therapy are NOT the patients to practice IVs on. Let the most experienced practitioner start the IV. Finally, watch for bleeding or hematomas at any injection site and control the bleeding with direct pressure if necessary. A pressure dressing should be applied to a site of potential bleeding in any patient who is a candidate for fibrinolytic therapy.

SUMMARY

Access to the venous circulation is a critical part of emergency management. Typically, the initial IV access is accomplished by cannulating a peripheral vein in the arm. If the patient is in cardiac arrest, select an IV site as close as possible to the central circulation. Preferably, place a large-bore catheter in the antecubital fossa and elevate the arm, or place the catheter in the external jugular vein. Following any drug administration, flush the line with at least 20 cc of saline and elevate the extremity to speed circulation to the cells.

In non-arrest situations, the veins in the dorsum of the hand, the wrist, and the forearm are the preferred IV sites. As a last resort, you can use the long saphenous vein in the leg.

In an emergency you must gain IV access quickly and may not be able to follow strict aseptic (sterile) technique. In these cases, remove the catheter as soon as possible after the emergency and replace it with an IV initiated with a strict aseptic technique.

REVIEW QUESTIONS

1. Which of the following types of catheters is most commonly used for peripheral venous cannulation?
   a. catheter over the needle
   b. catheter through the needle
   c. hollow needle
   d. intraosseous catheter

2. What is the preferred solution to be used to keep the vein open during cardiac arrest?
   a. 5% dextrose in water
   b. 5% dextrose in lactated Ringer's
   c. normal saline
   d. sterile water

3. Which of the following is **not** an advantage of peripheral IV cannulation (as compared to central IV cannulation)?
   a. It is easier to locate a larger number of suitable veins with peripheral cannulation.
   b. Delivery of medication to the central circulation is more rapid with peripheral cannulation.
   c. Peripheral cannulation is a relatively easy skill to master.
   d. Peripheral cannulation can be accomplished without interruption of CPR.

4. In cardiac arrest, which of the following would be the preferred site for peripheral IV cannulation?
   a. saphenous vein
   b. dorsum of the hand
   c. subclavian vein
   d. antecubital fossa

5. List two strategies for improving the delivery of medications to the central circulation in cardiac arrest.

   a. _____

   b. _____

6. What precaution should be taken when performing IV cannulation in a patient who is a possible candidate for fibrinolytic therapy?

   _____

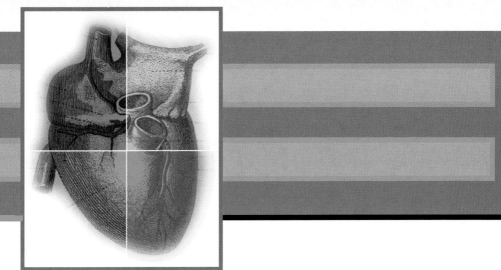

5

ECG Monitoring and Dysrhythmia Recognition

When treating a patient with an apparent cardiac problem, it is important to determine whether a mechanical or electrical dysfunction exists. Electrical activity and conduction malfunctions cause changes in the myocardial rhythm. An electrocardiogram can reveal the abnormal rhythm and provide information about the location and nature of the malfunction. This information is critical to treatment decisions you will make. Improper rhythm identification will almost certainly lead to improper management. So the ability to read and interpret an ECG is an essential skill in advanced cardiac life support.

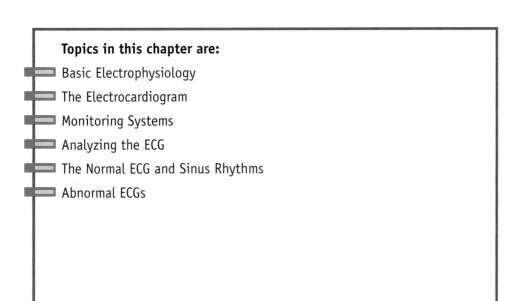

Topics in this chapter are:
- Basic Electrophysiology
- The Electrocardiogram
- Monitoring Systems
- Analyzing the ECG
- The Normal ECG and Sinus Rhythms
- Abnormal ECGs

CASE STUDY

You are a paramedic called to the house of Alma Brown, a 48-year-old woman who called 911 for a "fluttering sensation" in her chest. Upon your arrival, you find a conscious, alert female who is in no particular distress and who denies chest pain and shortness of breath but says that she feels like her heart is racing. This has happened a few times before, Mrs. Brown tells you, but it always ended within 2 or 3 minutes. She called for help when the sensation did not stop after 20 minutes.

The cardiac monitor shows the following:

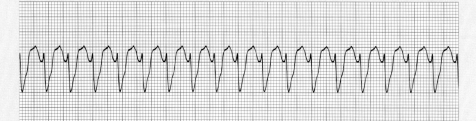

What additional assessment steps would you take to differentiate the origin of the dysrhythmia? What parameters would you use to determine the appropriate treatment? This chapter will discuss electrocardiograms and analysis of a variety of normal and abnormal cardiac rhythms. Later we will return to the case to see how these skills are applied.

INTRODUCTION

One of the critical aspects of assessing the status of a cardiac patient is determining the mechanical and electrical status of the heart. The patient's pulse and blood pressure are simple measures of myocardial function. Advanced diagnostics, such as the echocardiogram, give you information about heart wall movement. To assess the electrical activity of the heart, you need to know how to interpret the electrocardiogram (EKG or ECG). Analyzing the ECG is one of the most important skills of advanced cardiac life support.

It is worth emphasizing early that the ECG provides information only about the electrical activity of the heart, not about the mechanical function. It is possible for the ECG to be perfectly normal in the absence of mechanical contraction. Always remember the popular phrase: "Treat the patient, not the monitor."

BASIC ELECTROPHYSIOLOGY

Electrophysiology is often presented as complex, abstract, and frustrating. Many beginning students become so intimidated by the physiology that they never learn how to interpret ECGs. The intent of this chapter is to limit the amount of technical information to what you will need to identify the basic, life-threatening cardiac rhythms used in ACLS. Once you have mastered basic rhythm recognition, we encourage you to tackle electrophysiology, which will increase your understanding of cardiology and ACLS. Electrophysiology becomes less overwhelming once you have a grasp of the basics.

The heart is an unique organ. It is made up of muscle tissue that has the property of automaticity. Automaticity is the ability of the heart, or any of its individual muscle cells, to contract on its own—without any nervous system control. In fact, if you quickly remove the heart from the body, place it in a saline bath, and provide it with oxygen and glucose, the heart will continue to beat for quite some time. If you cut it into tiny pieces and separate them, each chunk of heart muscle will beat separately! This is an amazing physiological phenomenon and makes the heart dramatically different from any other organ in the body.

To contract, a myocardial cell must be depolarized. Depolarization is a process where a shift in the electrical properties of the cell occurs from the movement of electrically charged particles across the cell's membrane. When the electrical properties of the cell change, the cell is capable of contracting. Some areas of the heart have evolved to perform special functions. The three specialized types of myocardial cells are:

▶ Pacemaker cells

▶ Conduction cells

▶ Working cells

Working Cells

The physical contraction of the heart is caused by the myocardial working cells. These muscle cells are bundled into an interconnecting weave of muscle fibers. Contraction, or shortening, of these fibers causes a rapid decrease in the internal size of the atria and ventricles, which in turn ejects the blood from the chambers.

The actual contraction of the heart occurs when electrical depolarization is coupled with physical contraction. It is important to remember that the physical contraction is what generates blood flow—not the electrical activity. However, the physical contraction requires organized electrical activity. The organized electrical activity starts by the regular depolarization of pacemaker cells

Pacemaker Cells

Pacemaker cells are specialized cardiac tissue which depolarize regularly by controlling the flow of charged particles in and out of the cell. Pacemaker cells control the heart's rate and rhythm. Through influence from the autonomic (sympathetic and parasympathetic) nervous system, the rate of the depolarization can be altered.

The primary pacemaker of the healthy heart is the sinoatrial (SA) node. It is a bundle of cardiac tissue that is located on the inner wall of the heart near the junction of the right atrium and the vena cava. Without nervous control, the SA node will normally depolarize 60–100 times per minute. If the body demands changes in cardiac output, the autonomic nervous system can increase (as a sympathetic action) or decrease (as a parasympathetic action) the rate at which the SA node emits impulses.

If the SA node fails to emit an impulse, there are some backup functions that assure that the heart will continue to beat. If the SA node fails, the atrioventricular (AV) node at the junction of the atria and ventricles will take over as a pacemaker and will depolarize at a rate of 40–60 times per minute. If both the SA and AV nodes fail, the Purkinje fibers of the ventricles will depolarize at a rate of less than 40 times per minute.

Conduction Cells

The impulse from the pacemakers travels through the heart in a couple of ways. There are internodal pathways that connect the SA node to the AV node. In normal conduction, the AV node is the only electrical connection between the atria and the ventricles; therefore, any stimulation for the ventricles to contract that originates above the ventricles must pass through the AV node. Below the AV node the

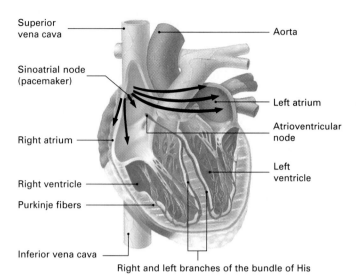

FIGURE 5–1
The cardiac conduction system.

Superior vena cava

Aorta

Sinoatrial node (pacemaker)

Left atrium

Atrioventricular node

Right atrium

Left ventricle

Right ventricle

Purkinje fibers

Inferior vena cava

Right and left branches of the bundle of His

impulse for contraction travels through the bundle of His, the bundle branches, and the Purkinje fibers.

The overall cardiac conduction pathway in the normal heart (Figure 5-1), therefore, is:

SA node → internodal pathways → AV node → bundle of His
→ right and left bundle branches → Purkinje fibers

THE ELECTROCARDIOGRAM

The body is a giant conductor of the electrical impulse transmission that occurs within the heart. These events can be detected by two electrodes, one positive and one negative, placed on the skin. Typically, the signal is amplified and then displayed on an oscilloscope or printed on graph paper. Theoretically, electrodes can be placed anywhere on the body, but this causes subtle differences in the relative size of each wave. For convenience and standardization, there are some conventional electrode placements that you should remember. Figure 5-2 shows typical ECG monitors with three-lead and four-lead placement. The polarity is changed to view Leads I, II, and III by activating a switch on the ECG monitor panel.

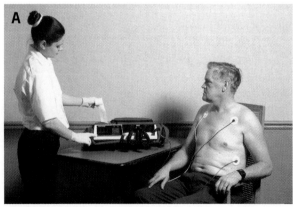

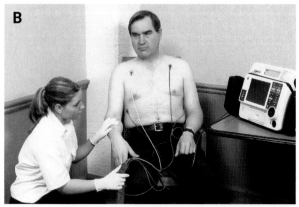

FIGURE 5–2
ECG placements: (A) three-electrode monitor lead placement and (B) four-electrode monitor lead placement.
(Carl Leet)

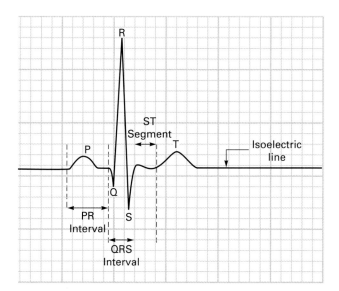

FIGURE 5–3
The electrocardiogram (ECG).

Because it is the most common monitoring lead, all of the rules and rhythm strips in this chapter are presented in Lead II. Other leads will be discussed in Chapter 6.

The electrical events of the heart rhythm produce waves that have been labeled alphabetically P through T. You should become familiar with these components of the normal ECG, as shown in Figure 5-3. In some cases, a U wave is seen following a T wave, the significance of which is unknown

Each wave represents the summation of the depolarization or repolarization of a mass of heart tissue. Atrial depolarization, which is associated with mechanical contraction of the atria, produces the P wave. Ventricular depolarization, which correlates with mechanical contraction of the ventricles, produces the QRS complex, and ventricular repolarization produces the T wave. Atrial repolarization is buried in the QRS complex (Figure 5-4).

Occasionally, there are variations in how the waves look and even if they are present. In fact, these alterations are how you will be able to recognize dysrhythmias. If you keep this in mind, dysrhythmia recognition becomes much easier.

▦ MONITORING SYSTEMS

There are many different cardiac monitors on the market. There are many features, with various configurations of switches and buttons, but basically all cardiac monitors are the same. They generally consist of a screen (or oscilloscope) and usually have a printer that will print a hard copy of the patient's cardiac rhythm.

Cardiac monitors print the ECG on a strip of graph paper (Figure 5-5). Since the paper exits the machine at a constant speed, the horizontal boxes represent time. (Each large box represents 0.20 seconds; each small box represents 0.04 seconds.) The vertical boxes represent the magnitude of the electrical impulse in millivolts. (Two large boxes represent 1 mV.) It is important to remember the time increments for each box, since they will be used extensively in ECG interpretation.

▦ ANALYZING THE ECG

Now that you know how to identify each wave of the ECG, analyzing the cardiac rhythm simply becomes a matter of looking at a number of parameters and applying

FIGURE 5–4
The relationship of the ECG (the heart's electrical activity) to the anatomical sequence of the heart's mechanical actions.

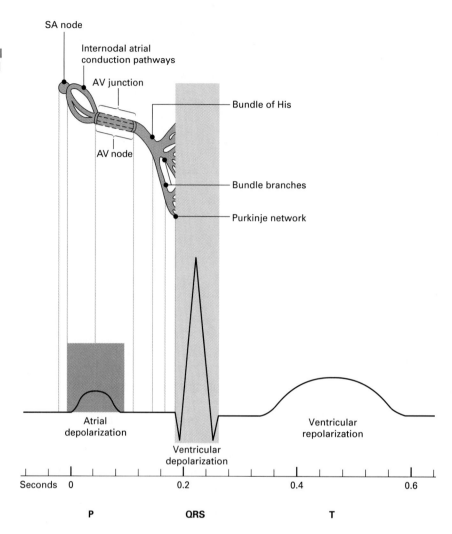

a couple of rules. We will use the "red flag" method of ECG interpretation. The "red flag" method looks at five parameters in each ECG and, by understanding what they mean, you will easily be able to interpret the ECG. The five parameters (Table 5-1) are:

- ▶ Rate
- ▶ Regularity
- ▶ QRS width
- ▶ P waves
- ▶ P-R interval

Rate

As we mentioned earlier, the SA node normally depolarizes 60–100 times a minute. This represents the normal range of heart rate. Any rate that is faster than 100 beats per minute is called *tachycardia* and any rate slower than 60 beats per minute is *bradycardia*. We assess the rate by looking at the number of QRS complexes in a given period of time.

There are two ways to determine the heart rate by looking at the ECG. The easiest way is to count the number of QRS complexes that occur in 6 seconds and multiply by 10. For your convenience, ECG paper is often marked in 3- or 6-second increments (Figure 5-6). This method is best used to count irregular rhythms.

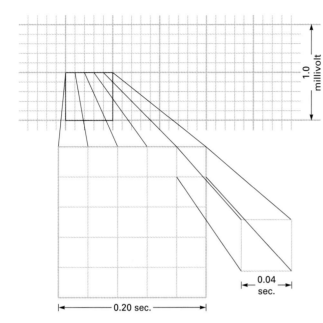

FIGURE 5–5
ECG graph paper. The horizontal axis represents elapsed time in seconds. The vertical axis represents the magnitude of the electrical impulse in millivolts.

The second way to determine the heart rate is to look for a QRS complex that falls on one of the heavy lines on the strip. You then count how many large boxes are between this and the next QRS complex. Then divide that number into 300—because 300 large boxes represent 60 seconds, or 1 minute. Therefore, if the next QRS fell exactly three heavy lines away, the rate would be 100 beats per minute (300 ÷ 3 = 100) (Figure 5-7).

Usually, you are not lucky enough to have the subsequent QRS fall directly on a heavy line, so this technique is often used just to estimate the heart rate. Study Figure 5-8. Can you see why the rate is estimated to be 70 on this strip?

Regularity

The next variable to analyze is the regularity of the rhythm. The normal heart rhythm is highly regular. A variance of more than 0.04 seconds, or 1 small box, between the complexes is considered abnormal. This is best analyzed using

TABLE 5–1	Five Parameters of ECG Analysis
Analyze	
Rate	■ What is the rate? (Normally 60–100 per minute)
Regularity	■ Is the rhythm regular? (Normally a variance of less than 0.04 seconds)
QRS Complex	■ Do all of the QRS complexes look alike? (Normally yes) ■ What is the width of the QRS complex? (Normally less than 0.12 seconds)
P Waves	■ Is there a P wave before every QRS complex? (Normally yes) ■ Is there a QRS complex after every P wave? (Normally yes) ■ Are the P waves upright and rounded? (Normally yes)
P-R Interval	■ What is the P-R interval? (Normally less than 0.20 seconds) ■ Is the P-R interval constant? (Normally yes)

FIGURE 5–6
You can determine the rate by counting the number of QRS complexes in 6 seconds and multiplying by 10.

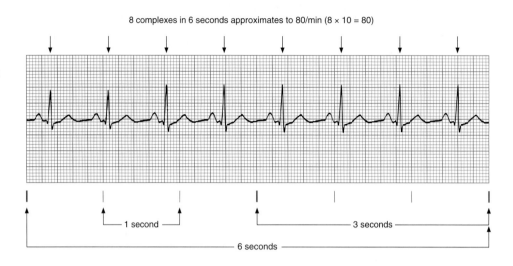

8 complexes in 6 seconds approximates to 80/min (8 × 10 = 80)

1 second

3 seconds

6 seconds

FIGURE 5–7
You can determine rate, or the regularity of rhythm, by counting the number of boxes between QRS complexes.

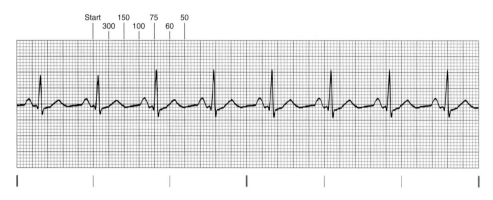

Start   150   75   50
    300   100   60

FIGURE 5–8
An ECG strip with a heart rate estimated at 70.

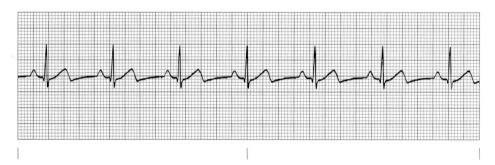

calipers. Simply measure the distance between two QRS complexes and then check the distances between others to determine if they are within 0.04 seconds of each other.

The QRS Complex

After evaluating the rate and the regularity of the rhythm, next analyze the QRS complexes. Remember that the QRS complex represents ventricular depolarization. Specifically, you are examining the QRS complexes to see if they have the same morphology (look the same) and if they are the same width. If all of the QRS complexes look alike, they are all following the same conduction pathways below the AV node and are termed monomorphic.

The width of the QRS complex has special significance. If the QRS complex is narrow, defined as less than 0.12 seconds (3 small boxes), the wave of depolarization must have followed the normal conduction pathways below the AV node. In other words, the beat did NOT originate in the ventricles. The rhythm is therefore referred to as *supraventricular,* i.e., "above the ventricles."

If the QRS complex is wide, the opposite is not necessarily true. If the QRS complex is greater than 0.12 seconds (3 small boxes), there are commonly three causes:

▶ The impulse may have originated in the ventricles.

▶ The impulse may have originated above the ventricles but circumvented the normal conduction pathway through the AV node. This is one form of *aberrant conduction.*

▶ The impulse may have originated above the ventricles and traveled through the AV node but experienced a delay in one side of the ventricular conduction system. This is called a bundle branch block. Bundle branch blocks are another type of aberrant conduction.

KEY POINT: Narrow QRS complexes are always of a supraventricular origin, whereas wide QRS complexes may have either a ventricular origin or a supraventricular origin with aberrant conduction.

The P Waves

Remember that the P wave represents atrial depolarization. There are three questions to ask about the P waves:

▶ Is there a P wave before every QRS complex?

▶ Is there a QRS complex after every P wave?

▶ Are the P waves upright and rounded?

The P-R Interval

The normal delay of conduction that occurs at the AV node is less than 0.20 seconds (1 big box or 5 small boxes). You need to know two things about the P-R interval to correctly interpret the ECG:

▶ Is the P-R interval less than 0.20 seconds?

▶ Is the P-R interval constant?

▦ THE NORMAL ECG AND SINUS RHYTHMS

Now that you know the five parameters for analyzing any ECG (rate, regularity, QRS complex, P waves, and P-R interval), interpreting and understanding cardiac rhythms simply becomes a matter of answering each question and applying a few rules. We call this the "red flag" method, because by knowing which of the five variables falls out of the normal range (raises a "red flag"), you can interpret any rhythm.

A WORD OF CAUTION: After you have analyzed many ECGs, you will have a tendency to "cut to the chase" and attempt to interpret the rhythm without going through each step of analysis. Although this will often result in a correct interpretation, you will sometimes miss important findings. We suggest that you use this sequential method of ECG analysis until you have gained considerable experience in ECG interpretation.

Normal Sinus Rhythm

Very simply, any rhythm where all of the variables fall within the normal limits is called normal sinus rhythm (NSR). There can be significant variations on how some of the waves look, but if the answer to every question falls within normal limits, the rhythm is normal (Table 5-2 and Figure 5-9).

TABLE 5–2 Normal Sinus Rhythm

Analyze	ECG
Rate	60–100 per minute
Regularity	Variance of less than 0.04 seconds
QRS Complex	
Do all of the QRS complexes look alike?	Yes
What is the width of the QRS complex?	Less than 0.12 seconds
P Waves	
Is there a P wave before every QRS complex?	Yes
Is there a QRS after every P wave?	Yes
Are the P waves upright and rounded?	Yes
P-R Interval	
What is the P-R interval?	Less than 0.20 seconds
Is the P-R interval constant?	Yes

FIGURE 5–9
Three variants of normal sinus rhythm.

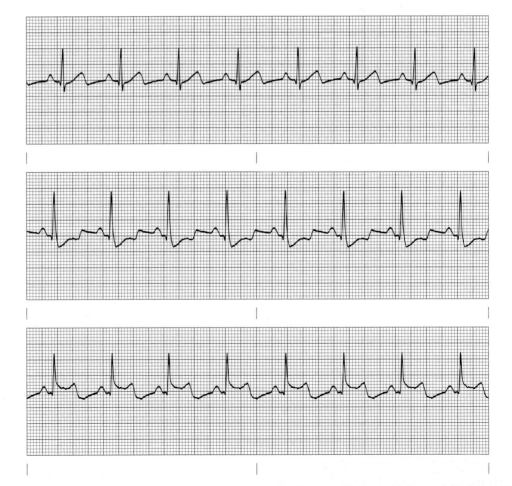

Sinus Tachycardia

Sinus tachycardia is a common variant of NSR where the only "red flag" is that the rate is over 100 (Table 5-3 and Figure 5-10). Every beat is stimulated by an impulse from the SA node. This is a common dysrhythmia caused by exercise, stress, fever, fear, or shock, or other conditions that stimulate the sympathetic nervous system.

TABLE 5–3 | **Sinus Tachycardia**

Analyze	ECG
Rate	**Greater than 100 per minute**
Regularity	Variance of less than 0.04 seconds
QRS Complex	
Do all of the QRS complexes look alike?	Yes
What is the width of the QRS complex?	Less than 0.12 seconds
P Waves	
Is there a P wave before every QRS complex?	Yes
Is there a QRS after every P wave?	Yes
Are the P waves upright and rounded?	Yes
P-R Interval	
What is the P-R interval?	Less than 0.20 seconds
Is the P-R interval constant?	Yes

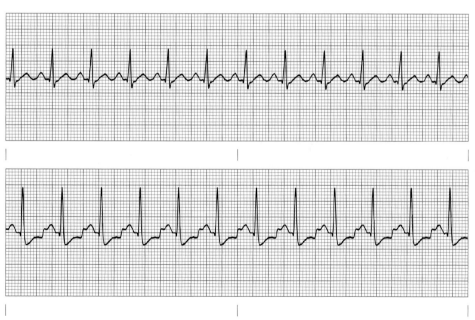

FIGURE 5–10
Two variants of sinus tachycardia.

Sinus Bradycardia

Sinus bradycardia is characterized by all of the variables falling within normal limits, except a rate that is less than 60 beats per minute (Table 5-4 and Figure 5-11). This is very common in well-conditioned athletes, but in an emergency it may be caused by a myocardial infarction or excessive parasympathetic stimulation.

TABLE 5–4 | **Sinus Bradycardia**

Analyze	ECG
Rate	**Less than 60 per minute**
Regularity	Variance of less than 0.04 seconds
QRS Complex	
Do all of the QRS complexes look alike?	Yes
What is the width of the QRS complex?	Less than 0.12 seconds
P Waves	
Is there a P wave before every QRS complex?	Yes
Is there a QRS after every P wave?	Yes
Are the P waves upright and rounded?	Yes
P-R Interval	
What is the P-R interval?	Less than 0.20 seconds
Is the P-R interval constant?	Yes

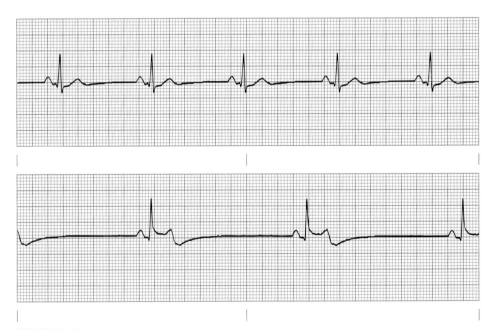

FIGURE 5–11
Two variants of sinus bradycardia.

Sinus Dysrhythmia

Sinus dysrhythmia is characterized by all variables being within normal limits except the regularity (Table 5-5 and Figure 5-12). Variation in the regularity is common and is normal in some people. It is thought that this results from the changes in venous return associated with breathing or the effects of caffeine and/or nicotine.

TABLE 5-5 **Sinus Dysrhythmia**

Analyze	ECG
Rate	60–100 per minute
Regularity	**Variance of more than 0.04 seconds** 🚩
QRS Complex	
Do all of the QRS complexes look alike?	Yes
What is the width of the QRS complex?	Less than 0.12 seconds
P Waves	
Is there a P wave before every QRS complex?	Yes
Is there a QRS after every P wave?	Yes
Are the P waves upright and rounded?	Yes
P-R Interval	
What is the P-R interval?	Less than 0.20 seconds
Is the P-R interval constant?	Yes

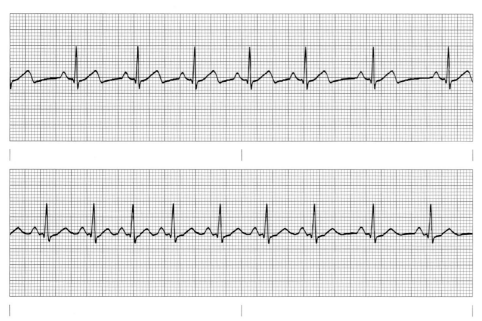

FIGURE 5–12
Two variants of sinus dysrhythmia.

⊞ ABNORMAL ECGS

There are some very confusing terms that are used when discussing ECGs. Technically, a dysrhythmia is an abnormality in the rhythm and arrhythmia is the absence of rhythm. In practice, however, the terms are used interchangeably.

There are only a few causes of abnormal ECGs and they are very easy to remember. If you think of cardiac dysrhythmias in terms of their causes, the interpretation becomes logical. Most textbooks teach dysrhythmia interpretation anatomically, i.e., atrial, junctional, and ventricular dysrhythmias. Although this is a convenient way to group dysrhythmias, it does not help to understand the causes of the rhythm disturbances.

In the "red flag" method of ECG interpretation, we evaluate each rhythm strip using the five criteria discussed. The answers to the questions direct us toward the correct interpretation. If you remember the questions, a little about the causes of the dysrhythmias, and a few rules, the pattern of abnormal findings leads you to the correct interpretation.

A brief word of caution: For clarity, we will only consider one dysrhythmia at a time in this chapter. In real life, patients can exhibit multiple dysrhythmias at the same time. When you are first learning, it is much easier to consider "textbook" ECG strips, which illustrate the concepts of dysrhythmia interpretation.

Fibrillatory Dysrhythmias

As we mentioned earlier, each cardiac muscle cell has the ability to initiate contraction on its own. Normally, this does not happen; instead, the heart produces a coordinated sequence of muscle cell contractions, which is required to pump blood. Unfortunately, there are some cases where the muscle cells of the heart lose their coordination and do not respond to the impulses from the heart's pacemakers. When this happens, the cells contract on their own, producing a chaotic, disorganized, completely uncoordinated myocardial rhythm referred to as *fibrillation*. If the ventricles fibrillate, there will be no blood pumped, no cardiac output, and no pulse—that is, cardiac arrest. This is the most common dysrhythmia producing cardiac arrest. Two fibrillatory dysrhythmias you must know are atrial fibrillation and ventricular fibrillation.

Atrial Fibrillation

When the tissue of the atria fibrillates, the atria do not contract. The patient will continue to have a pulse since the ventricles are still pumping, but the effectiveness of the myocardial contraction is decreased since the atria are not effectively filling the ventricles with blood. There are two primary ways to identify atrial fibrillation. First, there are no P waves, since there is no coordinated atrial depolarization. The millions of individual atrial cells depolarizing at random causes the baseline to be wavy with fibrillatory waves (fib-waves or f-waves).

The second identifying characteristic of atrial fibrillation is its irregularity (Figure 5-13). The ventricles will contract when enough fibrillatory impulses combine to send a signal through the AV node and down the conduction system. This does not occur at regular intervals and therefore causes an irregular ventricular response, represented on the ECG as a variance in the R-to-R interval of greater than 0.04 seconds (Table 5-6).

CLINICAL TIP: If you see a rhythm with no regularity whatsoever (that is irregularly irregular), think atrial fibrillation.

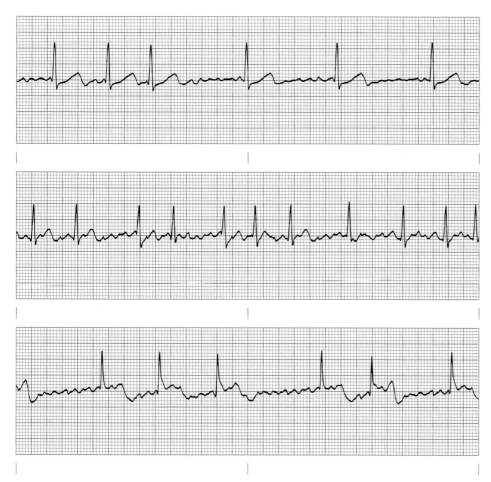

FIGURE 5–13
Three variants of atrial fibrillation.

TABLE 5–6 Atrial Fibrillation

Analyze	ECG
Rate	Ventricular rate varies but is usually faster in the unmedicated patient.
Regularity	**Variance of more than 0.04 seconds, irregularly irregular** ⚑
QRS Complex	
Do all of the QRS complexes look alike?	Yes
What is the width of the QRS complex?	Less than 0.12 seconds
P Waves	**There are no discernible P waves** ⚑
Is there a P wave before every QRS complex?	**The wavy baselines are called fibrillatory waves (f-waves).**
Is there a QRS after every P wave?	
Are the P waves upright and rounded?	NA (not applicable)
P-R Interval	
What is the P-R interval?	NA
Is the P-R interval constant?	NA

Ventricular Fibrillation

When the ventricular muscle tissue fibrillates, the ventricles cannot contract, resulting in no cardiac output and no pulse. Ventricular fibrillation is a cardiac arrest rhythm, but one that may be survivable with rapid defibrillation. It is also one of the easiest rhythms to identify, characterized by fibrillatory waves that may be fine, medium, or coarse and no discernible P waves, QRS complexes, or T waves (Table 5-7 and Figure 5-14).

TABLE 5-7	Ventricular Fibrillation
Analyze	**ECG**
Rate	**None**
Regularity	**NA**
QRS Complex	**Only fibrillatory waves are present.**
Do all of the QRS complexes look alike?	NA
What is the width of the QRS complex?	NA
P Waves	**Obliterated by the fibrillatory waves**
Is there a P wave before every QRS complex?	NA
Is there a QRS after every P wave?	NA
Are the P waves upright and rounded?	NA
P-R Interval	
What is the P-R interval?	**NA**
Is the P-R interval constant?	NA

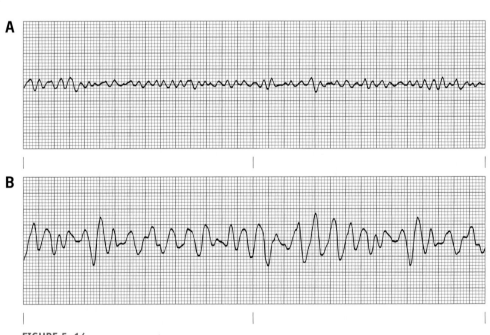

FIGURE 5-14
Two variants of ventricular fibrillation: (A) fine V-fib and (B) course V-fib.

Reentry and Atrial Dysrhythmias

Reentry and atrial dysrhythmias are those in which the site of impulse formation for the heart originates above the ventricles. This means that the rhythms will most likely have a narrow (< 0.12 sec) QRS complex, and also have a tendency to become rapid (or tachycardic).

The reentry phenomenon is very complex, but basically it represents a "short circuit" of the conduction system. This short circuit may be caused by local damage (infarct or ischemia) or a congenital defect. Typically, reentry involves a situation in which a portion of the conduction system will allow an impulse to travel in only one direction. When this occurs, a vicious cycle of very fast depolarization ensues as the impulse moves in a circle throughout the heart tissue (Figure 5-15). The characteristics of reentry dysrhythmias are that they are fast and they are comparatively easy to convert, either electrically or pharmacologically.

Atrial rhythms occur when the SA node fails to fire and a portion of the atrial tissue takes over as the pacemaker of the heart. If only one atrial site takes over, as is commonly the case, the P waves may be noted to be abnormally peaked, notched, or biphasic (above and below the isoelectric line), but they will all look the same (monomorphic) (Table 5-8 and Figure 5-16). If however, there are multiple atrial pacemakers trying to set the rhythm, the P waves may have a different morphology (polymorphic), and it usually results in some variance to the P-R interval (Table 5-9 and Figure 5-17).

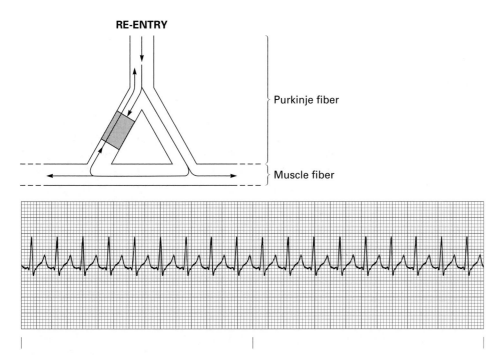

RE-ENTRY

Purkinje fiber

Muscle fiber

FIGURE 5–15
Reentry is a phenomenon usually created by a one-way block that causes a wave of depolarization to be rapidly propagated in a circular motion. Above: schematic drawing of reentry phenomenon. Below: ECG tracing of an atrial reentry rhythm.

TABLE 5–8 | Atrial Rhythms

Analyze	ECG
Rate	Usually 60–100 per minute
Regularity	Usually regular
QRS Complex	
Do all of the QRS complexes look alike?	Yes
What is the width of the QRS complex?	Less than 0.12 seconds
P Waves	
Is there a P wave before every QRS complex?	Yes
Is there a QRS after every P wave?	Yes
Are the P waves upright and rounded?	**No, may be peaked, notched, or biphasic**
P-R Interval	
What is the P-R interval?	Less than 0.20 seconds
Is the P-R interval constant?	Yes

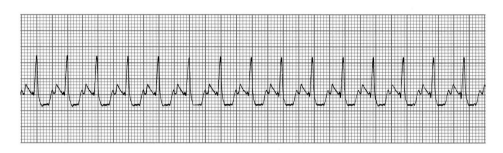

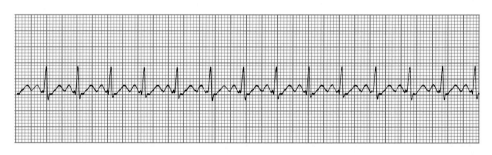

FIGURE 5–16
Two variants of atrial rhythms.

Atrial Flutter

Atrial flutter is another reentry dysrhythmia in which the reentry circuit is propagated through the atria. Atrial flutter is characterized by a baseline that looks like the top of a picket fence, commonly referred to as "picket-fence" or "saw-tooth" waves. These are flutter waves (abbreviated f-waves) and represent the rapid circle of depolarization of the atria (Table 5-10 and Figure 5-18).

Paroxysmal Supraventricular Tachycardia

Supraventricular tachycardia is a catch-all term that technically applies to any tachycardia rhythm that originates above the ventricles (Table 5-11 and Figure 5-19). There are quite a few causes of supraventricular tachycardia. By convention, if you are able to identify where the tachycardia is originating, you should be as specific as possible.

TABLE 5-9	Multiple Atrial Pacemaker Rhythms
Analyze	**ECG**
Rate	60–150 per minute
Regularity	**May have variance of more than 0.04 seconds** 🏳
QRS Complex	
Do all of the QRS complexes look alike?	Yes
What is the width of the QRS complex?	Less than 0.12 seconds
P Waves	
Is there a P wave before every QRS complex?	Yes
Is there a QRS after every P wave?	Yes
Are the P waves upright and rounded?	**No, may be peaked, notched, or biphasic and have varying morphology** 🏳
P-R Interval	
What is the P-R interval?	Less than 0.20 seconds
Is the P-R interval constant?	**Usually not constant** 🏳

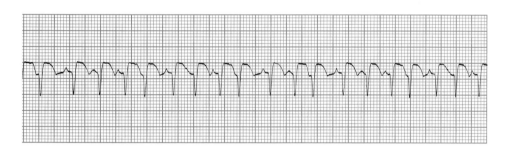

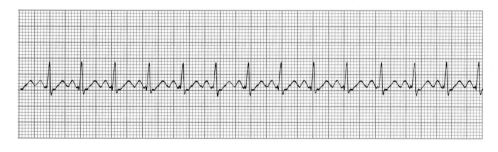

FIGURE 5-17
Two variants of multiple atrial rhythms.

You will recall that sinus tachycardia has a P wave which is evident. When the rate of sinus tachycardia gets above 160–170 beats per minute, the P wave gets buried in the previous T wave. Once this happens, it is impossible to tell if the tachycardia is created by rapid firing of the sinus node or by a reentry phenomenon. For narrow complex tachycardia from 150–200, it is important to look at the patient history to determine the electrophysiological cause of the dysrhythmia.

Shock, fear, fever, stress, or exercise usually indicates a sinus mechanism caused by sympathetic stimulation. Sudden onset and termination of tachycardia tend to be reentry in nature. A "run" of tachycardia that starts and stops abruptly is called *paroxysmal,* and is almost always a reentry mechanism. It is unusual for the SA node to discharge more than 200 beats per minute, so once the rate gets above 200, the dysrhythmia is probably caused by reentry.

TABLE 5–10　Atrial Flutter

Analyze	ECG
Rate	Can be any rate, depending on the ventricular response and presence of AV block.
Regularity	Variance of less than 0.04 seconds
QRS Complex	
Do all of the QRS complexes look alike?	Yes
What is the width of the QRS complex?	Less than 0.12 seconds
P Waves	**Flutter waves; no P waves discernible.** ⚑
Is there a P wave before every QRS complex?	NA
Is there a QRS after every P wave?	NA
Are the P waves upright and rounded?	NA
P-R Interval	
What is the P-R interval?	NA
Is the P-R interval constant?	NA

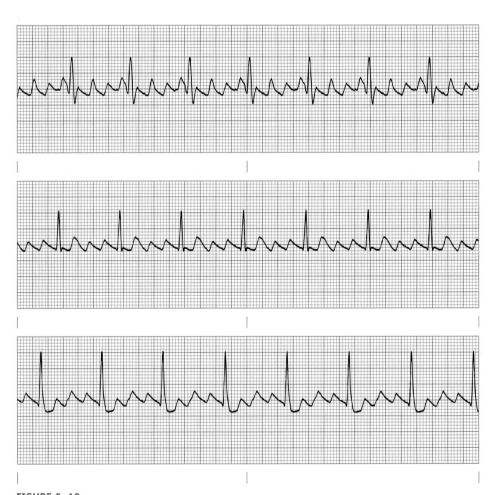

FIGURE 5–18
Three variants of atrial flutter.

TABLE 5–11 Paroxysmal Supraventricular Tachycardia

Analyze	ECG
Rate	**140–220 per minute** 🚩
Regularity	Variance of less than 0.04 seconds
QRS Complex	
Do all of the QRS complexes look alike?	Yes
What is the width of the QRS complex?	Less than 0.12 seconds
P Waves	**No P waves are identifiable** 🚩
Is there a P wave before every QRS complex?	NA
Is there a QRS after every P wave?	NA
Are the P waves upright and rounded?	NA
P-R Interval	
What is the P-R interval?	NA
Is the P-R interval constant?	NA

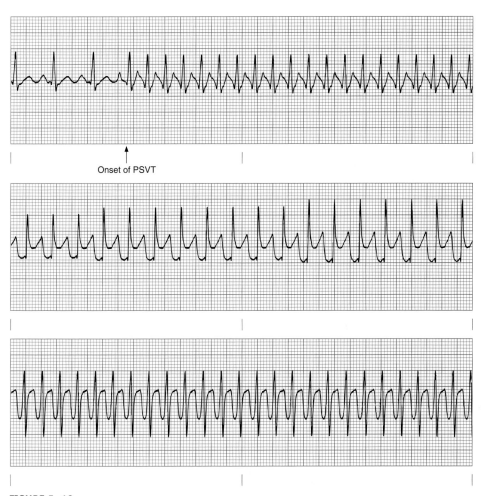

Onset of PSVT

FIGURE 5–19
Three variants of paroxysmal supraventricular tachycardia (PSVT).

Monomorphic Ventricular Tachycardia

Monomorphic ventricular tachycardia (VT or V-tach) is a reentry phenomenon occurring in the ventricles. Like other reentry dysrhythmias, it is regular and fast. Since the rhythm does not follow the normal conduction pathways of the heart, the QRS complexes are wide (Table 5-12 and Figure 5-20). Mechanically, V-tach may cause the ventricles to contract, but if it occurs in patients with underlying cardio-

TABLE 5–12	Monomorphic Ventricular Tachycardia
Analyze	**ECG**
Rate	**Greater than 100 per minute** 🚩
Regularity	Variance of less than 0.04 seconds
QRS Complex	
Do all of the QRS complexes look alike?	Yes
What is the width of the QRS complex?	**Greater than 0.12 seconds** 🚩
P Waves	**There are no P waves** 🚩
Is there a P wave before every QRS complex?	NA
Is there a QRS after every P wave?	NA
Are the P waves upright and rounded?	NA
P-R Interval	
What is the P-R interval?	NA
Is the P-R interval constant?	NA

FIGURE 5–20
Three variants of monomorphic ventricular tachycardia (V-tach).

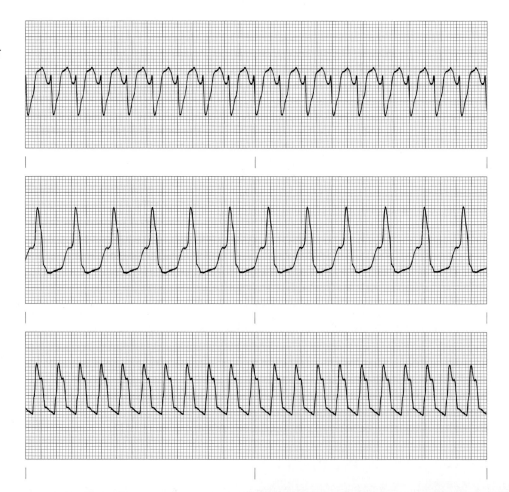

vascular disease, it is not well tolerated and may lead to ventricular fibrillation or pulselessness.

Polymorphic Ventricular Tachycardia

A variation of ventricular tachycardia is known as polymorphic ventricular tachycardia. This type of ventricular tachycardia has numerous other names such as torsades de pointes and multi-axial ventricular tachycardia. More specifically, polymorphic v-tach rhythms can be further subdivided into those with a normal QT interval, and those with a prolonged QT interval (or torsades). The characteristic of this rhythm includes wide QRS activity that has a varying morphology (unlike the similarly shaped QRS seen with monomorphic v-tach). With polymorphic ventricular tachycardia, the amplitude and direction of the QRS has a tendency to wax and wane around the baseline, creating an appearance as if the ventricular tachycardia is "turning" around a center point (Table 5-13 and Figure 5-21).

TABLE 5–13 **Polymorphic Ventricular Tachycardia**

Analyze	ECG
Rate	**Greater than 100 per minute**
Regularity	**Irregular rhythm**
QRS Complex	
Do all of the QRS complexes look alike?	**No**
What is the width of the QRS complex?	**Greater than 0.12 seconds**
P Waves	
Is there a P wave before every QRS complex?	**There are no P waves**
Is there a QRS after every P wave?	NA
Are the P waves upright and rounded?	NA
P-R Interval	
What is the P-R interval?	NA
Is the P-R interval constant?	NA

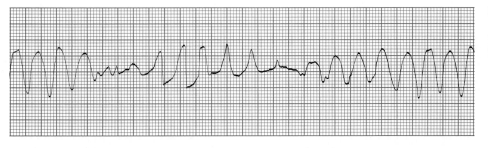

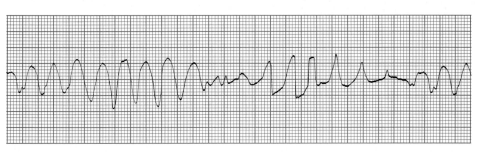

FIGURE 5–21
Two variants of polymorphic ventricular tachycardia.

Unlike monomorphic ventricular tachycardia, polymorphic is often caused by metabolic derangements such as drug toxicities or electrolyte abnormalities. Generally speaking, acceptable drugs to treat this rhythm include all of the agents listed for monomorphic ventricular tachycardia as well as consideration of overdrive pacing. In some cases, it may be difficult to distinguish supraventricular tachycardia with aberrant conduction from ventricular tachycardia. If uncertain, it is best to assume that the rhythm is V-tach.

CLINICAL TIP: In an emergency, consider any wide complex tachycardia to be ventricular tachycardia until proven otherwise.

The Absence of Rhythm: Asystole

Probably the easiest rhythm to interpret is asystole. Asystole is the absence of any ventricular contraction or QRS complexes. Occasionally, you may see isolated P waves or slow, wide QRS complexes that are generally called "agonal" beats (Table 5-14 and Figure 5-22).

TABLE 5-14 Asystole

Analyze	ECG
Rate	None
Regularity	NA
QRS Complex Do all of the QRS complexes look alike? What is the width of the QRS complex?	NA
P Waves Is there a P wave before every QRS complex? Is there a QRS after every P wave? Are the P waves upright and rounded?	NA
P-R Interval What is the P-R interval? Is the P-R interval constant?	NA

FIGURE 5-22
Two variants of asystole.

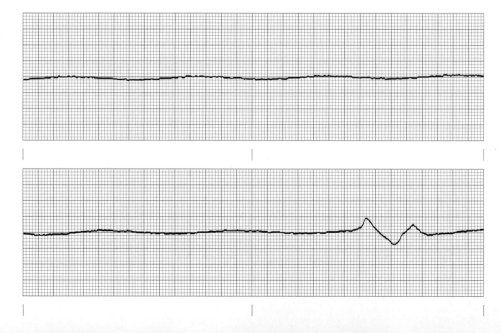

The Blocks

The atria and ventricles are isolated from each other electrically except for the atrioventricular (AV) node. The AV node, therefore, acts as a "gate" that any supraventricular signal must pass through if it is going to cause the ventricles to contract. Usually it takes less than 0.20 seconds for an impulse to pass through this gate. All of the blocks are caused by a delay at the AV junction. We will use the "gate" analogy to explain each of the blocks.

There are four AV blocks. It is easiest to consider the two ends of the spectrum, and then the intermediate situation. Therefore, we will start with a look at first- and third-degree blocks and then discuss the two types of second-degree block.

First-Degree AV Block

First-degree AV block represents a slight closing of the "gate." In first-degree AV block, the signal is delayed at the AV node, but all of the impulses get through. This is represented on the ECG as a constant P-R interval of greater than 0.20 seconds (Table 5-15 and Figure 5-23).

Third-Degree AV Block

Third-degree AV block is also called complete heart block. As the name implies, the "gate" is completely closed. There is no electrical connection between the atria and the ventricles; therefore, the atria and ventricles contract totally independently of each other. On the ECG, this is identified by a lack of relationship between the P waves and the QRS complexes (Table 5-16 and Figure 5-24). The P waves and QRS complexes have their own independent regular rates.

Second-Degree AV Block

Second-degree AV blocks represent some intermittent closing to the AV "gate." Since the gate does not remain closed, some of the beats get through and others do

TABLE 5–15 First-Degree AV Block

Analyze	ECG
Rate	60–100 per minute
Regularity	Variance of less than 0.04 seconds
QRS Complex	
Do all of the QRS complexes look alike?	Yes
What is the width of the QRS complex?	Less than 0.12 seconds
P Waves	
Is there a P wave before every QRS complex?	Yes
Is there a QRS after every P wave?	Yes
Are the P waves upright and rounded?	Yes
P-R Interval	
What is the P-R interval?	**Greater than 0.20 seconds**
Is the P-R interval constant?	Yes

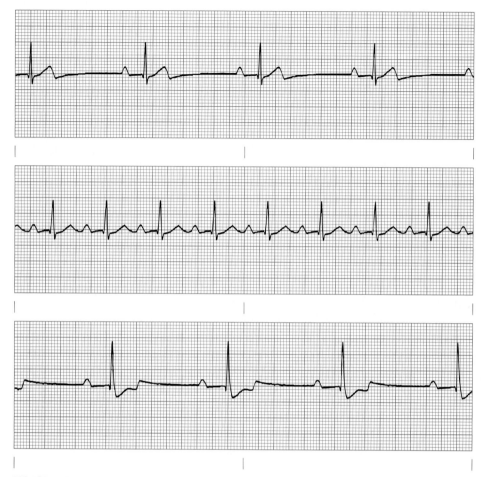

FIGURE 5–23
Three variants of first-degree AV block.

TABLE 5-16	Third-Degree AV Block
Analyze	**ECG**
Rate	Less than 60 per minute
Regularity	Variance of less than 0.04 seconds
QRS Complex	
Do all of the QRS complexes look alike?	Yes
What is the width of the QRS complex?	May be narrow or wide, depending on the location of the escape rhythm
P Waves	**There is no relationship between the P waves and the QRS**
Is there a P wave before every QRS complex?	**complex** 🚩
Is there a QRS after every P wave?	
Are the P waves upright and rounded?	Usually
P-R Interval	
What is the P-R interval?	**Variable** 🚩
Is the P-R interval constant?	**Variable**

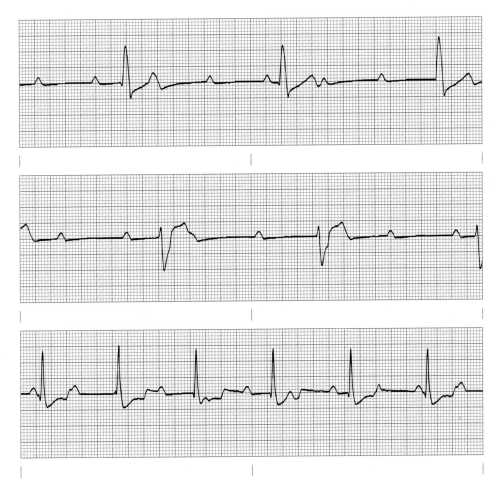

FIGURE 5–24
Three variants of third-degree AV Block.

not. In second-degree AV blocks, there are always more P waves than QRS complexes since some of the P waves are prevented from causing ventricular contraction by a gate that is opening and closing.

▶ **Type I.** Second-degree AV block, Type I (which is also called second-degree, Mobitz I or Wenckebach) is identified by a progressive prolongation of the P-R interval until one beat fails to get through, and then the pattern repeats itself (Table 5-17 and Figure 5-25).

▶ **Type II.** Second-degree AV block, Type II (also called second-degree, Mobitz II) is the intermittent closing of the "gate" at regular intervals. This leads to a pattern of grouped beats (P waves followed by QRS complexes) with pauses (P waves with no QRS complexes) (Table 5-18 and Figure 5-26). Typically, you can see the pattern developing if you look at a long-enough strip. Often, second-degree blocks are referred to by the ratio of P waves to QRS complexes. When compared to Mobitz I second-degree block, the interval between P wave and QRS complex does not lengthen in Mobitz II. It is also important to remember with this type of block that the intervals of the *transmitted* P waves are constant.

TABLE 5–17 | Second-Degree AV Block, Type I

Analyze	ECG
Rate	60–100 per minute
Regularity	**Missed beats, regularly irregular** 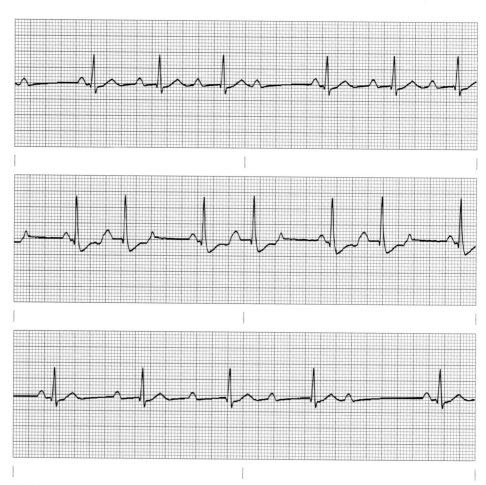
QRS Complex	
Do all of the QRS complexes look alike?	Yes
What is the width of the QRS complex?	Less than 0.12 seconds
P Waves	
Is there a P wave before every QRS complex?	Yes
Is there a QRS after every P wave?	**No**
Are the P waves upright and rounded?	Usually
P-R Interval	**The P-R interval is variable and progressively lengthens**
What is the P-R interval?	**until a QRS is dropped. Then the pattern repeats.**
Is the P-R interval constant?	

FIGURE 5–25
Three variants of second-degree AV Block, Type I.

TABLE 5–18 **Second-Degree AV Block, Type II**

Analyze	ECG
Rate	60–100 per minute
Regularity	**Dropped QRS complexes result in an irregular rhythm.** 🚩
QRS Complex	
Do all of the QRS complexes look alike?	Yes
What is the width of the QRS complex?	Less than 0.12 seconds
P Waves	
Is there a P wave before every QRS complex?	Yes
Is there a QRS after every P wave?	**No** 🚩
Are the P waves upright and rounded?	Usually
P-R Interval	**Non-conducted P waves are not followed by QRS complexes.**
What is the P-R interval?	**Conducted P waves have a constant P-R interval, typically**
Is the P-R interval constant?	**less than 0.20 seconds.** 🚩

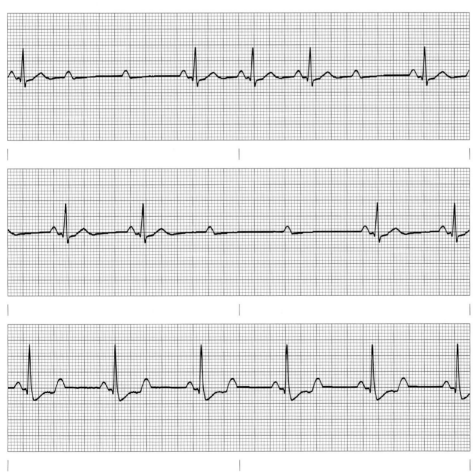

FIGURE 5–26
Three variants of second-degree AV Block, Type II.

Ectopic Beats

An ectopic beat occurs when a site *other than the primary pacemaker of the heart* depolarizes. Remember that myocardial cells have the property of automaticity, which may cause depolarization if the conditions are right. This can cause depolarization of the surrounding muscle tissue. If the ectopic beat originates above the ventricles, the impulse can follow the normal ventricular conduction system and result in the depolarization of the ventricles. If the ectopic focus is located in the ventricles, it will most likely depolarize just the ventricles and typically does not follow the normal conduction of the heart. If the ectopic beat comes earlier than the next-expected beat, based on the underlying rhythm, the ectopic beat is called "premature." If it comes after a pause in the underlying rhythm, it is referred to as an "escape" beat.

In the past, premature beats were thought to indicate increased cardiac irritability. Especially in the case of premature ventricular contractions, increased ectopic beats were thought to be a warning of sudden cardiac arrest from ventricular fibrillation and were typically treated aggressively. Routine treatment of PVCs has not been supported by scientific studies, but you should still consider the presence of ectopic beats in the setting of a suspected myocardial infarction significant.

The process for determining where ectopic beats are coming from is slightly different than interpreting the rhythm. Technically, ectopic beats are not dysrhythmias. All rhythms with premature beats are irregular, but the underlying rhythm that is interrupted by the premature beat may be regular.

You should think of the possibility of ectopic beats in the following two situations:

▶ When all of the beats do not look the same

▶ When there is some regularity to the rhythm, but none of the blocks seem to fit.

Once you suspect the presence of ectopic beats, you should do the following:

1. *Identify the underlying rhythm.* If the ectopic beats look different, this is very easy. Unfortunately, this is not always the case and you should look at the patterns of the rhythm.
2. *Determine where the ectopic beats are originating.* There are three possibilities: the atria, the AV node, or the ventricles. Determining the origin of the ectopic beat is accomplished by looking at the P wave, QRS complex, and the interruption of the underlying rhythm that is caused by the ectopic beat, as explained below.

Premature Atrial and Premature Junctional Contractions

Premature atrial contractions (PACs) are caused by an ectopic focus located somewhere in the atrial tissue. Premature junctional contractions (PJCs) are caused by the AV node firing prematurely. The difference between PACs and PJCs is minor and, in the setting of a cardiac emergency, considered to be clinically insignificant. We will therefore discuss PACs and PJCs together.

The PAC may have a P wave if the ectopic beat is high enough in the atria, but it will usually look somewhat different from the P wave of the underlying rhythm. If the premature beat originates lower in the atria, or in the AV junction, the P wave may be absent or upside down. The QRS complexes of PACs and PJCs are usually narrow, since the ectopic beats follow the normal ventricular conduction pathway (Figure 5-27).

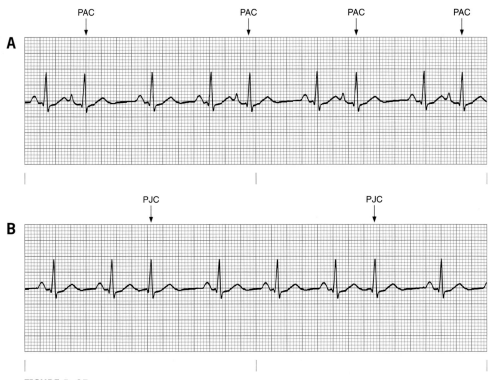

FIGURE 5–27
(A) premature atrial contraction (PAC); (B) premature junctional contraction (PJC).

TABLE 5–19   PACs and PJCs

Analyze	ECG
P wave of the ectopic beat	Usually looks different from the P waves of the underlying rhythm. May be upright if the ectopic foci are high in the atria. The P wave may be absent or upside down if it is low in the atria or in the AV junction.
QRS complex of the ectopic beat	Usually narrow. It is possible that the QRS is wide, even if the QRS of the underlying rhythm is narrow.
Interruption of the underlying rhythm that is caused by the ectopic beat	Non-compensatory pause

The SA node is reset by a premature atrial contraction and by most premature junctional complexes. Therefore the R-to-R interval for the beat immediately following the ectopic beat is usually the same as the R-to-R intervals of the underlying rhythm. If you measure the distance from the R wave of the last beat of the intrinsic rhythm to the R wave of the next beat after the ectopic beat, it is less than 2 R, the distance of two R-R intervals. This is called a non-compensatory pause (Table 5-19).

Premature Ventricular Contractions

Premature ventricular contractions (PVCs) are caused by an ectopic focus in the ventricles. Since the ectopic beat originates in the ventricles, there is no P wave.

FIGURE 5–28
Two variants of normal sinus rhythm with PVCs.

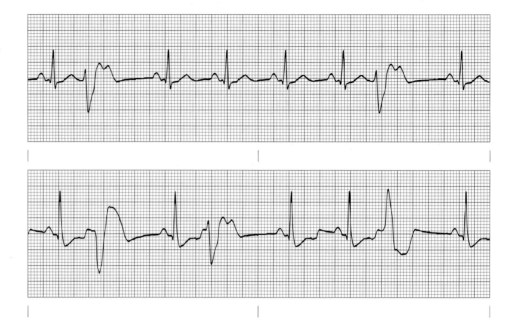

The ectopic beat does not follow the normal ventricular conduction pathway, and therefore the morphology of the PVC is always wide (Figure 5-28).

CLINICAL TIP: Not all wide premature beats are PVCs!

It is important not to make the mistake of assuming that all wide premature beats are PVCs. The underlying rhythm's QRS complexes can be narrow, and a PAC or PJC can be wide. Be sure to look at all the variables.

Since the PVC originates in the ventricles, the SA node is not affected by the ectopic beat. The SA node continues to fire uninterrupted and is not reset by a PVC. For that reason, the distance from the R wave of the beat immediately preceding a PVC to the R wave of the beat following the PVC will be 2R of the underlying beat. This is called a compensatory pause (Table 5-20 and Figure 5-29).

There are several types of PVCs with which you should become familiar.

▶ **Unifocal.** All of the PVCs look the same and probably come from one ectopic focus (Figure 5-30).

▶ **Multifocal.** The PVCs look different from each other and likely come from more than one ectopic foci (Figure 5-31).

▶ **Salvos or couplets.** Two or three PVCs in a row (Figure 5-32).

▶ **Bigeminy.** A PVC every other beat (Figure 5-33).

▶ **Trigeminy.** A PVC every third beat (Figure 5-34).

TABLE 5–20	PVCs
Analyze	**ECG**
P wave of the ectopic beat	Usually none
QRS complex of the ectopic beat	Always wide
Interruption of the underlying rhythm that is caused by the ectopic beat	Compensatory pause

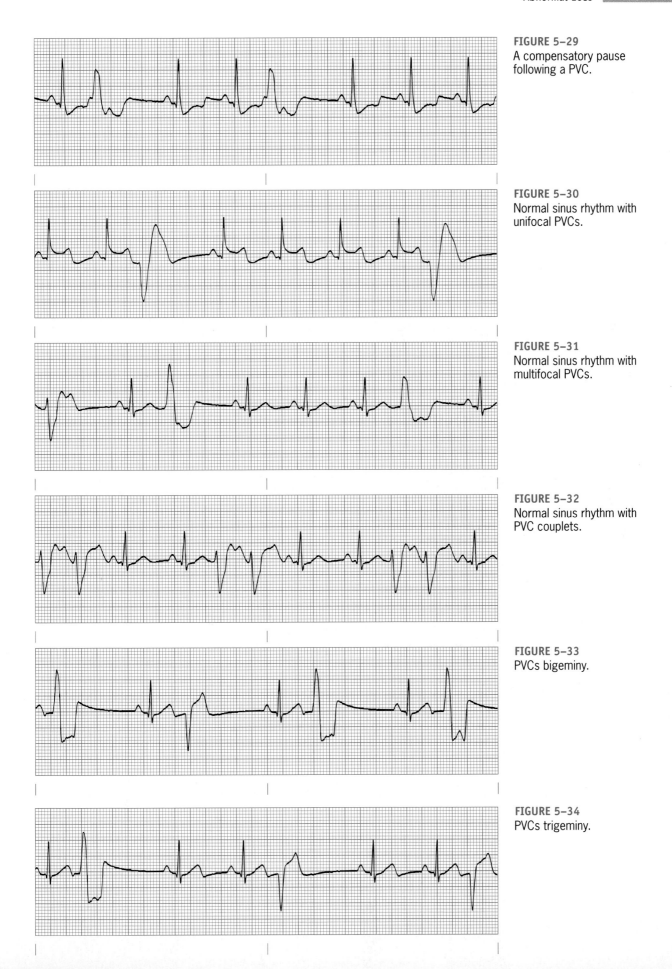

FIGURE 5–29
A compensatory pause
following a PVC.

FIGURE 5–30
Normal sinus rhythm with
unifocal PVCs.

FIGURE 5–31
Normal sinus rhythm with
multifocal PVCs.

FIGURE 5–32
Normal sinus rhythm with
PVC couplets.

FIGURE 5–33
PVCs bigeminy.

FIGURE 5–34
PVCs trigeminy.

Junctional and Ventricular Escape Rhythms

In the last section, you learned how an ectopic beat (QRS complexes) that occurred later than the next anticipated beat was an attempt by the heart to maintain some type of cardiac output when a higher pacemaker site failed to cause ventricular contraction. Understanding this, escape rhythms are simply those generated by a pacemaker site in either the junctional region (AV node) or the ventricles (Purkinje network) that becomes the primary pacemaker site because of failure of the normal site (SA node). One salient characteristic of escape rhythms is that they are regular.

Junctional escape rhythms, commonly referred to simply as junctional rhythms occur when the sinoatrial node fails to fire and the AV node takes over as the pacemaker of the heart. The "red flag" ECG change that occurs with junctional rhythms is that the P wave is either inverted, absent, or follows the QRS complex (Table 5-21 and Figure 5-35). The QRS complexes in junctional rhythms are still a normal width, since the impulse travels down the bundle branches and spreads throughout the Purkinje network normally. The rate of junctional rhythms is usually 40–60 beats per minute. If the junctional rhythm is 60–100 beats per minute, it is referred to as "accelerated junctional rhythm," and if it exceeds 100 beats per minute it is then termed "junctional tachycardia".

Ventricular escape rhythms, commonly referred to simply as ventricular rhythms occur when both the SA and AV nodes fail to cause ventricular depolarization, and the Purkinje fibers then become established as the only pacemaker site. The QRS complex is wider than normal, since the conduction must spread through out the ventricles outside the normal conduction pathway. Additionally, the normal rate for a ventricular escape rhythm is 20–40 beats per minute. Slower than 20 beats per minute is called an "agonal" rhythm, a rate of 40–100 beats per minute is called "accelerated ventricular rhythm," and, finally, a ventricular rhythm greater than 100 beats per minute is called "ventricular tachycardia" (Table 5-22 and Figure 5-36).

TABLE 5–21 Junctional Escape Rhythms

Analyze	ECG
Rate	**40–60 per minute**
Regularity	Usually regular
QRS Complex	
Do all of the QRS complexes look alike?	Yes
What is the width of the QRS complex?	Less than 0.12 seconds
P Waves	
Is there a P wave before every QRS complex?	Yes
Is there a QRS after every P wave?	Yes
Are the P waves upright and rounded?	**No, may be inverted or absent**
P-R Interval	
What is the P-R interval?	Less than 0.20 seconds
Is the P-R interval constant?	Yes

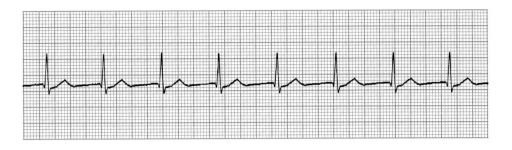

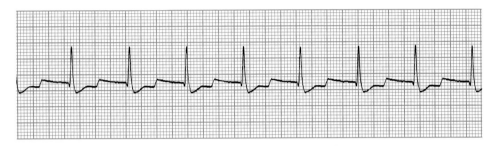

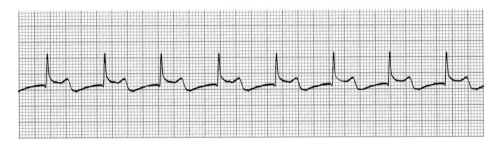

FIGURE 5–35
Three variants of junctional escape rhythms.

TABLE 5–22   Ventricular Escape Rhythms

Analyze	ECG
Rate	**20–40 per minute**
Regularity	Usually regular
QRS Complex	
Do all of the QRS complexes look alike?	Yes
What is the width of the QRS complex?	**Greater than 0.12 seconds**
P Waves	
Is there a P wave before every QRS complex?	**No**
Is there a QRS after every P wave?	**No**
Are the P waves upright and rounded?	NA
P-R Interval	
What is the P-R interval?	NA
Is the P-R interval constant?	NA

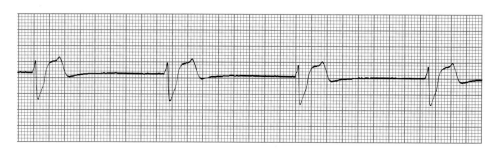

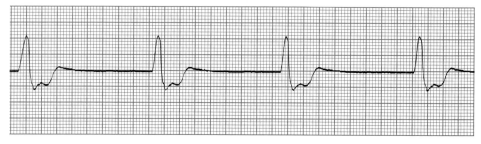

FIGURE 5–36
Two variants of ventricular escape rhythms.

⊞ SUMMARY

The recognition of dysrhythmias is one of the most important aspects of ACLS and a necessary component of the patient assessment for any cardiac patient. Many clinicians become intimidated by the electrophysiology of the heart and fail to learn a systematic method of evaluating ECGs. By using the "red flag" method and applying a few rules and an understanding of the etiology of dysrhythmias, dysrhythmia recognition becomes much easier.

CASE STUDY FOLLOW-UP

Assessment

Mrs. Brown is alert and oriented, she denies chest pain or shortness of breath, her pulse is 180, respirations 20 and unlabored, blood pressure 124/78. You remember that the majority of wide complex tachycardias are ventricular tachycardia. Often, you can get additional clues from the patient's history, but in this case it does not help, since she has not had the problem previously diagnosed. In this case, Mrs. Brown is stable and you are unsure of the origination of the dysrhythmia: This could be either ventricular tachycardia or a supraventricular tachycardia with aberrant conduction.

Treatment

You choose to administer lidocaine. The rhythm does not convert, and en route to the hospital, Mrs. Brown begins to complain of lightheadedness and dizziness. Reassessment reveals a pulse of 180, respirations of 22 and unlabored, and a blood pressure of 98/64. She is pale and diaphoretic.

Mrs. Brown is now unstable. You decide to abandon the pharmacological approach. You administer an intravenous sedative and cardiovert her at 100 joules. The rhythm converts to NSR and her blood pressure returns to 114/78.

Electrophysiology studies indicate that the rhythm was indeed ventricular tachycardia. Mrs. Brown is now taking Quinidine and doing fine.

REVIEW QUESTIONS

1. Myocardial cells possess the unique property of
   a. depolarization.
   b. repolarization.
   c. contractility.
   d. automaticity.

2. Which of the following is **not** one of the three specialized types of myocardial cells?
   a. pacemaker
   b. conduction
   c. depolarizing
   d. working

3. What is the purpose of pacemaker cells?
   a. to contract when a wave of depolarization reaches them
   b. to depolarize at regular intervals
   c. to repolarize contracted muscle tissue
   d. to delay the conduction from the atria to the ventricles

4. The main pacemaker of the healthy heart is the
   a. SA node.
   b. atrium.
   c. AV node.
   d. ventricle.

5. The AV node depolarizes spontaneously at what rate?
   a. greater than 100 times per minute
   b. 60–100 times per minute
   c. 40–60 times per minute
   d. less than 40 times per minute

6. The myocardial cells responsible for mechanical contraction of the heart are
   a. pacemaker cells.
   b. conduction cells.
   c. working cells.
   d. all of the heart cells.

7. What mechanical event corresponds to the QRS complex in the normal heart?
   a. atrial contraction
   b. the delay between atrial and ventricular contraction
   c. ventricular contraction
   d. reentry

8. A variance of greater than 0.04 seconds in the R-R interval is called
   a. irregularity.
   b. automaticity.
   c. ectopy.
   d. dysrhythmia.

9. Which of the following is a cause of wide QRS complexes?
   a. hypothermia
   b. bundle branch block
   c. hypernatremia
   d. acute myocardial infarction

10. What do we know for sure about a narrow QRS complex?
    a. It cannot have been generated by the SA node.
    b. The impulse was delayed at the AV node.
    c. It must have originated above the ventricles.
    d. It must have followed the internodal pathways.

11. What is the maximum normal P-R interval?
    a. 0.04 seconds
    b. 0.12 seconds
    c. 0.20 seconds
    d. 0.50 seconds

12. What is/are the "red flag(s)" in sinus tachycardia?
    a. rate
    b. regularity
    c. QRS complex
    d. P wave
    e. P-R interval
    f. If more than one "red flag," fill in the letters of the correct responses:

    _____

13. What is/are the "red flag(s)" in sinus dysrhythmia?
    a. rate
    b. regularity
    c. QRS complex
    d. P wave
    e. P-R interval
    f. If more than one "red flag," fill in the letters of the correct responses:

    _____

14. What dysrhythmia is **irregularly** irregular?
    a. second-degree, Type I heart block
    b. third-degree heart block
    c. sinus rhythm with PVCs
    d. atrial fibrillation

15. What is/are the "red flag(s)" in atrial fibrillation?
    a. rate
    b. regularity
    c. QRS complex
    d. P wave
    e. P-R interval
    f. If more than one "red flag," fill in the letters of the correct responses:

    _____

16. Which of the following is **not** a reentry dysrhythmia?
    a. atrial fibrillation
    b. supraventricular tachycardia
    c. atrial flutter
    d. ventricular tachycardia

17. What is/are the "red flag(s)" in atrial flutter?
    a. rate
    b. regularity
    c. QRS complex
    d. P wave
    e. P-R interval
    f. If more than one "red flag," fill in the letters of the correct responses:

    _____

18. What is/are the "red flag(s)" in supraventricular tachycardia?
    a. rate
    b. regularity
    c. QRS complex
    d. P wave
    e. P-R interval
    f. If more than one "red flag," fill in the letters of the correct responses:

    _____

19. What is/are the "red flag(s)" in ventricular tachycardia?
    a. rate
    b. regularity
    c. QRS complex
    d. P wave
    e. P-R interval
    f. If more than one "red flag," fill in the letters of the correct responses:

    _____

20. What is/are the "red flag(s)" in first-degree AV block?
    a. rate
    b. regularity
    c. QRS complex
    d. P wave
    e. P-R interval
    f. If more than one "red flag," fill in the letters of the correct responses:

    _____

21. What is/are the "red flag(s)" in third-degree AV block?
    a. rate
    b. regularity
    c. QRS complex
    d. P wave
    e. P-R interval
    f. If more than one "red flag," fill in the letters of the correct responses:

    _____

22. All PVCs are _____, but not all PACs and PJCs are _____.
    a. narrow, narrow
    b. wide, wide
    c. wide, narrow
    d. narrow, wide

23. Most PVCs have a _____ pause, and most PACs have a _____ pause.
    a. compensatory, compensatory
    b. non-compensatory, non-compensatory
    c. compensatory, non-compensatory
    d. non-compensatory, compensatory

24. What is the name for PVCs that occur "every third beat"?
    a. trigeminy
    b. bigeminy
    c. multifocal
    d. salvos

25. Identify the following rhythm.

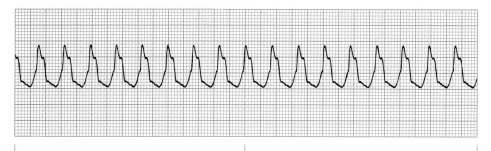

26. Identify the following rhythm.

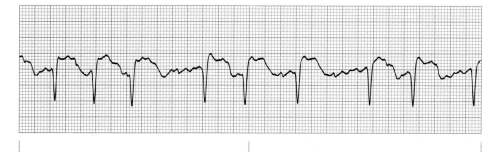

27. Identify the following rhythm.

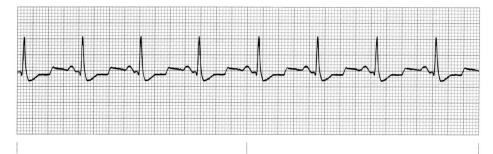

28. Identify the following rhythm.

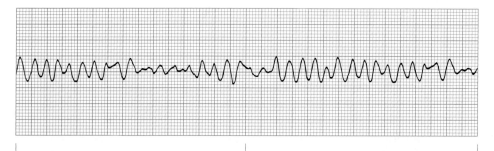

29. Identify the following rhythm.

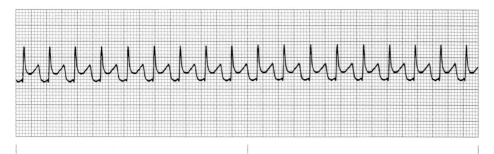

_____

30. Identify the following rhythm.

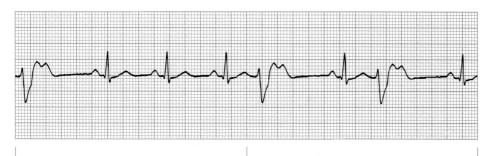

_____

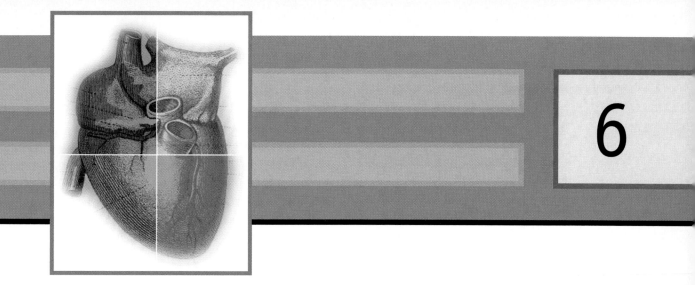

12-Lead Electrocardiographic Interpretation

The treatment of acute coronary syndromes has changed dramatically in the past 10 years. While prehospital care providers have teamed with emergency physicians and surgeons to rapidly deliver the patient with traumatic injuries to the operating suite for many years, patients with acute myocardial infarction are now being treated using a similar approach. Because of the progressive destruction of myocardial muscle during an infarction, the expression that should guide the emergency provider is "Time is Muscle."

Topics in this chapter are:

- Coronary Artery Anatomy
- ECG Leads
- Basics of 12-Lead ECG Interpretation
- Ischemia, Injury, and Infarction
- ECG Findings in Other Medical Conditions

CASE STUDY

"Medic 23 and Engine 34, first responder detail, please respond to 5612 Shady Grove for a 58-year-old female with arm and shoulder pain. Time out is 0934."

Upon your arrival, you find Mrs. Springer, an overweight 58-year-old female, who complains of moderate jaw, back, shoulder, and arm pain lasting for about an hour. She denies chest pain specifically, but you are concerned that she may be experiencing a cardiac event, so you perform a 12-lead ECG. The ECG shows ST-segment elevation in Leads II, III, and aVF, strongly suggestive of an inferior wall myocardial infarction. You phone the receiving emergency department and send them a 12-lead ECG before you leave the patient's house.

You begin rapid transportation, and upon arrival at the ED, the patient is taken quickly to the cardiac catheterization lab, where a 95% occlusion in her right coronary artery is opened with angioplasty and a stent is placed. Mrs. Springer is released from the hospital three days later with minimal myocardial damage, due in large part to your rapid identification of the crisis and initiation of chain of events that rapidly reperfused her dying heart tissue.

What would have happened if the patient did not call EMS so quickly, or if transportation was delayed?

INTRODUCTION

The previous chapter discussed the recognition of basic cardiac rhythms and dysrhythmias. This chapter focuses on the use of the 12-lead electrocardiogram (ECG) as an adjunct in the management of patients in the out-of-hospital setting. The most common use of 12-lead ECG is to help recognize emerging cardiac syndromes.

The ability to obtain and rapidly interpret a 12-lead ECG is essential to activating the emergency care system to respond to the cardiac patient. The first step in re-establishing blood flow in patients with acute myocardial infarction (AMI) is obtaining a diagnostic ECG. By recognizing the characteristic changes on the electrocardiogram, the emergency care provider can set in motion a series of steps designed to restore blood flow to the affected myocardium.

The primary purpose of this chapter is to familiarize the reader with the basic tenets of 12-lead ECG interpretation and recognition of the characteristic changes associated with an acute myocardial infarction. Combined with excellent physical exam and history-taking skills, the 12-lead ECG can also help to identify a variety of conditions, including pulmonary disease, hyperkalemia, hypocalcemia, and hypothermia.

CORONARY ARTERY ANATOMY

The heart is served by two major arteries: the right and left coronary arteries (Figure 6-1). Each of these arteries originates from the aorta just above the aortic root. The unique feature of coronary artery perfusion is that it occurs during *diastole* in contrast to other arteries in the body which fill during systole.

The left coronary artery (LCA) is typically the larger of the two major arteries serving the heart. It provides blood supply to the anterior wall, the lateral wall, and the posterior wall of the left ventricle, and the left interventricular septal wall. Almost immediately after leaving the aorta, the left coronary artery divides into the left anterior descending (LAD) artery and the left circumflex artery. The LAD supplies the anterior ventricular wall, whereas the circumflex artery provides cir-

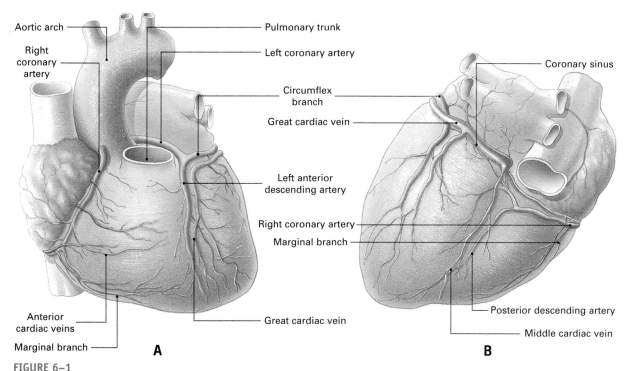

FIGURE 6–1
The coronary arteries: (A) anterior view, (B) posterior view.

culation to the posterior wall. A marginal branch of the LCA provides circulation to the lateral ventricular wall.

Understanding this portion of the coronary anatomy can help explain why patients who suffer an occlusion of the left coronary artery or its major branches develop an infarction of the anterior wall of the left ventricle (anterior MI). It also explains why patients with anterior MIs may have associated infarctions of the posterior or septal wall.

The right coronary artery (RCA) is typically smaller than the LCA. The RCA supplies blood to the right ventricle as well as the inferior portion of the left ventricle. It also supplies the upper portions of the conduction system (SA node, and AV node). Occlusion of the RCA is often associated with a right ventricular and/or an infarction of the inferior wall of the left ventricle (inferior MI). In addition, because the RCA supplies the conduction system, cardiac dysrhythmias such as bradycardia and heart blocks can occur in patients with inferior MIs.

ECG LEADS

The electrocardiogram is a representation of electrical events that are occurring within the heart as viewed by a variety of "cameras" placed on the surface of the body. These cameras provide different views of the same electrical events that occur during the cardiac cycle. On most calls, you are interested in determining only the patient's basic cardiac rhythm and will rely most often on Leads I, II, and III (collectively called *limb leads*) (Figure 6-2).

The limb lead electrodes are placed on the patient's trunk near the left arm, right arm, and left leg. This placement forms an imaginary triangle on the surface of the body referred to as Einthoven's triangle (Figure 6-3). These leads capture the ECG from the perspective of the frontal plane. By convention, Lead II is typically

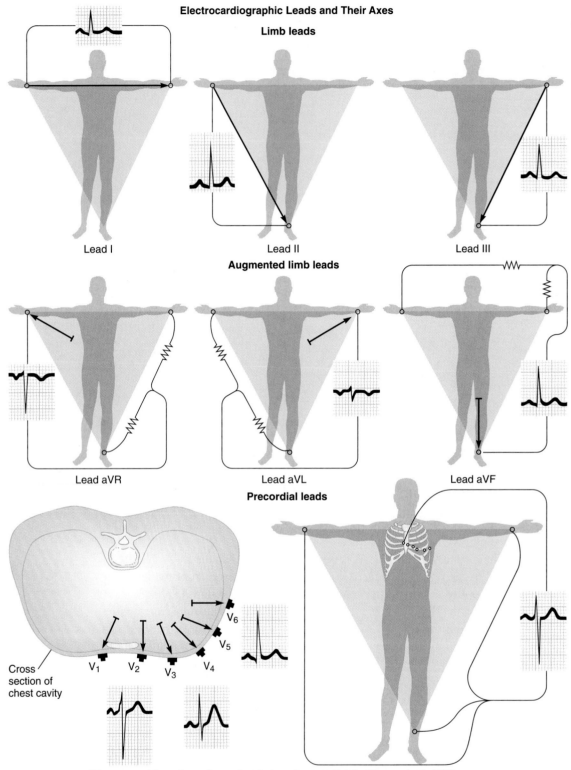

Electrocardiographic Leads and Their Axes

Limb leads

Lead I   Lead II   Lead III

Augmented limb leads

Lead aVR   Lead aVL   Lead aVF

Precordial leads

Cross section of chest cavity

V_1 V_2 V_3 V_4 V_5 V_6

When current flows toward arrowheads (axes), upward deflection occurs in ECG
When current flows away from arrowheads (axes), downward deflection occurs in ECG
When current flows perpendicular to arrows (axes), no deflection occurs

FIGURE 6–2
ECG leads and their axes.

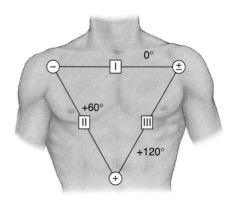

FIGURE 6–3
Einthoven's triangle as formed by the bipolar leads.

used when continuously monitoring the patient's cardiac rhythm. This is done because electrical evidence of atrial contraction (P waves) are best seen in Lead II.

The limb leads provide enough information for basic rhythm recognition but are generally inadequate to identify cardiac ischemia or infarction. When this information is necessary, nine additional leads (for a total of 12) are used. Three of these are referred to as *augmented limb leads* (review Figure 6-2) that view the electrical currents traveling from the center of the heart to the right arm (aVR), left arm (aVL), and left foot (aVF) (Figure 6-4). As you can see from the figure, Leads II, III, and aVF provide information about the inferior portions of the heart. Lead I and aVL are considered the lateral leads.

The six remaining views are obtained by examining the heart along the horizontal plane. These leads are referred to as the *precordial leads,* and the positive electrode for each lead proceeds from the right side of the chest (V_1) to the left chest (V_6) (review bottom of Figure 6-2). V_1 and V_2 provide information about the interventricular septum, V_3 and V_4 view primarily the anterior wall of the left ventricle, and V_5 and V_6 demonstrate the lateral wall of the left ventricle. The 12-lead electrocardiogram records the electrical activity of the heart from the perspective of each of the limb leads (3), the augmented limb leads (3), and precordial leads (6).

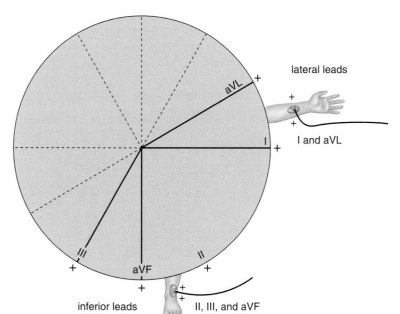

FIGURE 6–4
The conventional placement of limb lead electrodes. A positive left-arm electrode records lateral Leads I and aVL. A positive left foot electrode records inferior Leads II, III, and aVF.

⊞ BASICS OF 12-LEAD ECG INTERPRETATION

Twelve-lead ECG analyses typically occurs after you have determined that the patient has no immediate life-threatening condition or dysrhythmias. You will usually attach the cardiac monitor to the patient and continuously monitor his cardiac rhythm. In prehospital care, the 12-lead is most helpful in identifying patients who may be experiencing an acute coronary syndrome. It may also help you distinguish between possible causes of a dysrhythmia. For this purpose, you will look most closely at the axis and ST-segment changes.

Axis

Because of the fact that the left ventricle is larger than the right, the average electrical forces during ventricular contraction appear to be oriented toward the left side of the heart. As a result, cardiac leads that are directed toward the left side of the heart (such as Lead I, aVL, and precordial leads V_5 and V_6) will demonstrate a primarily positive QRS complex (large R wave). If you examine the precordial leads, you will notice that there is a tendency for the R wave to become more prominent as the tracing is viewed from V_1 through V_6 (called "R wave progression") (Figure 6-5).

    The cardiac axis describes the overall direction of ventricular depolarization. It can be thought of as an arrow pointing in the direction of the QRS complex (Figure 6-6). Since the larger left ventricle is oriented downward and to the left, in most normal patients the QRS axis points in that direction.

FIGURE 6–5

In the precordial leads, there is a tendency for the R wave to become more prominent as the tracing is viewed from V_1 through V_6.

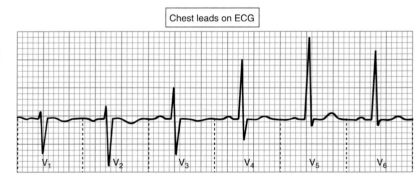

Chest leads on ECG

V_1 V_2 V_3 V_4 V_5 V_6

FIGURE 6–6

Cardiac vector (QRS axis).

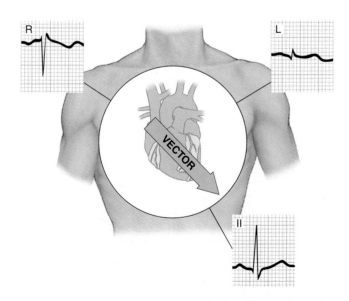

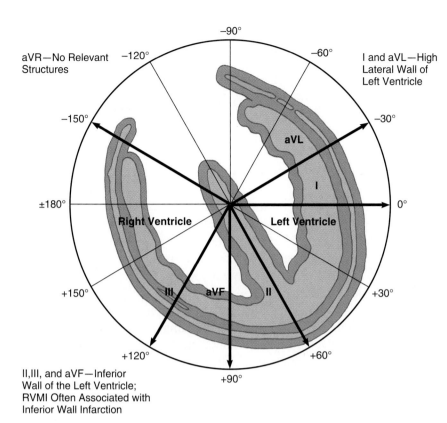

aVR—No Relevant Structures

I and aVL—High Lateral Wall of Left Ventricle

Right Ventricle

Left Ventricle

II,III, and aVF—Inferior Wall of the Left Ventricle; RVMI Often Associated with Inferior Wall Infarction

FIGURE 6–7
Detailed hexaxial reference system.
(Illustration courtesy of Ricaurte Solis, NREMT-P)

Picture the body as a 360 degree circle present along the frontal plane (Figure 6-7). If pointing due left on the patient is 0°, straight down is +90°, the right arm is at 180°, and the head is at −90°. The normal QRS axis is between 0° and +90°.

The easiest method of estimating the axis is by reviewing Lead I and aVF on the electrocardiogram (see below). Remember that a positive deflection of the electrocardiographic tracing indicates current flow in the direction of the lead. Therefore, a positive deflection of the QRS complex (large R wave) in both Lead I and aVF indicates that the major electrical depolarization is in the direction between 0° and +90°.

Axis	Lead 1	Lead aVF	Description
0° and +90°	+	+	normal axis
0° and −90°	+	−	left axis deviation
+90° and +180°	−	+	right axis deviation
−90° and −180°	−	−	extreme right axis deviation

If there is a positive deflection in Lead I (large R wave) and a large S wave in aVF, then the axis lies between 0° and −90°. This is called *left axis deviation*. A large S wave in Lead I and a large R wave in aVF indicates that the cardiac axis falls between +90° and +180°, and the patient has a *right axis deviation*. A patient with a calculated axis of between −90° and −180° (large S waves in both Lead I and aVF) has an *extreme right axis deviation*.

Left axis deviation is produced by those conditions that result in an abnormal enlargement of the left side of the heart. Such conditions as ischemic heart disease, hypertension, and aortic valve disease can lead to left axis deviation.

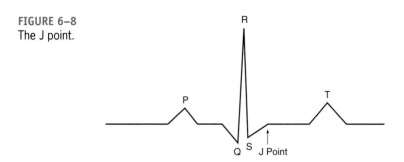

FIGURE 6–8
The J point.

Right axis deviation may occur in those conditions that strain the right side of the heart. Patients with COPD, pulmonary emboli, pulmonary hypertension, and cor pulmonale may have right axis deviation on their electrocardiogram. In addition, damage to the left ventricle from an acute myocardial infarction will cause the axis to shift toward the right, as there is a loss of forces from the left ventricle due to myocardial damage.

If the major positive deflection of the P wave is seen in the early V leads (V_1 and V_2), this suggests right atrial hypertrophy. This might occur in patients with tricuspid valve stenosis. If the major positive deflection is seen in the later V leads (V_5 and V_6), this suggests left atrial hypertrophy. In addition, you may see a large negative deflection in leads V_1 and V_2 with left atrial enlargement.

The ST Segment

Reviewing the ST segment and T wave is one of the most important aspects of interpreting the ECG in a patient with suspected cardiac disease. The ST segment begins at the J point and ends at the beginning of the T wave (Figure 6-8). The ST segment represents the initial phases of ventricular repolarization. Normally, the ST segment lies along the isoelectric line. In patients with cardiac disease, the ST segment may be either elevated or depressed. Other conditions, such as ventricular hypertrophy, conduction defects, drugs, hypothermia, pericarditis, and certain normal variants, may also alter the ST segment.

ISCHEMIA, INJURY, AND INFARCTION

Acute coronary syndromes occur when there is a difference between the oxygen requirements of the heart and the oxygen supplied to the heart by the coronary arteries. Findings can vary from transient symptoms, primarily angina (chest pain) caused by a temporary rise in the work of the heart, to permanent heart damage caused by a complete blockage of the blood supply to the heart from a thrombus (clot). The inciting event in all of these cases is most commonly atherosclerotic narrowing of the coronary arteries, which leads to a cascade of events that may ultimately cause complete obstruction of the blood supply to the heart. Early recognition of this process can minimize the damage to the heart muscle and lead to a better functional recovery.

Even in the setting of complete coronary occlusion, there are different areas of the heart that can be defined by their ultimate prognosis (Figure 6-9). While some areas are clearly permanently damaged by the lack of blood supply, other areas are potentially salvageable if there is prompt recognition and initiation of appropriate therapy.

Myocardial infarction produces a characteristic progression of changes in the ECG, particularly during the period of ventricular repolarization. As a result, initial

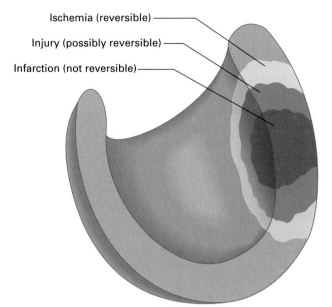

Ischemia (reversible)
Injury (possibly reversible)
Infarction (not reversible)

FIGURE 6–9
Sectors of myocardial damage resulting from coronary occlusion: ischemia, injury, and infarction (necrosis).

changes are found in the ST segment and T wave. Early recognition of these changes by emergency personnel can set in motion a series of steps designed to produce the best outcome of the patient suffering an acute myocardial infarction.

The earliest findings in patients with cardiac disease include *myocardial ischemia* in the area of involved blood supply (Figure 6-10). This is characterized by depression of the ST segment, T-wave inversion (opposite to the major direction of the QRS complex), and peaked T waves. ST-segment depression is considered significant when the ST segment (measured from the J point) is depressed at least 1 mm below the isoelectric line.

As the hypoxic insult progresses, evidence of *myocardial injury* is present (Figure 6-11). Myocardial injury is characterized by ST-segment elevation and T-wave inversion. Again, ST-segment elevation is considered significant when it is

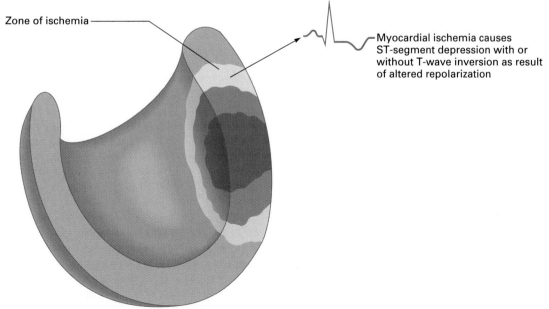

Zone of ischemia

Myocardial ischemia causes ST-segment depression with or without T-wave inversion as result of altered repolarization

FIGURE 6–10
ECG changes reflecting myocardial ischemia.

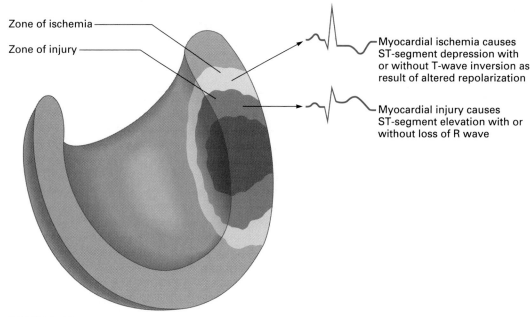

Zone of ischemia ——————————

Zone of injury ——————————

Myocardial ischemia causes
ST-segment depression with
or without T-wave inversion as
result of altered repolarization

Myocardial injury causes
ST-segment elevation with or
without loss of R wave

FIGURE 6–11
ECG changes reflecting myocardial injury.

greater than 1 mm above the isoelectric line. You should also note that when viewed in leads that are opposite in orientation to an ECG lead demonstrating ST elevation (for example, ST changes in aVR when there is ST elevation in Lead II), the ST segments may appear depressed. This is referred to as *reciprocal changes.*

Finally, as cellular death occurs following complete occlusion, ECG changes of *myocardial necrosis,* or tissue death, are seen (Figure 6-12). This is heralded by the presence of significant, or pathologic, Q waves. The Q waves are the first

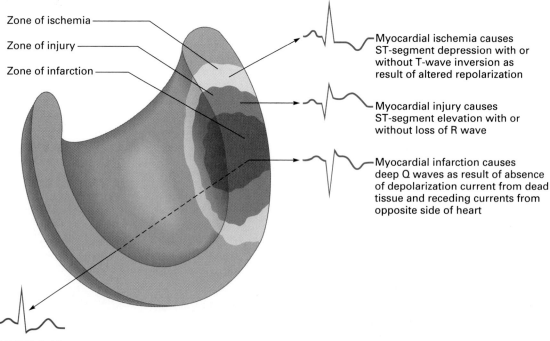

Zone of ischemia ——————————

Zone of injury ——————————

Zone of infarction ——————————

Myocardial ischemia causes
ST-segment depression with or
without T-wave inversion as
result of altered repolarization

Myocardial injury causes
ST-segment elevation with or
without loss of R wave

Myocardial infarction causes
deep Q waves as result of absence
of depolarization current from dead
tissue and receding currents from
opposite side of heart

FIGURE 6–12
ECG changes reflecting myocardial infarction (necrosis, or tissue death).

negative deflection of the QRS complex, signifying the initial unopposed depolarization away from the direction of the involved lead. A Q wave is defined as significant or pathologic if it is: (1) greater than 0.04 seconds (1 small box) and (2) more than 25 percent of the height of the R wave. Such pathologic changes in the Q wave result from the absence of a depolarization current from the necrotic tissue. These Q wave changes develop over the course of hours following an acute myocardial infarction and persist on subsequent electrocardiograms. As a result, it may be impossible to determine the age of myocardial necrosis based solely on the presence of significant Q waves unless there is some historical context for these findings.

You should also be aware that the classic ECG findings are consistent with those patients who experience a coronary artery occlusion that affects the entire wall of the heart. This is referred to as a *transmural MI* (*transmural* means "through the wall") since the damage occurs across all three layers of the heart: the epicardium, the myocardium, and the endocardium. These cases tend to develop the full progression of changes described above and are thus called "Q-wave MIs" or "transmural MIs."

Often the entire heart wall is not affected by an occlusion but only the most susceptible portions suffer damage. Since the endocardium has the highest oxygen demand, it is most likely to sustain injury. In these cases, the spectrum of ECG changes described above does not necessarily occur; such cases are called "non-Q wave MIs" or "subendocardial MIs." Patients with subendocardial MI tend to demonstrate ST depression rather than the classic ST elevation. In addition, these patients do not ultimately develop significant Q waves.

Findings in Inferior Wall MI

As we have stated at the beginning of this chapter, "Time is Muscle." Therefore, the emergency care provider must be efficient in obtaining a focused history that suggests an acute coronary syndrome but also be able to set in motion the series of steps that will lead to opening an occluded coronary artery in the shortest possible time. Perhaps the most important element of this process is the recognition of characteristic ECG findings of acute myocardial infarction. A familiarity with the coronary anatomy is essential and guides the clinician in understanding the two dominant patterns of acute myocardial infarction: *inferior myocardial infarction* and *anterior myocardial infarction.*

Remember that the right coronary artery (RCA) supplies the right ventricle, the posterior wall of the left ventricle, and the inferior wall of the left ventricle. The RCA also provides blood supply to portions of the conduction system including the SA node, AV node, and the His bundle.

The electrocardiogram simply represents the electrical activities of the cardiac cycle as viewed through several "cameras": the limb and precordial leads. Our basic understanding of the cardiogram reminds us that Lead II, Lead III, and Lead aVF view the inferior portions of the heart.

This tells us that if the patient has a history that is consistent with an acute coronary syndrome, we should also see evidence of ischemia, injury, or infarction in Leads II, III, or aVF (Figure 6-13). By convention, ST elevation is considered significant if it occurs in two or more of these leads and measures at least 1 mm in height. T-wave inversion may also be seen in conjunction with ST changes in the setting of an acute inferior myocardial infarction.

Also be aware of other ECG changes that may be found in association with an acute inferior MI. We have already noted the other areas supplied by the RCA.

FIGURE 6–13
Inferior myocardial
infarction with typical
ECG findings.

Inferior infarct

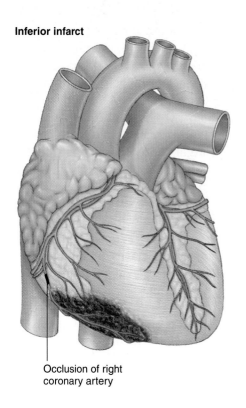

Occlusion of right
coronary artery

12-lead ECG consistent with acute inferior infarct

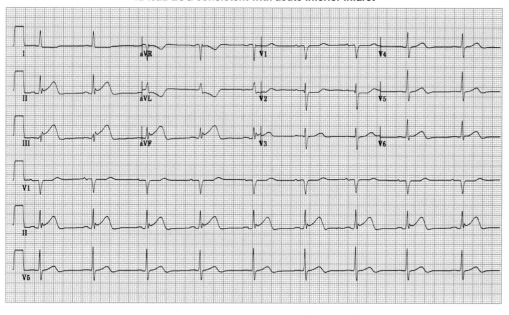

As stated earlier, right ventricular infarcts may be found in association with an acute inferior MI. These patients tend to present with hypotension that responds to fluid therapy, which increases right ventricular filling pressure. Preload-reducing agents such as morphine or nitrates can produce disastrous results when given to a patient with a right ventricular infarct. The classic ECG findings of RV infarct may be difficult to demonstrate. You must use special ECG leads placed on the right side of the heart in a position analogous to V_4 and V_5 (Figure 6-14).

Remember that the right coronary artery also supplies the posterior wall of the left ventricle. The difficulty in recognizing posterior MIs is that none of the

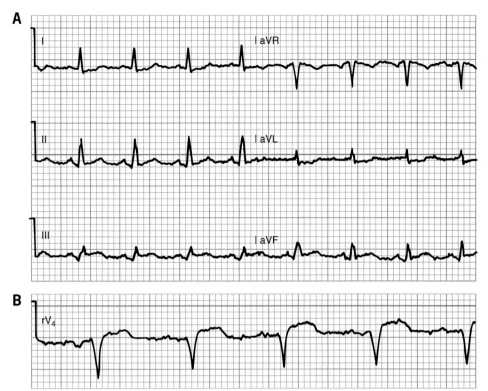

FIGURE 6–14
(A) ST elevation in Leads II, III, and aVF characteristic of an acute inferior myocardial infarction. (B) The rV_4 recording of the same patient showing the right-sided infarction.

ECG leads is directed posteriorly; therefore, none of our "cameras" will demonstrate the classic ECG findings of an acute posterior myocardial infarction. This leaves us with evaluating the leads that face in the *exact opposite* direction of the posterior wall: V_1 through V_4. Since these leads face in the opposite direction, then the findings of a true posterior MI would be "reciprocal" to the classic anterior MI pattern (Figure 6-15). As such, we will see ST depression in the involved leads. In the later stages, large R waves (the equivalent of deep Q waves) develop in the early precordial leads.

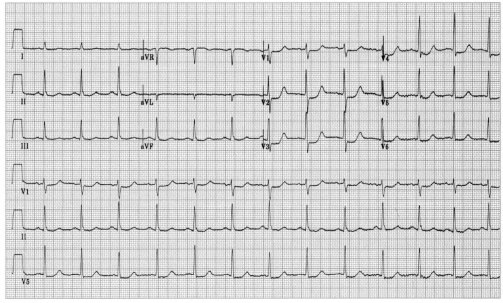

FIGURE 6–15
ECG findings consistent with posterior myocardial infarction.

FIGURE 6–16
Posterior V lead placement.
(Illustration courtesy of Ricaurte Solis, NREMT-P)

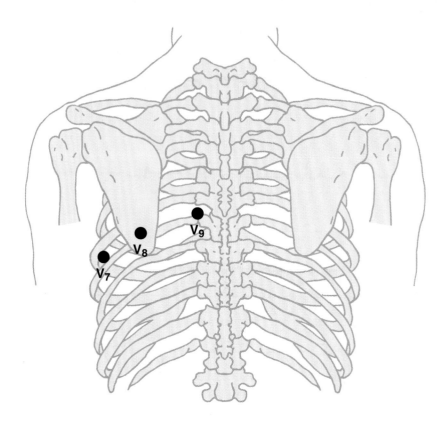

It has been suggested that a mirror can be utilized to determine posterior ST elevation by viewing the tracing with the ECG inverted. Alternatively, one could hold the ECG upside down and backwards toward bright light to visualize the classic ST pattern of acute MI.

Posterior V leads (also labeled V_7 through V_9) obtained with the patient in the right lateral decubitus position (right side down) have been suggested (Figure 6-16). Patients with a posterior MI in conjunction with an inferior MI tend to have more significant ventricular dysrhythmias in association with their disease.

In some patients with "right dominant" cardiac circulation, the right coronary artery also supplies the lateral wall of the left ventricle. In such cases, ST elevation may be seen in leads V_5 and V_6 in conjunction with an acute inferior MI.

Because the RCA provides blood supply to some portions of the conduction system, there are dysrhythmias that are seen in patients with acute inferior MI. Classically, first-degree AV block and second-degree Wenckebach (Mobitz I) AV blocks are seen. These are felt to be relatively benign dysrhythmias.

Findings in Anterior Wall MI

The left coronary artery (LCA) divides into the descending branch, which supplies the anterior wall of the left ventricle, and the circumflex branch, which supplies the lateral wall of the left ventricle (except in right-dominant circulation, as noted), portions of the posterior wall of the left ventricle, and the interventricular septum.

Occlusions of the left coronary artery can affect the septal (V_1 and V_2), anterior (V_3 and V_4), and lateral (V_5 and V_6) precordial leads. By convention, ST elevation of 2 mm or more in three contiguous precordial leads is diagnostic of an acute anterior MI (Figure 6-17). If the elevation is found in V_1 through V_4, the term *anteroseptal MI* is used. For leads V_3 through V_6, the term *anterolateral MI* is

Anterior infarct

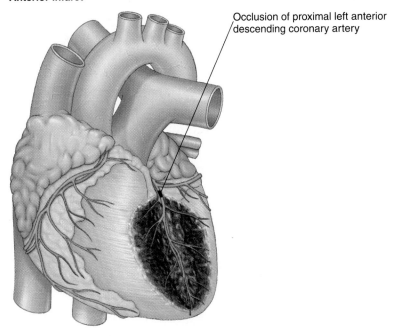

Occlusion of proximal left anterior
descending coronary artery

12-lead ECG consistent with anterior infarct

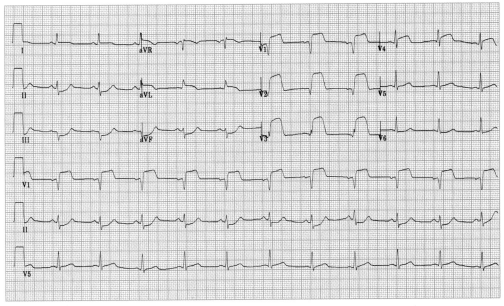

FIGURE 6–17
Anterior myocardial infarction with typical ECG findings.

applied (Figure 6-18). Here again, T-wave inversion may be associated with ST changes in the presence of an acute myocardial infarction.

Acute anterior MIs tend to involve a significant amount of cardiac damage. As a result, significant ventricular rhythm disturbances (ventricular tachycardia and ventricular fibrillation), cardiogenic shock, and severe conduction system blocks are associated with anterior MIs. In particular, second-degree Mobitz II AV block and complete heart block may be seen.

FIGURE 6–18
Anterolateral
myocardial
infarction.

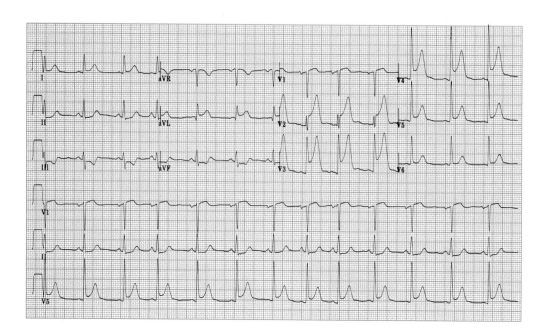

ECG FINDINGS IN OTHER MEDICAL CONDITIONS

There are characteristic patterns on the ECG that can suggest other significant diagnoses. However, these ECG patterns must be considered in the context of the patient's history and physical examination.

Bundle Branch Blocks

When the QRS complex is greater than 0.12 seconds, the conduction system may not be functioning appropriately. A condition known as a bundle branch block may have occurred. Under these circumstances, the electrical impulse is carried down the AV node through the bundle of His. From this point, there may be a blockage either in the left bundle branch or in the right bundle branch.

A right bundle branch block (Figure 6-19) is a fairly common finding on an ECG. It is often seen in patients who have suffered a myocardial infarction involving the anterolateral portion of the left ventricle. It is recognized by a widened QRS complex and a second positive deflection in the QRS complex (called an RSR′ [RSR prime] pattern) in the early precordial leads (V_1 and V_2).

In the case of a left bundle branch block (Figure 6-20), conduction proceeds into the right bundle and the right ventricle contracts. Conduction then proceeds through the cardiac muscle more slowly to the left ventricle which then contracts. Thus, the QRS complex is widened and reflects the non-simultaneous contraction of each ventricle.

A left bundle branch block is a more concerning problem than a right bundle branch block, since it is usually associated with significant cardiac damage. This pattern is recognized by a QRS duration of greater than 0.12 seconds and a broad, sometimes notched R wave in the lateral precordial leads. In addition to suggesting significant underlying cardiac disease, the presence of a left bundle branch pattern can make interpretation of the ECG difficult, especially in the setting of an acute

Right Bundle Branch Block

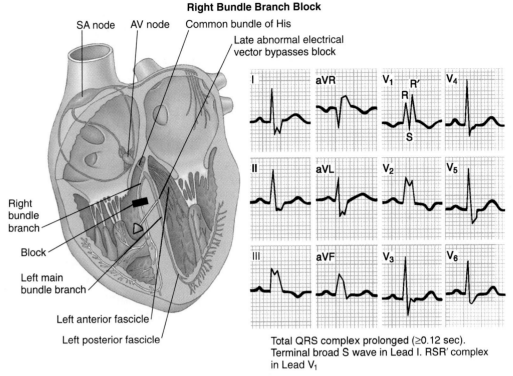

Total QRS complex prolonged (≥0.12 sec).
Terminal broad S wave in Lead I. RSR′ complex
in Lead V₁

FIGURE 6–19
Right bundle branch block.

Left Bundle Branch Block

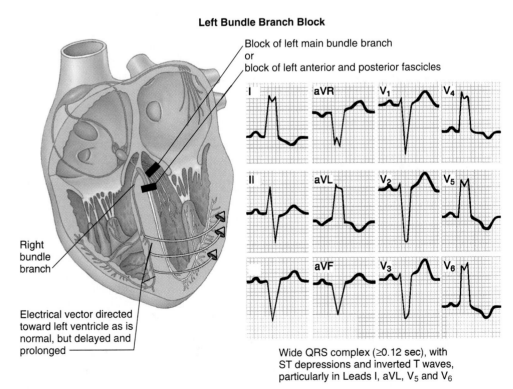

Wide QRS complex (≥0.12 sec), with
ST depressions and inverted T waves,
particularly in Leads I, aVL, V₅ and V₆

FIGURE 6–20
Left bundle branch block.

myocardial infarction. In fact, the presence of a new left bundle branch block in a patient with signs and symptoms consistent with cardiac chest pain is an indication to consider fibrinolytic therapy or immediate angioplasty. These patients are also at high risk of developing complete heart block and cardiogenic shock.

You should also be aware that the main two branches of the left bundle branch, the left anterior fascicle and left posterior fascicle, can become disrupted as well. A discussion of the ECG findings associated with these lesions is beyond the intent of this chapter.

Pericarditis

Pericarditis is an inflammatory condition involving the fluid surrounding the heart. This condition may be caused by a variety of bacterial or viral pathogens as well as other inflammatory mediators. Patients with acute pericarditis may present with diffuse ST elevation in most of the cardiac leads except aVR and V_1. The T waves are generally upright. ST-segment elevation is not limited to the a few isolated leads as with acute inferior or anterior myocardial injury. Also, the ST segments are classically described as having an initial flattened or concave appearance (Figure 6-21). The T wave may also appear to be elevated off of the isoelectric line. As the disease process continues, the ST segments return to baseline with the

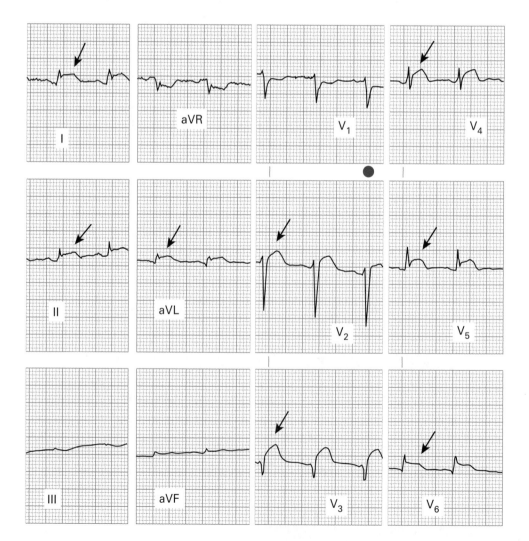

FIGURE 6-21
ECG of patient with acute pericarditis. Note the diffuse ST elevation in most of the cardiac leads except aVR and V_1.

T waves becoming flattened or even inverted. In the final stages, the ECG demonstrates a pattern of diffuse ST depression. With resolution of the disease, the ECG returns to normal.

Pulmonary Embolism

The most consistent finding in patients with a pulmonary embolism is an ECG demonstrating sinus tachycardia. However, there is a classic ECG pattern in patients with pulmonary embolism referred to as the "S1Q3T3" pattern (Figure 6-22). These patients will have a large S wave in Lead I, a Q wave in Lead III, and an inverted T

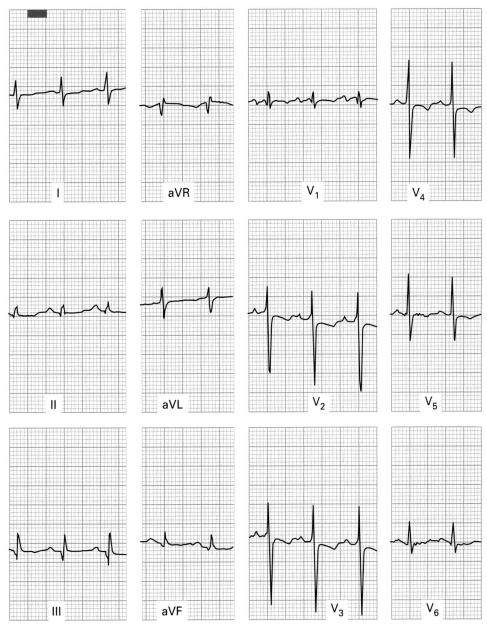

FIGURE 6–22
ECG of patient with pulmonary embolism. Note the characteristic S1Q3T3 pattern (large S wave in Lead I, Q wave in Lead III, and inverted T wave in Lead III).

wave in Lead III. Patients with pulmonary embolism may also demonstrate ST depression in Lead II. Finally, patients with this condition may also demonstrate T-wave inversion in leads V_1 through V_4 with a right bundle branch pattern.

Hyperkalemia

Potassium is one of the most important ions in regulating the electrical activity of the heart. As such, changes in potassium ion concentration will produce significant ECG findings. The most striking feature in patients with hyperkalemia (elevated serum potassium) is the appearance of tall peaked T waves (Figure 6-23). As the

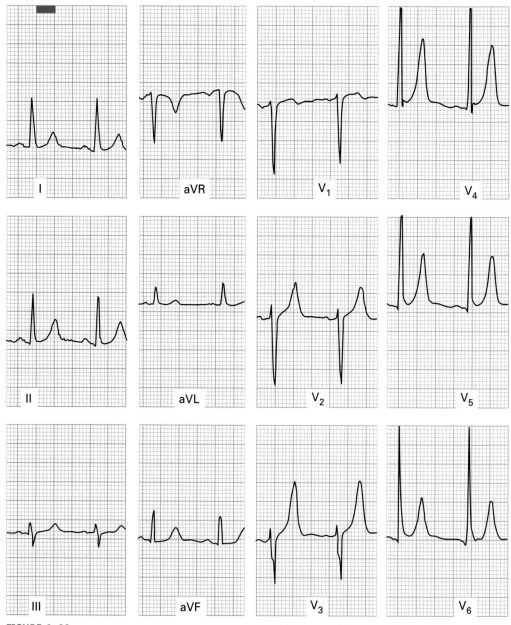

FIGURE 6–23
ECG of patient with hyperkalemia, showing characteristic tall peaked T waves.

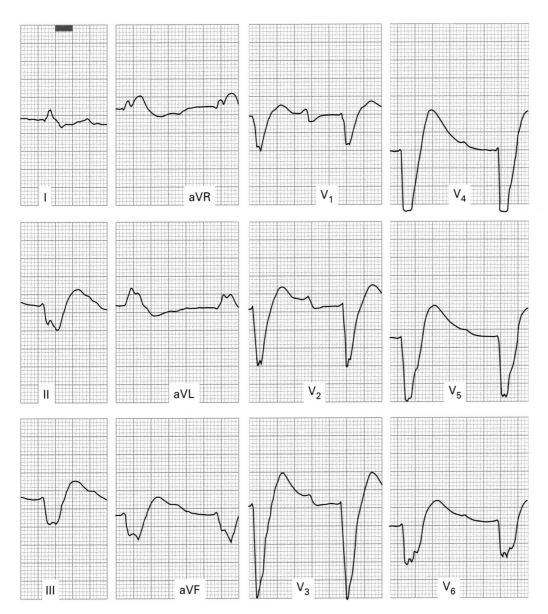

FIGURE 6–24
ECG of patient with hyperkalemia that has progressed to show widened QRS complexes blending into inverted T waves in a sine-shaped configuration.

level of potassium increases, the P waves begin to disappear and ventricular conduction slows. This results in a widening of the QRS complex into what are called "sine waves" (Figure 6-24). Eventually, with increasing serum potassium levels, marked bradycardia and cardiac arrest ensue.

Hypokalemia

Patients with low serum potassium demonstrate the opposite findings as those described for hyperkalemic patients. These patients will develop flattening of the

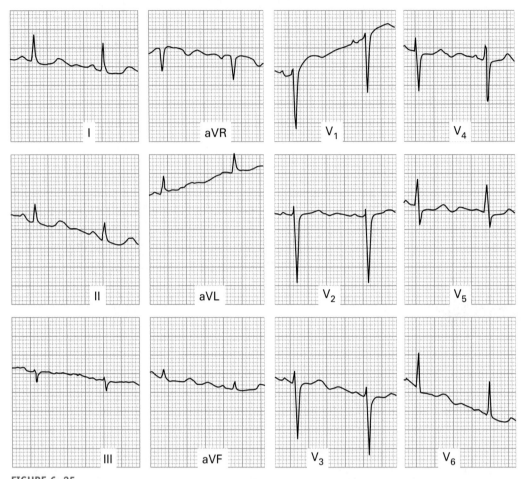

FIGURE 6–25
ECG of patient with hypokalemia with opposite findings as those for a hyperkalemic patient. Note the fattening of T waves and appearance of U waves.

T wave and may also develop prominence of the U wave (Figure 6-25). Finally, because hypokalemia increases ventricular irritability, ventricular dysrhythmias such as PVCs, ventricular tachycardia, ventricular fibrillation, and torsades de pointes can develop.

Hypocalcemia

Calcium is the major ion that contributes to cardiac repolarization. This is primarily reflected in the length of the QT interval, measured from the beginning of the QRS complex to the beginning of the T wave. Patients with hypocalcemia will demonstrate a prolonged QT interval, primarily due to a long ST segment (Figure 6-26). By definition, the QT interval is greater than 50 percent of the entire cardiac cycle. Conversely, patients with hypercalcemia will demonstrate a shortened QT interval.

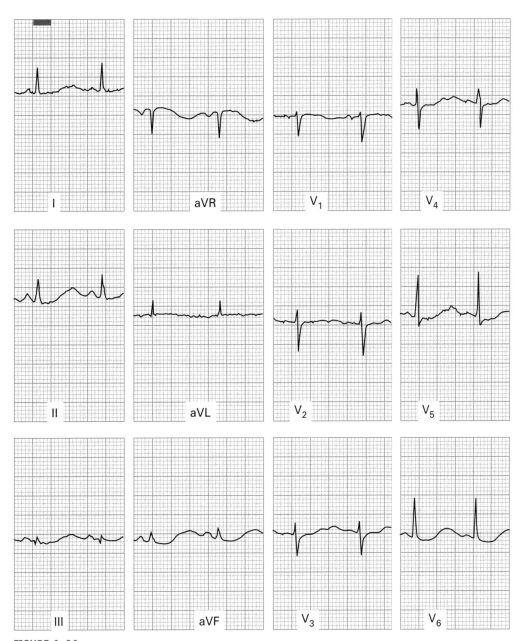

FIGURE 6–26
ECG of a patient with hypocalcemia showing a typical prolonged QT interval, primarily due to a long ST segment.

Hypothermia

Patients with hypothermia will demonstrate several different ECG findings, which often depend on the severity of the exposure. Initially, patients develop sinus tachycardia, which can progress to a profound bradycardia as the patient's core temperature drops. All types of atrial or ventricular dysrhythmias may be seen. The ECG pattern in hypothermia may be characterized by elevation of the J point, called a J wave or an Osborn wave (Figure 6-27). The J wave appears as a hump

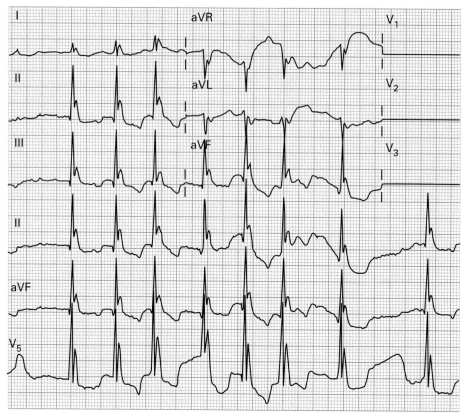

FIGURE 6–27
ECG of patient with hypothermia. Note the appearance of J waves just after the QRS complexes.

that occurs just after the QRS complex. It is most characteristically seen in Lead II or V_6 but can be seen in virtually all leads. The J wave may be confused with ST changes in acute myocardial infarction.

SUMMARY

For many patients, the 12-lead ECG is a valuable adjunct to your physical examination and history taking skills. It can provide important information about the possibility of an acute coronary event which may require rapid reperfusion. Being able to identify these patients and initiating the complex series of events that will lead to fibrinolysis or angioplasty is the hallmark of a well-coordinated and excellent EMS system.

CASE STUDY FOLLOW-UP

Mrs. Springer was given a second chance and heeded the advice of her cardiologist. She modified her diet, began an exercise program, and started to take statin medications to control her hypercholesterolemia. Over the next year she lost 38 pounds. Not only did she significantly reduce her risk of a myocardial event; she feels better, can do more, and has considerably improved her life.

REVIEW QUESTIONS

1. In the prehospital setting, the 12-lead ECG is most commonly used
   a. for basic cardiac rhythm recognition.
   b. to definitively diagnose a myocardial infarction.
   c. to identify patients who are likely candidates for rapid reperfusion.
   d. to distinguish between patients with angina from those experiencing an MI.

2. Which coronary artery perfuses the anterior wall?
   a. LAD
   b. Circumflex
   c. RCA
   d. RAD

3. Occlusion of the RCA is most likely to cause a(n) _____ MI.
   a. inferior wall
   b. intraventricular
   c. lateral wall
   d. anterior wall

4. Which of the following are referred to as the precordial leads?
   a. I, II, III
   b. aVR, aVL, and aVF
   c. $V_1 - V_6$
   d. II, III, and aVF

5. Which of the following represents right axis deviation?
   a. Lead I = large R wave; aVF = large S wave
   b. Lead I = large S wave; aVF = large R wave
   c. Lead I = large S wave; aVF = large S wave
   d. Lead I = large R wave; aVF = large R wave

6. Which of the following is a cause of left axis deviation?
   a. left ventricular hypertrophy
   b. right ventricular hypertrophy
   c. pulmonary hypertension
   d. pulmonary embolism

7. Which ST-segment change is most suggestive of myocardial ischemia?
   a. ST-segment depression in the corresponding leads
   b. ST-segment elevation in the corresponding leads
   c. peaked T waves
   d. Q waves

8. Q waves suggest
   a. old injury.
   b. myocardial ischemia.
   c. hypothermia.
   d. transmural MI.

9. ST elevation in which of the following leads would suggest an anterior wall MI?
   a. V_1, V_2
   b. V_3, V_4, V_5
   c. II, III, and aVF
   d. aVR, aVL, and aVF

10. Right bundle branch blocks most commonly manifest as widened and notched QRS complexes in
    a. V_1, V_2.
    b. V_3, V_4, V_5.
    c. II, III, and aVF.
    d. aVR, aVL, and aVF.

11. Which condition is associated with tall peaked T waves?
    a. hyperkalemia
    b. hypokalemia
    c. hypercalcemia
    d. hypermagnesemia

12. What is the unique ECG finding in hypothermia?
    a. Q wave
    b. Osborn wave
    c. peaked T waves
    d. flattened QRS complex

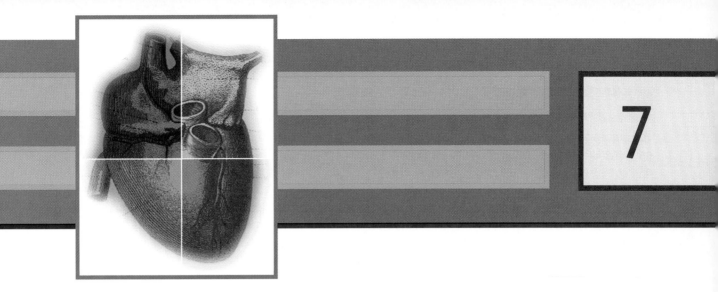

Electrical Therapy: Defibrillation, Cardioversion, and Cardiac Pacing

O ccasionally you will encounter a patient whose cardiac problem is likely to deteriorate before drug treatment would have time to be effective. In other cases, the patient may be suffering from a dysrhythmia that is unresponsive to any currently known drug therapy. In these situations, a form of emergency electrical therapy may be the most appropriate intervention.

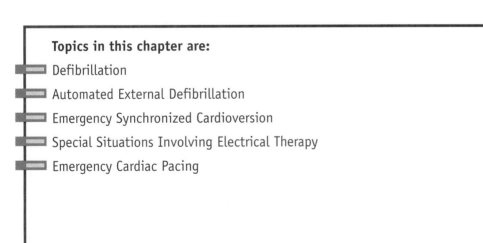

Topics in this chapter are:

- Defibrillation
- Automated External Defibrillation
- Emergency Synchronized Cardioversion
- Special Situations Involving Electrical Therapy
- Emergency Cardiac Pacing

CASE STUDY

You are working a night shift for a rural EMS system. The night has been quiet, and you have been catching up on some light reading between the sparse calls. As you near the end of your shift, dispatch tones you out for a patient experiencing chest pain. When you arrive on scene 7 minutes later, you find an anxious middle-aged man sitting on his couch, his left hand clenched over his sternum.

Upon questioning, the patient—Mr. Griffiths—tells you that the chest pain started about 4 hours ago when it woke him from his sleep. He adds that, shortly thereafter, he started having trouble breathing and became "sweaty." As you initiate oxygen therapy, your partner obtains a set of vitals that reveal a blood pressure of 102/62 mmHg, a heart rate of 220 per minute and regular, and a respiratory rate of 36 per minute with slight retractions. With an anxious look and a scared voice, Mr. Griffiths asks you, "Am . . . I . . . going to be O.K.?"

How would you proceed to assess and care for this patient? This chapter will describe the assessment and necessary treatment of a patient with a cardiac emergency that requires the use of electrical therapy. Later, we will return to the case and apply the procedures learned.

INTRODUCTION

During the course of emergency cardiac care, the prehospital advanced life support provider may encounter a patient for whom traditional treatment with pharmacology may be ineffective or require more time to exert the desired physiologic action than is available. As well, there are certain cardiac dysrhythmias that are generally unresponsive to any type of drug therapy. It is in these specific instances that the most appropriate choice of therapeutic intervention may well be electrical therapy.

Electrical therapy can be used to terminate specific cardiac dysrhythmias. Depending on the type of dysrhythmia, you may need to apply defibrillation, synchronized cardioversion, or transcutaneous pacing. While all of these interventions require the administration of electricity to the patient's body, their delivery methods and indications differ significantly.

In this chapter, each method of administering electrical therapy will be discussed with its rationale, indications, and procedures. We will also discuss the current role of the automated external defibrillator, a device designed to reduce the incidence of out-of-hospital deaths from sudden cardiac arrest, and the expanding role biphasic defibrillators are occupying in emergency cardiac care.

DEFIBRILLATION

The therapeutic benefit of electrical defibrillation (also known as asynchronous cardioversion) is its ability to terminate a fibrillating heart by passing a current of electricity through it.

As a reminder, ventricular fibrillation is a life-threatening dysrhythmia in which a grave disruption in the normal conduction system has occurred. Multiple cells within the heart are discharging and repolarizing independently of other cardiac cells. Since there is no organized depolarization wave spreading through the myocardium to cause muscle contraction, there can be no cardiac output. Ventricular fibrillation is a self-propagating and self-defeating dysrhythmia, as the varying degrees of depolarization prohibit organized repolarization. Thus, ventricular fibrillation will eventually degrade into asystole as the heart becomes damaged from ensuing acidosis and hypoxia. Without correction, the heart's ability to propagate any impulse will eventually cease.

There are two theories about how electrical defibrillation works. By passing a large amount of electrical current through the heart over a brief period of time, the first theory maintains, a "critical mass" of ventricular cells are depolarized as a unit, thereby allowing repolarization to occur more uniformly—after which, it is hoped, when a normal pacemaker in the heart provides its electrical impulse, the impulse can now travel down a repolarized (and ready) conduction system.

The second theory views the multiple depolarizations of ventricular fibrillation as mini "wave fronts" passing through the heart in search of repolarized tissue. In this second theory, the act of passing a large current of energy through the heart will depolarize all primed (repolarized) muscle tissue, subsequently leaving nowhere for the "wave front" to spread next, eliminating the fibrillatory impulses.

Regardless of the exact mechanism of defibrillation, however, the fact remains that if ventricular fibrillation is left untreated, the patient will die. It is important to understand that electrical defibrillation is currently the most effective method of terminating ventricular fibrillation. CPR does not terminate fibrillation, nor do intravenous drugs, intubation, or IV fluids. While these may make a more favorable environment in which to achieve successful defibrillation, a fibrillating heart must receive early electrical therapy. Pulseless ventricular tachycardia (VT, or V-tach) will rapidly degrade into ventricular fibrillation (VF, or V-fib), so either of these rhythms should receive immediate defibrillation.

Currently, there are two methods by which the defibrillatory energy (or current) can be administered to the patient. These are referred to as "waveforms" and their importance is worth mentioning. The traditional waveform, used for defibrillators for decades, is termed "monophasic." This means that the energy is delivered to the heart via the current traveling in one direction from one paddle to another in one phase, with the hopes that when it passes through the heart positioned between them, the ventricular fibrillation or ventricular tachycardia is terminated.

A newer method, although not as thoroughly researched, delivers the energy via a "biphasic" waveform. With this configuration, during the period when the energy is leaving the electrode paddle, the current initially flows in one direction during the first phase of the shock and then reverses for the second phase (Figure 7-1).

This biphasic waveform for energy delivery has been shown to be more successful in terminating ventricular fibrillation than the traditional monophasic waveform. There are, however, many unknowns about this new technology. For

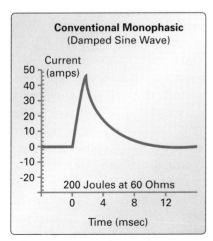

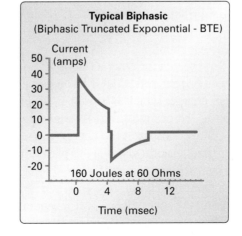

FIGURE 7-1
Defibrillation waveforms.

example, several studies have cited how lower energy levels using a biphasic waveform are more apt to terminate fibrillation than the traditional monophasic defibrillation at 200 joules. But the exact energy level *most* appropriate is not yet known, nor for that matter are what biphasic energy levels would be too high and potentially harmful. Additionally, the studies using biphasic technology did not use an escalating energy level for termination of fibrillation (as is the current practice with monophasic waveform defibrillation). But one important clinical fact is known—biphasic waveform *is* more effective in terminating fibrillation at lower levels; it also allows for more uniform delivery of energy to patients that have various amounts of resistance to electrical flow due to the composition of the thorax. Other theoretical advantages include less damage to the myocardium from lower energy levels and potentially longer battery life.

Based on these studies, and others that are ongoing, the FDA has approved the marketing and use on patients of biphasic defibrillators. You will want to keep attuned to future changes in this technology and procedure. At this time, the only recommendation made is that when delivering a defibrillatory charge to a patient, the provider should use the recommended monophasic energy level or its equivalent biphasic energy dose.

Importance of Defibrillation

A significant portion of all heart-related deaths can be classified as *sudden cardiac death,* which is defined as cardiac arrest occurring within hours of the onset of cardiac signs and symptoms. The most frequent rhythm underlying sudden cardiac death is ventricular fibrillation. Prehospital providers, then, can make a significant impact in reducing the number of sudden cardiac deaths by providing rapid defibrillation.

Defibrillation is inextricably time dependent. For example, the likelihood of successfully resuscitating a person in ventricular fibrillation is highest (greater than 90%) if defibrillation is delivered within the first minute of cardiac arrest. However, after only 9 minutes of cardiac arrest, a successful resuscitation occurs in less than 1 out of every 10 attempts. While CPR is effective and necessary in a cardiac arrest situation, studies indicate that the main benefit of CPR is not in converting ventricular fibrillation but rather in maintaining coronary and cerebral blood flow until a defibrillator is available.

Components of a Defibrillator

The defibrillation unit may be a stationary device requiring an external power source, a portable device that can be carried to the patient's side, or an integral part of a cardiac monitor.

Irrespective of type, all defibrillation machines share common components. A direct-current defibrillator has a variable transformer that will generate a high-voltage charge, which is stored in an electrical capacitor to be delivered to the patient at the desired time. To complete the circuit, the defibrillator is equipped with connections from the energy capacitor to the patient via defibrillation electrodes (paddles or pads) that are placed in contact with the patient's thorax.

Defibrillators manufactured today have numerous energy-level settings which the prehospital care provider selects before charging the capacitor and delivering the energy. The specific amount of energy is selected based upon patient needs and is measured in *joules,* or watt-seconds.

What is a watt-second? How much energy is that? Try to picture the following analogy between a defibrillator and a light bulb. A common energy level used in monophasic defibrillation is 360 watt-seconds. Now picture putting four fingers into four empty light sockets specifically designed only for 90-watt light bulbs. Now, if someone turns on the light switch to these sockets for one full second and then shuts it back off, the amount of energy you just received (i.e., were shocked by) totals 360 watt-seconds (four 90-watt light sockets turned on for one second equals 360 watt-seconds). This is certainly not an experiment the authors recommend that you try at home! It is intended solely to help illustrate the amount of energy you are delivering when you defibrillate your patient.

Transthoracic Resistance to Energy Flow

Electricity, as is well known, will travel along the pathway of least resistance. This is why electrical cables and high tension wires are constructed of the materials they are—because these materials conduct electricity well. However, the materials that conduct electricity best are not found within the human body. In fact, the chest can offer a high resistance to electrical flow (termed *transthoracic resistance*) during defibrillation attempts.

Because it is typically not possible to defibrillate the heart directly during emergency cardiac care in the prehospital setting, the energy must pass through the chest wall and associated structures before it reaches the heart. Since a portion of the energy delivered is used up in overcoming the high transthoracic resistance of the chest, the amount of current available for defibrillation, once the current reaches the heart, is less than that initially delivered through the paddles. The concern is that, if transthoracic resistance (the resistance to current flow) is not lowered during the defibrillation process, a subtherapeutic amount of energy may reach the heart and be unable to defibrillate a "critical mass" of the myocardium.

Many factors determine the amount of transthoracic resistance to current flow. These include electrode size, electrode position, electrode-skin interface material, phase of ventilation, electrode contact pressure, time interval of previous countershocks, and selected energy level (Table 7-1).

TABLE 7–1	Methods of Reducing Transthoracic Resistance During Defibrillation
Electrode Size	8.0–12 cm adult 8 cm child 4.5 cm infant
Electrode Position	anterior-apex placement anterior-posterior placement
Electrode-Skin Interface Material	electrode gel pads electrode paste
Phase of Ventilation	end expiration
Electrode Contact Pressure	25 pounds (11 kg) of muscular pressure on paddles
Time Interval of Previous Countershocks	deliver shocks in rapid succession
Selected Energy Level	For monophasic waveform defibrillator, start 200 J, then 200–300 J, 360 J from then on For biphasic waveform, defibrillator equivalent biphasic (non-escalating) energy level

The following sections outline these factors and describe methods to decrease the resistance to current flow.

Electrode Size

The size of the electrode applied to the patient's chest can decrease resistance if the proper size is used. For an adult, the defibrillation electrode should be 8 to 12 cm in diameter. Infant paddles, when needed, typically clip onto the adult paddle and have a smaller surface area that a child under 1 year of age can accommodate. Infant defibrillation paddles are typically 4.5 cm, and a child's size would be about 8 cm. The most important aspect to choosing electrode size is to use the size that can comfortably and appropriately fit on the patient's chest and that does not allow for large gaps under the paddle.

Electrode Position

Placement of the defibrillation electrodes in one of two recommended positions will assure that the maximum amount of electricity will flow through the myocardium. The anterior-apex placement will put the negative electrode to the right of the sternum, just beneath the clavicle. The positive electrode will then be placed to the left of the nipple of the left thorax, positioned midaxillary (left apex). The anterior-posterior placement will find the anterior (negative) electrode over the left precordium, with the posterior (positive) electrode in the infrascapular space of the left scapula, on the midscapular line. Either method is equally effective in enhancing the amount of energy reaching the heart. The anterior-apex placement is more commonly used because it is the easier of the two to use during a cardiac arrest (Figure 7-2).

The prehospital care provider may also encounter situations where the patient has had a permanent pacemaker or defibrillator surgically implanted in the thorax. The presence of such a device does not, however, preclude defibrillation when necessary. In these and other situations where other medical devices are in close proximity to your defibrillation landmarks, common sense dictates repositioning your electrodes slightly to avoid defibrillating directly over the top of one of these devices. Defibrillations over the implanted device may contribute to an ineffective flow of energy to the myocardium. If necessary, change the position of the monitor electrodes to gain additional space.

FIGURE 7–2
The anterior-apex position for placement of defibrillation electrodes.

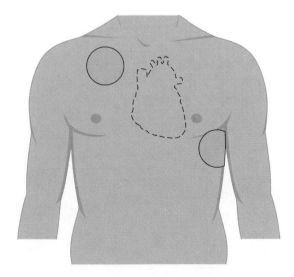

Electrode-Skin Interface Material

Some type of commercially available gel pad or electrode gel is necessary to eliminate the resistance between the bare chest and the dry metal electrode. You must ensure that there are adequate amounts of conductive medium after repeated defibrillations. It is also important to ensure that there is no contact between the mediums of each paddle, which would make the electricity flow across the chest rather than through it. Arcing between paddles is also a potentially dangerous complication of improperly performed defibrillations and may occur when the paddles are inappropriately placed too close together, when there is a gap between the electrode and skin, or when the conductive mediums used for each paddle are allowed to come into contact with each other.

Phase of Ventilation

The phases of ventilation will change the distance between the electrodes and the heart as the size of the thorax increases and decreases with inspiration and expiration. Delivering the defibrillation during the end-expiratory phase will eliminate resistance caused by an expanded thorax. This will not be a factor in the cardiac arrest patient, who has no spontaneous respiration.

Electrode Contact Pressure

Contact pressure is also an important aspect to successfully defibrillating a patient. By applying about 25 pounds of muscular pressure, you will ensure good contact of the paddle to the conductive medium against the chest. This will also help eliminate the chance for arcing of the electricity.

How much is 25 pounds of muscular pressure? Try placing a standard bathroom scale on the floor and applying pressure to it until you achieve 25 pounds on the display. Practice exerting *only* the muscular strength of your arms and *not* using the weight of your body. If you rely on your body weight to apply the pressure and wind up slipping while leaning over a patient, you run the risk of shocking yourself, a bystander, or another care provider near the patient.

Time Interval of Previous Countershocks

Transiently, the degree of transthoracic resistance will decrease with successive countershocks as long as they are administered rapidly. (The terms *countershock* and *shock* are used interchangeably.) After the first defibrillation, the body becomes "polarized," and subsequent discharges flow against reduced resistance. This allows more electricity to be delivered to the heart.

Selected Energy Level

Naturally, the higher the amount of energy selected, the more energy that will be delivered to the heart. However, anytime you defibrillate someone you run the risk of causing myocardial damage. Therefore, you start with an energy level that is likely to convert the rhythm from fibrillation but is not so high that it will cause unnecessary damage. A setting of 200 joules with a monophasic defibrillator is appropriate for the initial defibrillation attempt in a patient with pulseless VF or VT. The second countershock can be 200–300 joules (remember that the chest resistance drops with the first shock); the third and highest energy level is 360 joules. Successive defibrillations for persistent VF or pulseless VT are delivered at 360 joules. And if the VF/VT recurs after previously being successfully converted, select the energy level that was previously successful.

STEPS OF DEFIBRILLATION

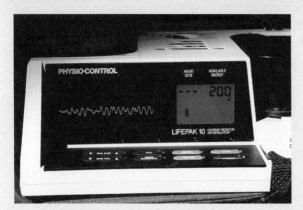

FIGURE 7–3A
Identify ventricular fibrillation on the cardiac monitor.

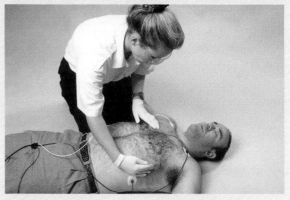

FIGURE 7–3B
Apply electrode gel to the paddles or place commercial defibrillation pads on the patient's exposed thorax.

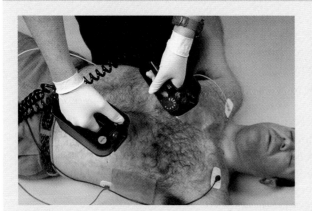

FIGURE 7–3C
Charge the defibrillation paddles.

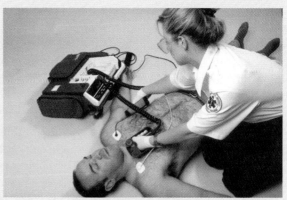

FIGURE 7–3D
Reconfirm the rhythm on the cardiac monitor.

Procedure for Defibrillation

Once the decision for defibrillating the patient is made, follow these steps to perform defibrillation (Figures 7-3A to 7-3G).

1. Confirm ventricular fibrillation or pulseless ventricular tachycardia on the cardiac monitor.
2. Place the patient in a safe environment if initially in contact with some electrically conductive material (e.g., metal, water).
3. Apply electrode gel to the paddles, or place commercial defibrillation pads on the patient's exposed thorax.
4. Turn on and charge the defibrillator to 200 J for the first shock (or the clinically equivalent biphasic energy dose).
5. Ensure that the electrodes are appropriately placed on the patient's thorax with proper pressure.

STEPS OF DEFIBRILLATION *(continued)*

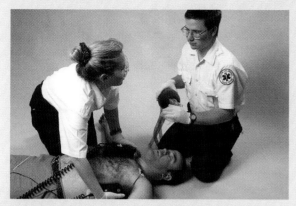

FIGURE 7–3E
Verbally and visually clear everybody from the patient (including yourself).

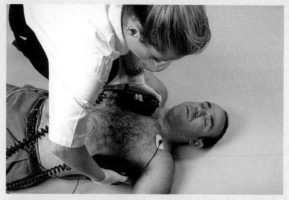

FIGURE 7–3F
Deliver a defibrillatory shock by depressing both buttons on the defibrillator paddles simultaneously.

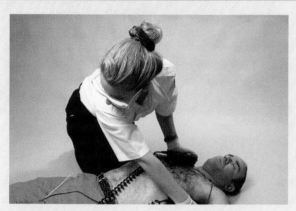

FIGURE 7–3G
Reconfirm the rhythm on the cardiac monitor.

6. ENSURE THAT NO ONE ELSE IS IN CONTACT WITH THE PATIENT. Verbally and visually clear everybody prior to any defibrillation attempt (including yourself).

7. Deliver a defibrillatory shock by depressing both buttons on the defibrillator paddles simultaneously (depressing only one button will not result in the shock being delivered).

8. Reconfirm the rhythm on the monitor screen; if still VF/VT, recharge and repeat steps 5–7, using higher energy levels (when using monophasic defibrillators).

See Figure 10-2 in Chapter 10, the ventricular fibrillation/pulseless ventricular tachycardia (VF/VT) algorithm.

Newer style monitors allow the prehospital provider to defibrillate the patient without having to physically hold the defibrillation paddles. This adds a degree of safety in that there is a lower risk for accidental shocks to the provider. The only difference between defibrillating a patient manually or with "hands-free" or "hands-off" defibrillation is the application of the patches to the chest wall. All other components and steps stay the same. Refer to Figure 7-4A–C.

FIGURE 7–4
"Hands-free" or "hands-off"
defibrillation with LifePak 12.
(A) Identify ventricular
fibrillation on the monitor.
(B) Ventilate patient and
place defibrillation pads
on patient. (C) Deliver
hands-free shock.

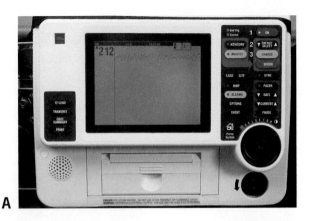

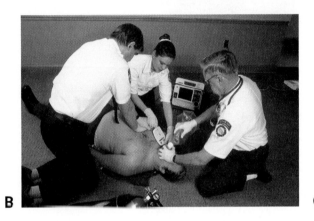

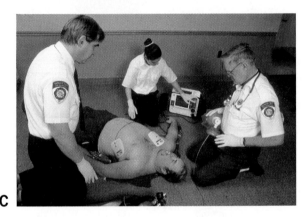

Defibrillation and Asystolic Hearts

When you recognize asystole on the heart monitor, you should confirm it in two different leads, since fine ventricular fibrillation may "hide" or be "masked" in one lead but not another. And if asystole does in fact turn out to be fine VF in another lead, you should manage the rhythm as VF and carry out defibrillation attempts as previously discussed.

However, if asystole is truly asystole in multiple leads, defibrillation attempts are not warranted. Randomly shocking an asystolic heart under the premise that "no harm can be done" is inaccurate. The defibrillation attempt actually induces a profound increase in vagal tone, which can inhibit the natural pacemakers of the heart to an extent that any chance for recovery is eliminated.

Current-Based Defibrillation: "Smart Defibrillators"

Also under investigation is an alternative approach to defibrillation called current-based defibrillation. With current-based defibrillation, you can select the desired electrical current to be delivered to the heart (in amperes), rather than the customary energy level delivered from the defibrillator (in joules). Then, the defibrillator determines the degree of resistance offered by this specific patient's thorax by passing a small amount of energy through it from electrode to electrode. Once it has determined the amount of energy required to overcome the resistance, the defibrillator adjusts the current flow to allow the exact energy selected to be delivered to the heart. This technology will be beneficial to patients with varying degrees of resistance due to differences in the size and/or integrity of the thorax.

⊞ AUTOMATED EXTERNAL DEFIBRILLATION

Defibrillation was once a skill reserved specifically for those health care providers capable of identifying the appropriate rhythms by reading and interpreting ECGs and trained in the use of manual defibrillation. However, the success of conversion from ventricular fibrillation is directly related to the speed with which defibrillation is provided. Unfortunately, there has often been a delay in getting a team trained in ECG interpretation and manual defibrillation to the patient's side.

Fortunately, with advances in medical technology, devices were invented that could distinguish between rhythms that are or are not ventricular fibrillation. After this, it was easy to create the computer programming that could deliver sequential countershocks independent of human interpretation. Thus, the device known as the automated external defibrillator (AED) was created. Because the AED is so simple to operate, laypersons, first responders, and EMT-Basics can now be trained to provide early defibrillation in a variety of settings, reducing the number of deaths from out-of-hospital cardiac arrests.

Components of an Automated External Defibrillator

There is striking similarity between an AED and a standard manual defibrillator. With both, a power source charges the capacitors to a specified amount of energy. They both have cables that attach to electrodes that are in contact with the patient's chest in order to deliver the defibrillation. (The AED also interprets the ECG through the electrodes attached to the chest.) The main difference between the two is how the rhythm is detected.

While the manual defibrillator requires a person to interpret the rhythm on the monitor, the AED has an internal rhythm analysis system capable of identifying VF, or VT above a preset rate. Its rhythm analysis system does not determine every dysrhythmia known; rather it looks simply for the presence of VF/VT. If the criteria it analyzes (amplitude, frequency, and slope of the ECG) fit the requirement for VF/VT, a shock is recommended. If not, no shock is advised.

Semi-automated AEDs

Although AEDs are designed to do much of the work themselves, they still rely on human involvement. The provider must confirm that the patient is pulseless and apneic before attaching the AED. With semi-automated AEDs, the provider may be required to activate the "analyze" button for the unit to interpret the rhythm. If the unit identifies VF/VT, it will emit an audible tone or voice synthesizer, alerting the care provider to depress the "discharge" or "shock" button after verifying the rhythm and charging the capacitors to the appropriate level. This allows the provider to visually and verbally clear the patient prior to the shock. The major advantages are that the AED provides ease of use with a great amount of safety since it never enters the analysis or discharge mode without the operator's direction.

AED Use in Children Less than 8 Years of Age

It has been found that ventricular fibrillation is far more common in children than once thought. Previously, automated external defibrillators were not approved for children under 8 years of age or 25 kg. Now, some manufacturers have modified their adult AED equipment to include pediatric cables and pads that reduce the energy level delivered by the AED by about 50 to 70 joules, thus, making the adult AED available for use in children above 1 year of age. If an AED is used in a pediatric patient, it is highly recommended that an adult AED with the pediatric pad/cable system be used to deliver more appropriate energy levels. However, if a pediatric pad/cable system is not available and you are confronted with a child between the ages of 1 year and 8 years of age who is in confirmed cardiac arrest, it is appropriate to apply and use the adult AED. If only one rescuer is on the scene, one minute of CPR should be performed on the child. Then attach the adult AED and defibrillate. Application of the AED and defibrillation is only indicated in ventricular fibrillation and pulseless ventricular tachycardia. Do not apply the AED if the patient has a pulse or other signs of circulation. **Do not** apply or use the AED in infants less than 1 year of age. In an infant less than 1 year old, immediately initiate CPR and contact an ALS unit. Even though an adult AED can be applied to a child older than 1 year of age who is in confirmed cardiac arrest, it is still advisable and preferred that a manual defibrillator with the feature of setting variable lower energy levels be used to defibrillate a child less than 8 years of age.[1]

Procedure for Defibrillation with an AED

AEDs from various manufacturers have a multitude of different options available. For example, a basic unit may have just an audible tone and lights to alert the operator to defibrillate. Other models may have paper strip recorders, an oscilloscope for rhythm interpretation, tape back-up of the cardiac arrest events, voice synthesizer, and more. Become familiar with the operational steps of the AED used in your service or unit, especially when as a provider of advanced cardiac life support, you will have to back up a BLS unit which is using their own AED.

Although they vary, the basic steps for use of all AEDs (Figures 7-5A to 7-5F) are as follows:

1. Initiate and maintain CPR until the defibrillator is available. Once it is available, immediately attach the AED.
2. Apply the device to the patient confirmed to be pulseless and apneic.
3. Turn the main power switch on.
4. Apply the self-adhesive monitoring/defibrillation electrodes to the thorax in the standard "anterior-apex" or "anterior-posterior" location.
5. Clear the patient for "hands-off" analysis of the patient's rhythm.
6. With some models you may have to initiate analysis of the rhythm.
7. Be sure everyone is clear of the patient and deliver the defibrillation shock, if advised.

Refer to Figure 7-6 for the AED treatment algorithm

The sequence of defibrillation for an AED is also slightly different than when using a manual defibrillator. With AEDs, after the first stack of three shocks is delivered (200 J, 200–300 J, 360 J), pulselessness should be reconfirmed and CPR instituted for 1 minute. After one minute of CPR, the rhythm is reanalyzed, and if VF/VT is persisting, another stack of three shocks is delivered (200 J, 200–300 J, 360 J). So the overall sequence when using an AED is a stack of three

[1]Samson RA, Berg RA, Bingham R, et al. "Use of Automated External Defibrillators for Children: An Update." *Circulation*. 2003; 107:3250.

USING A SEMI-AUTOMATED AED

Ideally, at least two practitioners should be present when defibrillation is to be performed with a semi-automated AED—one to operate the AED, the other to perform CPR. The AED should be placed near the patient's head, but is placed differently in these photographs to make the AED's screen and controls visible.

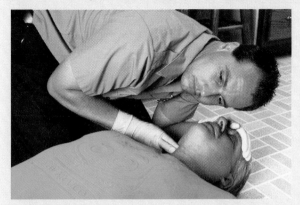

FIGURE 7–5A
Perform initial assessment and verify absence of pulse and breathing.

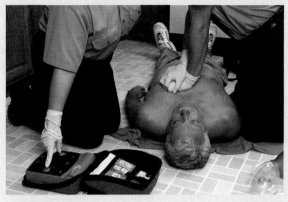

FIGURE 7–5B
One practitioner should initiate CPR while the other prepares the AED.

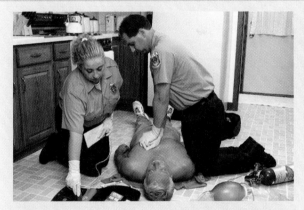

FIGURE 7–5C
Turn on the defibrillator. (Note: These photos show a biphasic AED, which is turned on before the electrodes are placed. For other types of AEDs, the electrodes are placed before the defibrillator is turned on. Always follow the manufacturer's instructions.)

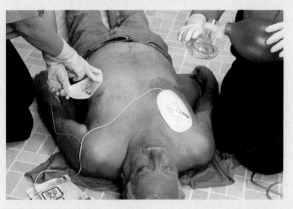

FIGURE 7–5D
Place the defibrillator electrodes on the patient's chest.

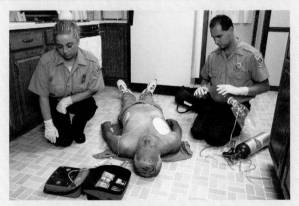

FIGURE 7–5E
Stop CPR and begin the rhythm analysis.

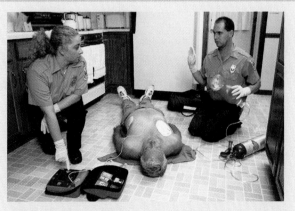

FIGURE 7–5F
If a shock is advised, clear all people from the patient and deliver the shock.

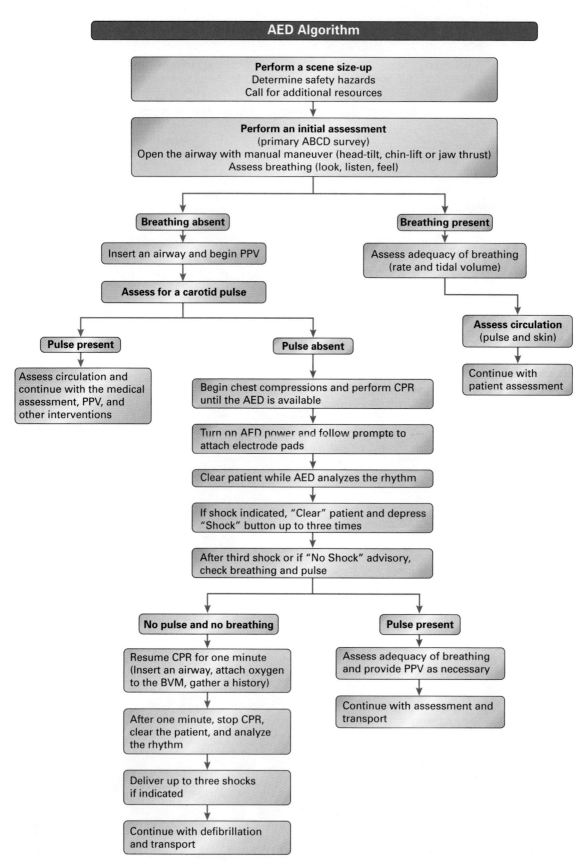

FIGURE 7-6
Algorithm for automated external defibrillation.

shocks followed by 1 minute of CPR, then another stack of three shocks followed by 1 minute of CPR.

This sequence will continue until the "no shock indicated" message is received. If the providers receive "no shock indicated" three times in a row (with intervening periods of CPR), the likelihood of successful defibrillation is extremely low. As such, the rhythm analysis can occur on a 1–2 minute cycle.

Coordination of ACLS with AEDs

With the widespread acceptance and use of AEDs by laypersons and emergency response personnel (e.g., police, fire personnel, EMT-Bs), the likelihood of responding to a patient in cardiac arrest with an AED attached is rapidly increasing. To promote a smooth transition from initial care using an AED to the provision of ACLS, the following guidelines are recommended:

▶ The prehospital advanced cardiac life support provider with the greatest amount of emergency cardiac care education always assumes responsibility as team leader.

▶ The team leader should ask for a brief summary of the arrest situation and the number of defibrillations that have been delivered by AED. If the personnel are still completing their stacked countershocks using the AED, the team leader should allow them to proceed with their protocol.

▶ As long as the AED has a monitoring screen that will allow the team leader to interpret the underlying rhythm, you can consider leaving the AED device on and use it to deliver any additional defibrillations as appropriate. The personnel familiar with the AED should be allowed to operate the device. However, if the unit has no monitoring screen, the AED should be rapidly removed and replaced with a conventional monitor/defibrillator.

▶ Factor any defibrillations administered by the AED into your algorithm for the treatment of VF/VT. In other words, if the last defibrillation delivered was at 360 J, any subsequent defibrillations by the prehospital advanced cardiac life support provider should be at 360 J rather than starting back at 200 J. The same applies for the first three stacked defibrillations in the ventricular fibrillation algorithm. There is no need to repeat the stack of three defibrillations (200 J, 200–300 J, 360 J) if they were already delivered using the AED.

▶ During transport with an AED in place, special considerations must be made. While it is not inherently dangerous to transport a patient attached to an AED, it is required to bring the vehicle to a complete stop before reanalyzing the rhythm. Some services also recommend turning the engine off prior to reanalyzing the rhythm. This is to avoid any rhythm disturbance caused by the moving vehicle. En route, be sure to maintain CPR, airway management, and drug therapy as appropriate.

▶ A patient with an AED (or manual defibrillator, for that matter) who has been defibrillated into a perfusing rhythm may refibrillate. In this case, verify pulselessness, immediately resume the analysis mode, and deliver additional defibrillations as necessary.

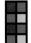 EMERGENCY SYNCHRONIZED CARDIOVERSION

As stated in the chapter introduction, there may be certain dysrhythmias in which the unstable patient is decompensating so rapidly that there may not be the luxury of time to wait for a specific drug therapy to exert its action. Or, on occasion, the patient may display a rhythm that is not responsive to routine drug therapy but has the potential to decompensate into a fatal dysrhythmia. It is in these instances that synchronized cardioversion may be the best option available.

Synchronized cardioversion is actually a "controlled" form of defibrillation that is reserved for those patients who still have organized cardiac activity with a pulse. Within the defibrillator, there is a synchronizing circuit that, when activated, will interpret the QRS cycle and deliver the electrical discharge during the "R" wave of the QRS complex. This reduces the likelihood of delivering the cardioversion on the vulnerable period of the QRS cycle, which is known to precipitate ventricular fibrillation. Additionally, synchronizing also permits the use of lower energy levels and reduces the potential for secondary dysrhythmias.

Indications for Synchronized Cardioversion

Synchronized cardioversion is used for tachydysrhythmias that, as discussed above, are unstable. Table 7-2 outlines the indications for synchronized cardioversion.

Procedure for Synchronized Cardioversion

Essentially, the procedure for defibrillation and synchronized cardioversion are the same, with the exception of activating the synchronizing circuit during synchronous cardioversion. As with defibrillation, transthoracic resistance can result in subtherapeutic energy levels reaching the myocardium in synchronized cardioversion. To reduce this problem, take the necessary measures to reduce transthoracic resistance so that you may increase the potential for success in terminating the dysrhythmia.

TABLE 7–2   Indications for Synchronized Cardioversion
Tachydysrhythmias necessitating emergency synchronized cardioversion:
▪ Hemodynamically unstable* ventricular tachycardia with a pulse ▪ Hemodynamically unstable* supraventricular tachycardia
Hemodynamically unstable is defined as a patient presenting with one or more of the following signs and/or symptoms, and the cause of the signs/symptoms is from the tachydysrhythmia:

SIGNS:
• pulmonary edema
• rales
• hypotension
• jugular venous distension
• ischemic EKG findings on 12-lead

SYMPTOMS:
• significant dyspnea
• severe chest pain (cardiogenic in nature)
• altered mental status

The following steps are necessary to successfully and safely provide synchronized-cardioversion to a patient:

1. Confirm the symptomatic tachydysrhythmia on the monitor.

2. Place the patient in a safe environment if initially in contact with some electrically conductive material (e.g., water, metal).

3. Time permitting, administer a sedative agent (such as diazepam, midazolam, barbiturate, etomidate, or ketamine).

4. Apply electrode gel to paddles, or place gel pads on the patient's exposed thorax.

5. Activate the synchronizing circuit by depressing the "synch" button before each cardioversion. Assure proper capture of the QRS complex.

6. Turn on and charge the capacitor to the appropriate energy level.

7. Ensure appropriate placement and pressure of electrodes on the patient's thorax.

8. ENSURE THAT NO ONE IS IN CONTACT WITH THE PATIENT. Verbally and visually clear everybody prior to any cardioversion attempt (including yourself).

9. Deliver synchronized cardioversion by depressing and holding both buttons on the defibrillation paddles simultaneously. (Depressing only one will result in no shock being delivered.) You may experience a brief pause while the unit identifies the appropriate moment to discharge. Keep the paddles firmly placed on the chest until the energy is discharged.

10. Reconfirm the rhythm on the monitor screen; if still present, recharge and repeat steps 5 to 7, using higher energy levels.

Refer to Figure 7-7 for the algorithm for synchronized cardioversion.

SPECIAL SITUATIONS INVOLVING ELECTRICAL THERAPY

Manual defibrillation, AED defibrillation, and synchronized cardioversion all share the same fundamental principle of operation. The following section discusses specific situations in which the care provider may need to slightly alter the treatment regimen or care for the device in a certain way. While these situations are not that frequently encountered, their importance makes them worthy of mention.

Defibrillation of Hypothermic Patients

Chapter 13 specifically discusses cardiac arrest in a hypothermic patient, but a few points should be mentioned here. A hypothermic heart is more likely to go into ventricular fibrillation from the cold temperature; however, it is much less responsive to defibrillation. The cardiac monitor or AED should be applied as usual, and the rhythm analyzed. However, if ventricular fibrillation or pulseless ventricular tachycardia is present and a shock is indicated, provide only the first three defibrillations. If defibrillation is unsuccessful, resume CPR, airway management, and rewarming efforts, and transport the patient to a more advanced medical facility, ideally one with cardiac bypass capabilities. Defibrillation should be continued only after adequate rewarming has been achieved.

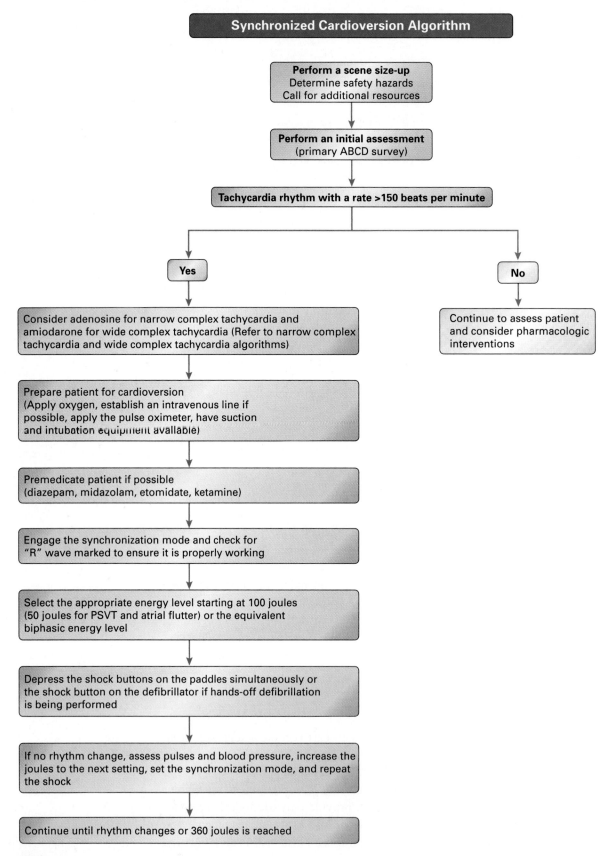

FIGURE 7–7
Algorithm for synchronized cardioversion.

Defibrillation of Patients with Automatic Implantable Cardioverter/Defibrillator (AICD)

An AICD is, in essence, a mini version of a fully automated AED that is implanted and attached to the heart. AICDs are implanted in persons at high risk for cardiac arrest due to VF or VT. These devices continually analyze the heart rhythm via electrodes attached to the heart and, upon identification of ventricular fibrillation or ventricular tachycardia, they will deliver a specific amount of energy to the heart. With regard to this, you should know the following:

▷ If the unit discharges while you are in contact with the patient, you may feel the current flow, but it is not dangerous. If the AICD is in the process of shocking a patient, allow it 30 to 60 seconds to complete its treatment cycle.

▷ If VF or VT is present despite the AICD, external transthoracic defibrillations are still warranted. In these instances, the AICD has either malfunctioned or exhausted its preprogrammed number of countershocks.

▷ Since the AICD electrodes are attached to the myocardium by patches, the patches may block the conventional defibrillation and reduce the amount of electricity that reaches the myocardium. If you find a patient with an AICD who is in ventricular fibrillation that is unresponsive to repeated defibrillatory shocks, consider changing from anterior-apex electrode placement to anterior-posterior placement (or vice versa), and attempt defibrillation again. By doing this, you may avoid the area of the myocardium covered by the AICD patches.

Interruption of CPR

During patient transport, considerable patient-handling and moving may have to take place. It is imperative that there be a concerted effort to avoid unnecessary delays in or interruption of CPR during these movements. As a guideline, CPR should not be interrupted more than 5 seconds at a time. The only exception to this is while the AED is analyzing and charging for each of its stacked shocks. During this time period, not to exceed 90 seconds, the benefits of the AED unit providing defibrillation to a fibrillating heart outweigh the negative effects of temporarily stopping CPR.

Monitor/Defibrillator and AED Maintenance

While the ACLS provider will probably not have the biomedical technical expertise to troubleshoot and repair a broken defibrillator, there are basic maintenance steps that should be completed daily to ensure the unit is operating at peak performance when it is needed. While a specific checklist are usually provided from the device manufacturer, the following highlights the points that should be checked daily.

▷ No breaks or cracks in the casing or wires

▷ Paddles are clean, non-pitted, release easily from housing

▷ Adequate defibrillation supplies are available (batteries, gel, strip paper, etc.)

▷ Device works properly on AC or battery power

▷ All indicator lights work

▷ Paper recorder works (if present)

▷ Device charges appropriately on AC and battery power

■ EMERGENCY CARDIAC PACING

Emergency cardiac pacing is a concept that has been around in a variety of forms since the 19th century. However, the "modern age" of cardiac pacing began about 45 years ago, and this therapy has rapidly developed into one of the mainstay treatments for certain bradydysrhythmic and tachydysrhythmic patients over the past 15 years.

Its concept is simple: The heart is a muscle that will contract when stimulated with an electrical impulse. The heart is not particularly interested in where the impulse originated. Therefore, delivering an artificial electrical impulse to a heart that is mechanically capable should result in a contraction and propulsion of blood.

There are actually several different types of cardiac pacemakers; their names reflect the impulse delivery mode. Table 7-3 lists the various types. Of these, the type of pacing used most often in emergency cardiac care is transcutaneous pacing because of its minimal complications, speed of initiation, and effectiveness.

Components of a Cardiac Pacemaker

The first portion of a cardiac pacemaker is the pulse generator. This is the device that initiates the impulse and controls its rate and strength. Its location will either be outside the body or implanted within the body, depending on the type of pacemaker. The impulse created by the cardiac pacemaker then travels through the electrodes. The impulse exits the electrode and enters the body tissue at the site where the electrode is positioned. Again refer to Table 7-3 to review various electrode locations.

Indications for Emergency Cardiac Pacing

Although there are numerous pathological changes to the conduction system of the heart that may necessitate placement of an internal pacemaker, here we will only

TABLE 7–3 Types of Cardiac Pacemakers			
Name	**Electrode Location**	**Pulse Generator Location**	**Synonyms**
Transcutaneous	Skin (anterior chest wall and back)	External	External Noninvasive
Transvenous	Venous (venous catheter with tip in right ventricle or right atrium or both)	External	Temporary transvenous Permanent transvenous
Transthoracic	Through the anterior chest wall into the heart	External	Transmyocardial
Transesophageal	Esophagus	External	
Epicardial	Epicardium (electrodes placed on the surface of the heart during surgery)	External or Internal	
"Permanent"	Venous or epicardial	Internal	Implanted Internal

From *Textbook of Advanced Cardiac Life Support,* 1994. © American Heart Association.

be concerned with emergency transcutaneous cardiac pacing. Primarily, emergency cardiac pacing is indicated for those individuals who are decompensating physiologically from poor cardiac output secondary to a slow or absent heart rate. Typically, in these situations, the primary problem is simply the inability of the heart to maintain a sufficient heart rate to sustain normal cardiac output and systolic blood pressure.

Unless there is previous damage to the myocardium, stimulation of the heart to contract with an artificial rate and impulse will increase the cardiac output. Put another way, pacing is most effective in those patients who have a primary rate problem but whose myocardial contractility is effective.

Symptoms of a hemodynamically unstable patient secondary to a rate problem include hypotension (systolic <80 mmHg), pulmonary edema, an altered mental status, severe chest pain, congestive heart failure, and pulmonary congestion. If these signs and symptoms of hypoperfusion are present, emergency cardiac pacing can be considered either prior to drug therapy, or in conjunction with drug therapy, or in bradycardia, which is refractory to traditional drug therapy. As mentioned earlier, transcutaneous pacing is the preferred method for pacing in emergency cardiac care because it can readily be applied, is non-invasive, doesn't interfere with other treatments being rendered, has minimal complications, and is usually effective.

Transcutaneous pacing has also been used in the past to terminate tachydysrhythmias. While not the preferred treatment for rate control (drug therapy still is), by pacing the heart at a faster rate (termed "overdrive" pacing) than the intrinsic tachydysrhythmia, you can achieve "capture" of the rhythm, and then slow down the pacer rate with hopes that the normal conduction system will eventually take over.

Finally, pacing has been shown to have some limited success in capture for patients who have been in asystolic cardiac arrest for less than 10 minutes. However, survival numbers did not change. The problem is that by the time the heart is asystolic, it has suffered prolonged periods of hypoxia and acidosis, which limits the heart's ability to contract. In patients with prolonged periods of asystole (>10 minutes), some studies have indicated no benefit whatsoever to emergency transcutaneous pacing, especially in the prehospital environment.

Transcutaneous Pacing Equipment

Many of the newer cardiac monitor/defibrillators have a built-in cardiac pacing device. This allows the device to be portable enough so that pacing can be conducted at the patient's bedside. While various manufacturers of pacing units offer different features, the following list illustrates basic components of a transcutaneous pacemaker.

- ▶ External pulse generator (typically housed within the monitor)
- ▶ Cables that connect the pacer to the electrodes on the thorax
- ▶ Self-adhesive pacing electrodes, some of which are capable of serving several functions (i.e., cardiac monitoring, pacing, "hands-off" defibrillation)
- ▶ Fixed-rate or demand-mode pacing option
- ▶ Adjustable amperage control
- ▶ Adjustable rate control

Procedure for Transcutaneous Pacing

After you provide oxygenation, ventilation, and intravenous access, you can then ready the patient for transcutaneous pacing.

1. If the patient has excessive body hair that interferes with adhesion of the pads, rapidly shave or clip off hair at points of contact. (Clipping of hair rather than shaving will reduce the likelihood of irritation from small nicks to the skin.)

2. Attach the pacing electrodes to the patient's thorax by placing the anterior electrode to the left of the sternum, as close to the point of maximal impulse as possible (approximately the fifth intercostal space, midclavicular line). Place the posterior electrode directly behind the anterior electrode, lateral to the spine on the left thorax.

3. Set the rate of pacing to the physiologically desirable number, typically 80/min.

4. Set the unit to either the demand or the asynchronous mode. In demand mode, the pacemaker operates whenever the intrinsic heart rate drops below the designated rate; the asynchronous mode delivers pacemaker impulses regardless of the intrinsic rate of the heart. The demand mode is beneficial when performing standby pacing (discussed below).

5. Turn the unit on, and adjust the milliamps (mA):
   – For bradycardia, start at 0 mA, and slowly increase in increments of 5–10 mA until capture occurs.
   – For asystolic hearts, start at maximal mA, and decrease mA if capture is achieved.

6. Assess for capture two ways:
   – First, look for the characteristically wide QRS following the pacer spike (Figure 7-8).
   – Assess the carotid pulse to see if the artificial rhythm is producing a pulse.

7. Continue pacing at an mA level about 10% higher than needed minimally for capture.

8. Consider an analgesic or sedative for possible pain should the patient be responsive.

9. Monitor vitals and level of consciousness, and constantly assure capture.

   If the unit fails to capture (Figure 7-9), the failure may be related to electrode placement or the characteristics of the patient's thorax. Be sure that you are using as many methods as possible to reduce transthoracic resistance.

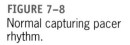
FIGURE 7–8
Normal capturing pacer rhythm.

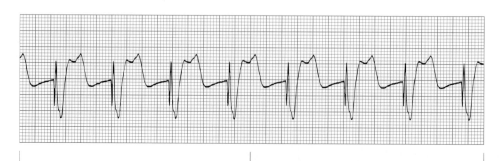

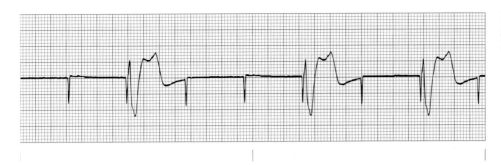

FIGURE 7-9
Abnormal pacer function; loss of capture.

Standby Pacing

Standby pacing is indicated for the patient who is hemodynamically stable but is displaying a bradydysrhythmic rate with the potential for rapid deterioration. Table 7-4 lists those rhythms requiring emergency cardiac pacing and those rhythms needing standby pacing in case the patient deteriorates before the dysrhythmia can be eliminated. By setting up the pacer and momentarily switching it on to assure capture, you will be ready to immediately institute transcutaneous pacing should the patient suddenly decompensate (become symptomatic) while emergency care is being rendered. As preparation, you should become familiar with the asystole and bradycardia algorithms, Figures 10-4 and 10-5, in Chapter 10.

Complications of Transcutaneous Pacing

The most common complication of transcutaneous pacing is pain. Fortunately, with more current revisions in pacing technology, the discomfort created by pacing is usually tolerable. If not tolerable, then it may be controllable by administration of analgesics.

Two other complications are failure to recognize if the pacemaker spike is capturing, and failure to recognize ventricular fibrillation due to the influence of the pacer spikes. These two problems can be eliminated if the monitoring is done with a special filtration process that will allow the care provider to accurately assess the underlying rhythm.

TABLE 7-4　Transcutaneous Pacing
Indications for Emergency Transcutaneous Pacing:
■ Hemodynamically unstable bradycardic rhythms 　– Any bradycardic rhythm that results in hemodynamic instability in the patient 　　should receive TCP as early as possible.
■ Asystolic cardiac arrests 　– Pacing may be beneficial in asystole, but do not institute TCP prior to 　　compressions, tracheal intubation with PPV, oxygen, IV therapy, and at least one 　　trial of epinephrine and atropine.
Indications for Preparing to Provide Transcutaneous Pacing:
■ Bradycardic patient who does not currently present as symptomatic, but whose 　rhythm or condition is likely to deteriorate 　– Mobitz heart blocks (2nd-degree Types I and II) 　– Complete heart blocks (3rd-degree with junctional or ventricular escape rhythms) 　– Recent onset of bundle branch block in light of a potentially evolving myocardial 　　infarction

Ventricular fibrillation is a potential complication once pacing is instituted, but it is probably rare since the energy level necessary to disrupt the conduction system is greater than the energy delivered by the pacing device. Be cautious, however; that potential does exist.

Contraindications to Transcutaneous Pacing

As discussed earlier, asystolic cardiac arrest is not ordinarily responsive to external transcutaneous pacing. For this reason, it is considered a relative contraindication. If, during the cardiac arrest management, there are adequate personnel to apply the pacer while CPR, intubation, IV access, and drug therapy are being done concurrently, then it may be attempted. However, do not withhold these interventions in the asystolic patient in an attempt to pace the heart.

Hypothermia causes diminished responsiveness of the myocardium to the pacing impulse as with the defibrillation stimuli discussed earlier. Remember also that bradycardia is thought to be a protective function as the general metabolic activity decreases in hypothermia. Management of hypothermic patients is aimed toward rewarming and ensuring adequate ventilation. Since the heart becomes unstable due to hypothermia, the irritation caused by the pacing impulse could result in ventricular fibrillation.

Pediatric bradycardia results from hypoxia and hypoventilation and responds favorably when the hypoventilation is corrected with oxygenation and adequate alveolar ventilation. Therefore, initial management of bradycardia in pediatric patients is aimed at reversing the hypoxia. Only when the bradycardia exists within known congenital defects, drug overdose, or recent heart surgery should external pacing be considered.

Other Pacing Techniques

Several other methods are available to achieve emergency cardiac pacing in the symptomatic patient. These methods include transvenous pacing, transmyocardial transthoracic pacing, transesophageal pacing, and epicardial pacing, as listed previously in Table 7-3. The first three have been shown to be beneficial in specific situations; however, transcutaneous pacing should be performed until these methods are implemented. The last method (epicardial pacing) is performed under direct visualization of the heart during open chest surgery, so it is not a viable option to prehospital bradycardic patients.

▦ SUMMARY

Within this chapter we have covered diverse medical interventions necessary to emergency cardiac care. However diverse the methods discussed, the common thread is that they all utilize electricity therapeutically to eliminate a dysrhythmia.

A fundamental understanding of defibrillation, synchronized cardioversion, AED use, and external pacing allows the prehospital care provider to appropriately and safely use these interventions in the symptomatic patient.

However beneficial these therapies are when used appropriately, they can certainly be fatal if used inappropriately. It is the responsibility of the prehospital provider of advanced cardiac life support, then, to be thoroughly familiar with the indications for and proper uses of these therapies. It is equally important to stay abreast of the changes and developments in the usage of electrical therapy in emergency cardiac care.

CASE STUDY FOLLOW-UP

Assessment

During your initial assessment of Mr. Griffiths, your impression is of a middle-aged male experiencing a cardiac emergency. In addition to the vitals you obtained (blood pressure 102/62 mmHg, heart rate 220 per minute and regular, respiratory rate 36 per minute with slight retractions), you also hear fine inspiratory crackles upon lung auscultation. You recall that extremely tachycardic rates can diminish cardiac output and drop coronary artery perfusion—both of these contributing to the chest pain.

You reassure Mr. Griffiths as you administer a high concentration of oxygen.

Treatment

Since Mr. Griffiths is dyspneic and has chest pain, you elect to administer oxygen via a nonrebreather face mask at 15 lpm and apply the pulse oximeter. You remove his shirt to apply the cardiac monitor while you ask your coworker to initiate an IV.

While monitoring Lead II, you identify an extremely rapid narrow-complex rate. Currently, there are no P waves distinguishable from the T waves, but the QRS complex is narrow and regular at 220/minute. Since you consider Mr. Griffiths to be an unstable patient in supraventricular tachycardia, you ask your partner to prepare and administer 6 mg of adenosine while you ready the defibrillation paddles. At this point, Mr. Griffith's orientation is diminishing and his respiratory distress is increasing.

With no effect from the adenosine, you elect to administer a synchronized countershock at 100 joules. You place the gel pads in the anterior apex position on the thorax, apply about 25 pounds of pressure to the paddles, and charge the unit. While assuring that the synchronizing circuit is activated, and after being sure everyone else is clear, you cardiovert the patient during exhalation.

With no success from the initial cardioversion, you rapidly administer a subsequent synchronized countershock at 200 joules. After this countershock, Mr. Griffiths becomes apneic and pulseless. Ventricular fibrillation is identified on the monitor.

You charge the paddles to 200 joules, assure that the synchronization mode is turned off, and deliver an asynchronous monophasic countershock to the patient. With no change in the rhythm, you complete the "stacked three" shocks by administering asynchronous monophasic defibrillations at 300 joules, then 360 joules. CPR is initiated, the airway is intubated, and 1 mg epinephrine is administered.

Approximately 2 minutes later, ventricular fibrillation persists on the monitor. You again defibrillate at 360 joules, and fortunately this converts the patient into a bradycardia identified as a third-degree block with a pulse; however, he is hypotensive. The external pacer is applied and it captures, causing both the rate and the systolic pressure to increase.

As you prepare Mr. Griffiths for movement to the ambulance, your back-up arrives on scene and says, "So, is everything under control here?"

REVIEW QUESTIONS

1. Defibrillation is used to manage
   a. life-threatening bradydysrhythmias.
   b. asystolic dysrhythmia.
   c. ventricular fibrillation.
   d. chronic atrial fibrillation.
   e. c and d are both correct

2. Which of the following scenarios will most likely result in immediately successful cardioversion?
   a. applying the electrical therapy 25 minutes after onset of symptoms
   b. cardioverting only after epinephrine and/or other drugs have been administered
   c. timing the cardioversion with the end-expiration phase of ventilations
   d. utilizing synchronous cardioversion for a patient in VF

3. Which of the following statements about asynchronous cardioversion is true?
   a. It is also known as defibrillation.
   b. It is the preferred method to terminate symptomatic tachydysrhythmias.
   c. The initial energy level is 50–100 joules.
   d. It does not require the use of gel pads or electrode paste.
   e. It is never used in pediatric patients.

4. Defibrillating an asystolic heart may
   a. initiate spontaneous rhythms.
   b. make the heart more susceptible to the effects of the IV drugs.
   c. be performed only after assuring the heart is in asystole in two leads.
   d. inhibit the natural pacemakers of the heart.

5. Which of the following energy dose regimes is correct for monophasic defibrillation?
   a. 50–100 joules, 200 joules, 360 joules
   b. 100 joules, 200 joules, 300 joules, 360 joules
   c. 200 joules, 200–300 joules, 360 joules
   d. 50–100 joules, 200 joules, 300 joules, 360 joules

6. AEDs are used for
   a. cardiac arrest victims in VF.
   b. cardiac arrest victims in asystole.
   c. cardiac arrest victims over 1 hour away from the hospital.
   d. cardiac arrest victims suffering from severe trauma only.

7. The difference between the countershocks delivered by the AED and those administered manually is the AED:
   a. repeatedly delivers "stacked shocks" of three, whereas manually they are delivered only one at a time.
   b. uses lower energy levels than manual defibrillators.
   c. uses higher energy levels than manual defibrillators.
   d. is not as effective as manual defibrillation.

8. Synchronized cardioversion delivers the countershock
   a. during expiration.
   b. during the R wave of the cardiac cycle.
   c. during the T wave of the cardiac cycle.
   d. immediately upon depressing the discharge buttons of the paddles.

9. The greatest benefit of using synchronous versus asynchronous countershocks for an unstable patient in supraventricular tachycardia is
   a. lowest possible chance for causing VF.
   b. faster delivery of energy.
   c. lower risk of damage to the myocardium.
   d. a and c are correct.
   e. a, b, and c are correct.

10. Which of the following findings would indicate a hemodynamically unstable patient in ventricular tachycardia with a pulse?
    a. extreme diaphoresis
    b. chest pain
    c. mild respiratory distress
    d. cyanosis
    e. tachycardia

11. You have just delivered a synchronous cardioversion at 300 joules, and the patient goes into VF. You should immediately
    a. resume CPR.
    b. defibrillate at 200 joules.
    c. intubate the trachea.
    d. administer epinephrine.
    e. administer lidocaine.

12. AED utilization for pediatric patients less than age 8 is acceptable.
    a. true
    b. false

13. It is inappropriate to defibrillate a patient with an AICD.
    a. true
    b. false

14. External cardiac pacing is the preferred treatment for
    a. bradycardia.
    b. asystole.
    c. tachycardia.
    d. ventricular fibrillation.
    e. a and b are correct

15. How do you confirm that the external pacemaker is "capturing"?
    a. Assess for a QRS complex after the pacer spike.
    b. Palpable pulse in conjunction with the pacemaker.
    c. The presence of a blood pressure.
    d. The patient will complain of pain or discomfort.
    e. a and b are correct

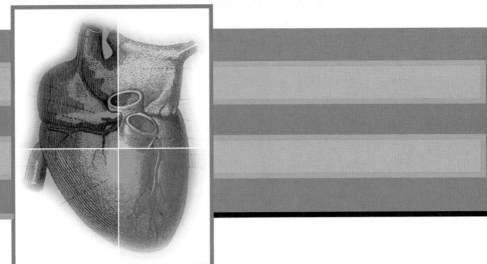

Pharmacological Therapy

In conjunction with proper oxygenation, ventilation, compressions, and defibrillation, pharmacological therapy is an integral component of successful cardiac arrest management. Additionally, caring for patients experiencing any one of many non-arrest cardiovascular emergencies will certainly include the administration of cardioactive drugs. This chapter will provide an introduction to the drugs that are most commonly used during advanced cardiac life support.

Topics in this chapter are:

Cardiovascular Pharmacology

Note: An index to the drugs discussed in this chapter appears on page 210.

CASE STUDY

One night you are relaxing at home after a hard day's work. And, as on every other Tuesday night, you find your-self in front of the TV so you can watch your favorite program from 9:00 to 10:00 PM. This show, which you never miss, is titled *Code Blue, Stat!* It is a show about the heroic efforts of emergency health care providers as they do battle with cardiovascular disease, trauma, and death on a daily basis. Your interest in the show stems from your knowledge of prehospital emergency care—and your curiosity about the appropriateness of their treatment.

This week's program immediately catches your attention, since the first patient is a middle-aged man with chest pain and bradycardia—almost the identical presentation to the man you treated just a few hours ago at work. You lean back in your recliner and say out loud to the TV screen, "OK, folks, impress me."

The TV character, Mr. Hedger, has summoned EMS because of severe chest pain, diaphoresis, and dizzi-ness. As the TV medics start to assess him, one applies the pulse oximeter and monitor. The TV screen flashes a saturation of 91% with a sinus bradydysrhythmic rate on the monitor. Appropriately, the second paramedic orders oxygen administration and the initiation of an IV of 0.9% sodium chloride.

How would you proceed to assess and care for this patient? This chapter will describe the assess-ment and pharmacologic treatment of patients experiencing a cardiovascular emergency. Later, we will return to the case and apply the procedures learned.

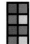 # INTRODUCTION: CARDIOVASCULAR PHARMACOLOGY

Pharmacological therapy is an integral part of advanced cardiac life support, and the prehospital health care provider must become completely familiar with the most commonly used drugs. Admittedly, this is not an easy task, nor one of the most pleasant portions of this text to read, but it is a necessity for optimal patient outcome. The need is obvious: Quality patient care depends on the prehospital advanced cardiac life support provider, who is therefore obligated to learn and stay abreast of current medications and their dosages.

What you must *not* do is allow yourself to become complacent and rely on charts or pocket references to guide your drug therapy during patient management. Books and charts cannot interpret the special circumstances that are part of every cardiac emergency, nor can they offer all the differential approaches to drug ther-apy that may be required. Proper management of the patient will only occur when the prehospital provider understands the pathophysiology behind the patient's con-dition, understands the physiological actions of drugs, and can then apply this knowledge to provide the appropriate pharmacological care for the patient.

To aid the learning process, the authors of this text have made every effort to present the information about each drug in a logical, easy-to-read format. However, it will take an investment of time on your part to comprehend and apply the information. One word of advice: Do not try to simply "memorize" the indica-tions, side effects, and contraindications. Information learned by rote memory is likely to be lost from lack of use or because of stress during an emergency. Rather, by learning and understanding *how a drug works,* its indications, side effects, and contraindications become obvious. Thus, the only thing left to memorize is the specific drug dose—*and there is no shortcut to memorizing drug doses.*

You will notice as you read through this chapter, that some drugs are explained in great detail with guidelines for prehospital administration of the drug. Other drugs however, lack this specificity and are discussed in only general terms.

The reason for the delineation is this: prehospital providers need to become intimately familiar with only a certain number of all drugs used for cardiovascular care. These drugs are those most commonly administered in the prehospital setting that you must be responsible for. The second category of drugs are those that are mentioned mainly from an informative standpoint. The prehospital provider of advanced cardiac life support does not commonly administer these drugs. However, the provider may come across them during inter-hospital transports or within a mobile intensive care (sometimes called critical care) environment (e.g., med-evac or ground transport). If, however, you are working in the latter environment, where you have the medical direction to administer these medications, it then becomes your responsibility to familiarize yourself with specific doses. Finally, some medications used in cardiac care, which are usually third or fourth line agents or those that necessitate concurrent hemodynamic monitoring, have been excluded since they are beyond the scope of this text.

Take the time necessary to become familiar with the drugs discussed in this chapter. They are integral to successful resuscitation, and any one of them has the potential to help, or harm, the patient.

Organization of This Chapter

The drugs in this chapter are arranged in nine categories (chapter parts) according to their common actions and indications. This classification is designed to help you comprehend the information.

However, you will note that certain drugs found in one category may also have indications in another category (for example, oxygen or atropine). Also be aware that while a given drug may have numerous applications in the prehospital setting (for example, the use of epinephrine in cardiac arrest *or* anaphylaxis), *only the indications in cardiovascular care will be discussed here.* It is the authors' contention that arranging the drugs in these categories and keeping the information specific to cardiac emergencies will help you grasp how these drugs apply in advanced cardiac life support.

As a further aid to comprehension, the information about each drug is presented in a consistent format. First you will read about the drug's *action,* followed by the *indications, side effects/precautions, contraindications,* and finally *dosage.*

On page 210 is an index of the drugs discussed in this chapter to aid you in finding and reviewing the information for any specific drug.

Part One: Oxygen

Oxygen is one of the most important and most-often-administered drugs for the patient experiencing a cardiovascular crisis. Oxygen is an essential requirement for the body to maintain its metabolic activities. Since any cardiovascular crisis can result in inadequate oxygenation at the cellular level, you must be acutely aware of the need to initiate oxygen therapy or to increase the amount and concentration of oxygen already being administered.

Oxygen

Oxygen: Mechanism of Action
Oxygen is a colorless and odorless gas that is necessary for life. Oxygen rapidly diffuses across the alveolar walls and binds to hemoglobin in the red blood cells.

Index By Categories

Alphabetical Index

After hemoglobin saturation, the blood circulates the oxygen throughout the body, and it is taken into the cells where it promotes the breakdown of glucose into adenosine triphosphate (ATP), a usable energy substance. (This process is known as *aerobic* metabolism, meaning metabolism that occurs in the presence of oxygen.) Without oxygen, glucose is broken down ineffectively, resulting in the development of lactic acidosis. (This process is known as *anaerobic* metabolism, or metabolism that occurs in the absence of oxygen.)

Oxygen: Indications

Oxygen is indicated whenever there is known or suspected hypoxia, regardless of the etiology. Therefore, oxygen should be administered to any patient with chest pain, a medical emergency, a traumatic or surgical emergency, respiratory distress, or in any instance where you believe that the patient is or has the potential to become hypoxic.

Oxygen: Side Effects/Precautions

The major precaution with administering high concentrations of oxygen is to ensure that there is sufficient gas available to meet the patient's inspiratory volume.

There is some concern that patients with chronic obstructive pulmonary disease (COPD) may experience depressed ventilations with the administration of high flow oxygen. (COPD patients' respiration tends to be regulated by a "hypoxic drive"—in which respiration is stimulated by the brain's perception of a low oxygen level, rather than by a high CO_2 level, as in normal patients. Therefore, there is concern that the COPD patient will react to the administration of oxygen with depressed respiratory effort.) However, even high flow oxygen to these patients will not have a clinically significant effect on ventilatory effort during the brief time it is used during acute cardiopulmonary resuscitation.

Additionally, there is a fear that neonates may suffer retinal damage from high flow oxygen; but again, this is not a concern in the acute situation in view of the short period of time that oxygen will be administered.

Oxygen toxicity, as a side effect, usually does not occur until a patient has spent days on high flow oxygen and ventilatory support. But the emergency patient may complain of nasal irritation from drying the mucosa or may experience epistaxis (a nosebleed) if non-humidified oxygen is administered for a long period of time.

Oxygen: Contraindications

In the emergency setting, there are no contraindications to the use of oxygen. Additionally, despite the known side effects and precautions, OXYGEN SHOULD NEVER BE WITHHELD FROM ANY PATIENT KNOWN (OR SUSPECTED) TO BE HYPOXIC.

Oxygen: Dosage

There is no concern about overdosing with oxygen. It can be administered relatively liberally. The general guideline about oxygen administration during the pre-hospital phase of an emergency is simply this: Administer oxygen in the highest concentration available based upon the patient's clinical condition and ventilatory status. (Review the Chapter 3 discussion of oxygenation devices.) Eventually, as pulse oximetry and capnography indicate proper oxygenation and normal levels of exhaled CO_2, administration of oxygen may be readjusted.

Arterial blood gases (ABGs) may also guide administration of oxygen. Although not a prehospital skill, any care provider must be cautious about contemplating an arterial puncture for a patient who may receive fibrinolytic therapy for reperfusion, because of the potential for uncontrollable bleeding at the site. (See the discussion on reperfusion therapy later in this chapter.).

Part Two: Sympathomimetics

By definition, a *sympathomimetic* is a substance that "mimics" the actions of the sympathetic nervous system. As such, these drugs either directly stimulate the adrenergic receptors of the sympathetic nerve fibers, or indirectly stimulate the sympathetic nervous system by causing certain hormones (catecholamines) to be released within the body (Figure 8-1). These agents may either be naturally occurring in the body (endogenous) or synthetically derived.

FIGURE 8–1
Activity at nerve synapses (spaces) of the sympathetic
nervous system. Catecholamines are released from
pre-synaptic nerve endings, travel across the synapse,
and stimulate receptors on the post-synaptic nerves.
Subsequently, the catecholamines are either
deactivated by enzymes in the synapse or taken up
by the pre-synaptic nerve.

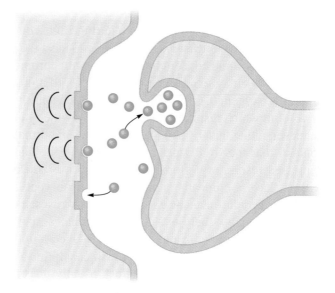

The final result of either mechanism is an increase in sympathetic tone.
(Recall that the autonomic nervous system has two divisions: the sympathetic and
the parasympathetic. The sympathetic nervous system is responsible for the
excited effects of the "fight or flight" response. The parasympathetic system tends
to have opposite, calming effects. See Figure 8-2.)

Administered sympathomimetics have effects that are similar to the actions
of the sympathetic nervous system. Common effects of sympathomimetic drugs
are *positive inotropic effects* (increasing the heart's contractile force), *positive
chronotropic effects* (increasing the heart rate), and *positive dromotropic effects*
(increasing electrical conduction velocity through the heart).

FIGURE 8–2
Organization of the nervous system. Many
drugs stimulate or mimic actions of the
sympathetic or parasympathetic nervous
system.

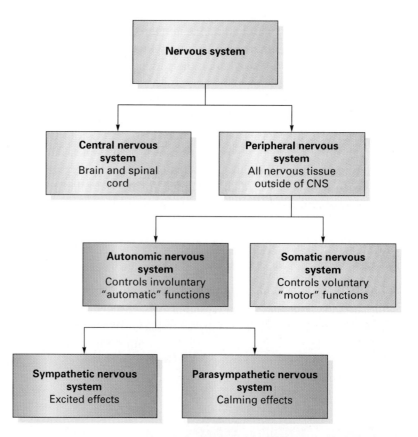

Epinephrine

Epinephrine: Mechanism of Action

Epinephrine is an endogenous catecholamine. This means it is a hormone that is normally produced, secreted, and utilized by the body. A catecholamine is a substance that acts on the autonomic nervous system. Administered epinephrine has effects that result from stimulation of the sympathetic nervous system.

Epinephrine (known casually as *epi*) achieves its therapeutic benefits by stimulating the alpha and beta adrenergic receptor sites of the autonomic nervous system. (If these concepts are unfamiliar to you, any physiology text should explain them in detail. Understanding how the autonomic nervous system, hormones, and alpha and beta adrenergic receptors work is integral to an appreciation of the complex actions of epinephrine.) By stimulating the beta 1 and beta 2 receptor sites, epinephrine increases the activity of the heart and causes dilation of the bronchioles. By stimulating alpha receptor sites, epinephrine increases vascular tone, which helps increase blood pressure. The cardiac effects of epinephrine are summarized below.

Cardiac Effects of Epinephrine

▶ Increased heart rate (positive chronotropic effect from beta 1)

▶ Increased contraction strength (positive inotropic effect from beta 1)

▶ Increased conduction velocity (positive dromotropic effect from beta 1)

▶ Increased arterial tone (i.e., vascular resistance from alpha stimulation)

▶ Increased blood pressure (by way of enhanced cardiac output and increased systemic vascular resistance, mixed beta and alpha effects)

▶ Increased coronary and cerebral perfusion during CPR (increased vascular tone from alpha stimulation)

▶ Increased electrical activity in the heart (beta 1 effects)

▶ Increased myocardial oxygen demand (as a result of the myocardium working harder)

In the cardiac emergency setting, the alpha properties are the chief reason for the use of epinephrine: Because it increases vascular tone, it will increase blood flow to the heart and brain during compressions. But its beta effects are also beneficial, since it may initiate electrical activity in a heart that has none. In addition, epinephrine is also thought to increase the coarseness of ventricular fibrillation, lending it more receptive to defibrillation attempts.

A final important consideration is that epinephrine normally degrades rapidly in the body. For this reason, it is necessary to administer epinephrine to the patient at continuous short intervals to keep the blood levels in a therapeutic range.

Epinephrine: Indications

Epinephrine is indicated in any patient who requires extensive cardiopulmonary resuscitation. And since the alpha properties are so desirable, it is commonly the first drug (after oxygen) that is administered to every patient in complete cardiac arrest—regardless of the underlying rhythm causing the arrest. The only current exception to this is when vasopressin (to be discussed later) is administered following the first three defibrillations in ventricular fibrillation. Despite this, in the overwhelming majority of times, epinephrine is still the first medication to administer.

Epinephrine: Side Effects/Precautions

As mentioned in the beginning of this chapter, when you understand how a drug works, you can also understand the potential side effects and/or precautions. If you bear in mind the strong alpha and beta effects of epinephrine, it will be obvious why the side effects are those that are typical of strong sympathetic stimulation. The awake patient may demonstrate palpitations, tremors, anxiety, headache, dizziness, even nausea and vomiting. More severely, the patient may complain of chest pain if the sympathetic effects of epinephrine increase myocardial oxygen demands beyond the ability of the coronary arteries to supply oxygenated blood. There are few side effects from epinephrine in the cardiac arrest patient. The post-arrest patient may experience hypertension and tachycardia.

Epinephrine, like other catecholamines, can be deactivated if mixed with an alkaline solution. Thus, do not mix epinephrine with drugs like sodium bicarbonate. Also be aware of other medications the patient is taking or receiving. For example, if the patient takes an antidepressant, the effects of epinephrine may be intensified by the synergistic actions of the two drugs.

Since epinephrine increases the workload of the heart it may precipitate additional cardiac dysrhythmias and/or ischemia. Be prepared to manage these emergencies if they should occur.

Epinephrine: Contraindications

Since the administration of epinephrine is mainly reserved for the patient with severe cardiovascular instability, there are no real contraindications in the emergency setting when it is administered via intravenous bolus. Be aware, however, that epinephrine may also be given via infusion, and with that mode of administration there are additional considerations.

Epinephrine: Dosages

There is a very important delineation to make here: Parenteral epinephrine is commonly packaged in two strengths, each containing the same amount of drug. The 1:10,000 concentration has one milligram of epinephrine in 10 ml of solution in a prefilled syringe. This is the common packaging for intravenous use. Epinephrine also comes packaged as a 1:1,000 ampule, which is one milligram of drug in 1 ml of solution. Obviously then, the latter packaging has the same dose but is more concentrated (1 mg in 1,000 parts of water versus 1 mg in 10,000 parts of water.)

The 1:1,000 ampule form gives the care provider the ability to administer the same amount of drug with less fluid, or high amounts of the drug with relatively small amounts of fluid. For example, if you were to administer 10 mg of epinephrine using the 1:1,000 concentration, you would administer a total of 10 ml of fluid. Administering the same dose of epinephrine with 1:10,000 would mean administering 100 ml of fluid. As stated above, 1:10,000 is the common strength for intravenous administration. Epinephrine 1:1,000 is more commonly used for administration by tracheal tube when higher dosages are given and when additional fluid may be undesirable.

As mentioned earlier, there are enzymes in the body that constantly degrade epinephrine and decrease its effects. For this reason, epinephrine boluses must be repeated frequently.

The following list identifies the dosing regimen of epinephrine in cardiac arrest. Please note when the different concentrations are applicable.

Cardiac Arrest

▶ 1 mg every 3–5 minutes intravenous push. Consider higher doses of epinephrine (0.2 mg/kg) if several attempts of the traditional dose fail.

▶ When administering the drug via IV push, follow the dose with a 20 cc flush and raise the arm to speed venous return to the core circulation. If doses are administered via the tracheal route, use 2–2.5 times the normal IV dose. A 1:1,000 concentration should be used, diluting the dose to 10 cc prior to administration. If possible, use the tracheal route only when no IV is available and only until a patent IV is established.

Symptomatic Bradycardia

▶ 1 µg/min titrated to the desired hemodynamic response (2 to 10 µg/min). Prepare the infusion by adding 1 mg of 1:1,000 epi to 500 ml of normal saline.

Vasopressin

Vasopressin: Mechanism of Action

Vasopressin normally acts as an antidiuretic hormone that occurs naturally in the body. But studies have shown that when administered at a much higher dose, it has the additional property of causing vascular smooth muscle contraction which would elevate systemic vascular resistance. Although it has a clinical response similar to that of alpha stimulation, it does not cause vascular vasoconstriction via direct adrenergic stimulation of alpha receptor sites. It does stimulate V_1 receptor sites in vascular smooth muscle which promotes this elevation in systemic vascular resistance. Its vasoconstrictive properties affect primarily blood vessels found in the skin, muscle, intestinal system, and adipose tissues, and to a minimal extent, the coronary vascular beds. Vasopressin was found to have a beneficial effect in maintaining coronary blood flow during CPR, which is conducive to successful arrest management.

Vasopressin: Indications

Studies have shown that vasopressin can be a useful agent to pharmacologically promote vasoconstriction during periods of cardiac arrest. It should not be used concurrently with epinephrine during arrest management. Vasopressin's use is considered to be an alternative to epinephrine administration during initial management of ventricular fibrillation in the cardiac arrest patient. It has also seen some utilization as a vasoconstrictive agent in hemodynamically unstable vasodilatory shock (for example, septic shock), refractory to more traditional therapy. However, this last indication is not warranted in the prehospital environment.

Vasopressin: Side Effects and Precautions

Side effects would be those consistent with increased vascular tone, and include nausea, intestinal cramps, possible vomiting, urge to defecate, and potentially bronchial vasoconstriction. Additionally, the increased systemic vascular resistance promoted by this drug may increase myocardial workload, which in turn, increases the demand for oxygen. In the absence of adequate coronary perfusion following administration, this could elicit cardiac ischemia or infarction.

Vasopressin should be used with caution in patients who are either pregnant, (it can produce uterine contraction) or who have coronary artery disease (because the vasoconstrictive action would further reduce blood flow in these patients whose arteries are already partially blocked). Fortunately, when administered in the prehospital setting to a patient in ventricular fibrillation, neither of the aforementioned precautions apply.

Vasopressin: Contraindications

As with any drug, hypersensitivity would obviously be a contraindication. Otherwise, in the emergent prehospital setting, no other contraindications exist.

Vasopressin: Dosage

Currently, the prehospital administration of vasopressin is reserved exclusively as an alternative agent for epinephrine in the patient in ventricular fibrillation. In this situation it is used, like epinephrine, for its vasopressive properties. Vasopressin should not, however, be administered concurrently with epinephrine. Since the half-life of vasopressin is thought to be about 10–20 minutes, the continued administration of epinephrine should come 10–20 minutes after vasopressin in the absence of any clinical response. Finally, since the use of vasopressin has not been clinically studied for other arrest rhythms (asystole, PEA), it is only to be administered to the patient in ventricular fibrillation/pulseless ventricular tachycardia.

Specifically, the dosage of vasopressin is a single dose of 40 U via intravenous push for a patient in cardiac arrest with a presenting rhythm of V-fib or pulseless V-tach. Ten to twenty minutes following the administration of vasopressin, revert back to the IV dose of epinephrine (1 mg) every 3–5 minutes for the duration of the rhythm.

Norepinephrine

Norepinephrine: Mechanism of Action

Norepinephrine is an endogenous catecholamine similar to epinephrine. Norepinephrine is a potent vasoconstrictor (arterial and venous) that achieves this effect by profoundly stimulating the alpha receptors of the sympathetic nervous system. Norepinephrine also exhibits some stimulation of the beta receptors and may, therefore, increase the heart rate and contractility of the myocardium. However, such stimulation is slight and is not considered the primary action of norepinephrine.

Norepinephrine: Indications

Norepinephrine is indicated for severe cardiogenic shock and hemodynamically significant hypotension (B/P < 70 mmHg) that is refractory to other means of stabilization. In these situations this drug is considered to be a last resort. As a result of norepinephrine's ability to promote arterial and venous vasoconstriction, norepinephrine facilitates a desirable increase in blood pressure. As mentioned, norepinephrine is considered in cases of cardiogenic shock or hypotension that do not respond to other agents such as dopamine or fluid challenges. Rarely, then, will norepinephrine be used by the prehospital provider of advanced cardiac life support.

Norepinephrine: Side Effects and Precautions

When norepinephrine is being administered, it is paramount to monitor the blood pressure throughout administration (every 5 to 10 minutes) so as to prevent a dangerous hypertensive state. In the case of hypertension, norepinephrine is traditionally titrated down to a dosage that results in a more desirable blood pressure.

Norepinephrine stimulates the sympathetic nervous system. Side effects include nervousness, anxiety, tremors, headache, dizziness, nausea, and vomiting. As with other sympathomimetic drugs, norepinephrine is deactivated when mixed in any alkaline solution.

Conversely, the effects of norepinephrine can be potentiated when administered with other drugs that promote similar action. For example, a dangerous state of hypertension can be induced when delivering norepinephrine concomitantly with beta blockers. Recall that blocking the beta receptors located on the arterial blood vessels will cause vasoconstriction and increase blood pressure. As norepinephrine accomplishes the same effect through a different mechanism, administration of both agents can prove devastating.

Norepinephrine predominantly stimulates the alpha receptors, but some beta receptor stimulation may occur. While this is not the primary mechanism of action, it may promote an increased myocardial workload. Consequently, it is prudent to administer supplemental oxygen to patients with profound hypotension who are receiving norepinephrine to counteract any myocardial ischemia that might result from an increase in heart rate and contractility. Similarly, dysrhythmias may also occur and should be addressed on an individual basis.

Norepinephrine: Contraindications

As discussed under "Indications," norepinephrine is a *late* intervention used in the treatment of hypoperfusion. This means that more appropriate, less invasive means of treating hypotension should be attempted prior to the administration of norepinephrine. Norepinephrine is never used in the long-term treatment of hypoperfusion.

Volume depletion should be addressed with volume replacement. Decreased vascular tone is first treated by the administration of dopamine rather than norepinephrine. If these interventions fail, norepinephrine can then be tried. Some authorities allow for the use of norepinephrine in cases of volume-related hypotension, but only as a temporary measure until adequate volume is achieved.

Norepinephrine: Dosage

Norepinephrine is delivered by intravenous infusion. Norepinephrine may cause tissue necrosis (tissue death) and should be administered into the largest vein possible so as to avoid infiltration.

Norepinephrine should be given within the dose range of 0.5 to 30 µg/minute. Mixing 4 mg of norepinephrine in 250 cc of D_5W or normal saline yields a concentration of 16 µg/cc. Initially, norepinephrine should be infused at 0.5 to 1.0 µg/minute. From this beginning point, the dose can be titrated upward to the desired effect.

If more than 20 to 30 µg/minute are needed, using dopamine with norepinephrine is permissible. A mechanical infusion pump should be used to achieve precise delivery of norepinephrine.

Isoproterenol

Isoproterenol: Mechanism of Action

Isoproterenol is a sympathetic agonist that can be used in the treatment of refractory bradycardic emergencies. As a synthetic catecholamine, isoproterenol primarily stimulates the beta 1 and beta 2 receptors of the sympathetic nervous system.

When stimulated, beta 1 receptors produce an overall increase in the rate and contractile strength of the heart. In response, cardiac output increases and improved perfusion should ensue. Isoproterenol also affects the beta 2 receptors located in the bronchiole and vascular smooth muscle. Stimulation of the beta 2 receptors promotes vasodilation and relaxation of the pulmonary bronchioles. Characteristically, this permits more oxygen to flow through the pulmonary tree. The increase in cardiac output is usually enough to offset the slight drop in vascular resistance that results from the peripheral vasodilation in lower doses.

In the treatment of bradycardic emergencies, isoproterenol has generally been replaced by more reliable interventions with fewer negative side effects. Such agents include atropine, dopamine, and transcutaneous pacing.

Isoproterenol: Indications

After other interventions prove ineffective, isoproterenol should be used in the temporary treatment of hemodynamically significant bradycardia. Direct stimulation of the cardiac beta 1 receptors will increase the rate and stroke volume of the heart and facilitate a greater cardiac output.

Isoproterenol has shown some promise in the treatment of bradycardia as it pertains to the transplanted heart. A problem with transplanted hearts is a relative lack of innervation from the autonomic nervous system. In this situation, giving a drug that will directly stimulate the heart rather than stimulating the autonomic nervous system may be beneficial. Also as a result of its direct stimulatory properties, isoproterenol may be effective in the stabilization of bradycardia that occurs secondary to a more serious heart block. However, it must be emphasized that other interventions have proven more reliable and must be tried prior to the administration of isoproterenol.

The other indication for isoproterenol is for refractory torsades de pointes which is unresponsive first to magnesium sulfate.

Isoproterenol: Side Effects/Precautions

Any drug that increases the workload of the heart also increases the heart's oxygen demands. Isoproterenol is no different. By increasing rate and contractility, isoproterenol causes the heart to require more oxygen to function. If oxygen is not available, myocardial ischemia can present itself. For this reason, be cautious about administering isoproterenol to anyone with ischemic heart disease, in whom it is prone to promote dysrhythmias. Also, isoproterenol can lead to shifts in potassium, resulting in hypokalemia. If profound, this electrolyte disturbance can manifest itself with dysrhythmias. This is most likely to occur with protracted use of the drug in the non-acute setting. Therefore, when isoproterenol is delivered, the electrical rhythm of the heart must be monitored. Should a dysrhythmia develop, deal with it by reducing the dosage of isoproterenol and administering the appropriate drug therapy.

As stated above, beta 2 stimulation can cause vasodilation and lower blood pressure. A drop in blood pressure leads to a decrease in coronary artery perfusion. The concern is that if the refractory bradycardic patient is hypotensive (which is usually the case), isoproterenol may aggravate the blood pressure. Despite this, when used with extreme caution in lower doses, it may be beneficial. It is paramount to remain vigilant to blood pressure when isoproterenol is used.

Isoproterenol: Contraindications

As with any bradycardia, the slow rhythm should never be treated pharmacologically unless it is hemodynamically significant. Treat the patient, not the monitor!

Additionally, isoproterenol should *never* be used as a *first-line* intervention in the treatment of hemodynamically significant bradycardia. Newer agents and interventions with fewer negative side effects than isoproterenol have proven more effective in the treatment and stabilization of bradycardic emergencies.

Isoproterenol: Dosage

Isoproterenol is administered as an IV infusion and is constituted by mixing 1 mg of the drug in 250 cc of D_5W. This mixture yields a concentration of 4 µg/cc and should be delivered through a microdrip administration device or with an infusion pump.

Isoproterenol should be administered within the range of 2–10 µg/minute. The higher the dosage, the greater opportunity for adverse side effects. Therefore, the administered dosage should be titrated to the lowest possible amount that achieves the desired hemodynamic effect. Often, this equates to a heart rate of approximately 60 beats per minute or a blood pressure of >90 mmHg. As with other infusions, administration of isoproterenol must be precise and requires an infusion pump for exact delivery.

The dosing of isoproterenol in refractory torsades de pointes follows the same infusion range; however titration of the medication upwards should only occur until the VT is suppressed or a maximum of 10 µg/minute is given.

Dopamine

Dopamine: Mechanism of Action

Dopamine is a naturally occurring catecholamine that is a chemical precursor to norepinephrine. Dopamine stimulates the sympathetic nervous system by interacting with the dopaminergic, alpha, and beta receptor sites. By doing so, dopamine promotes vasoconstriction and increased myocardial contractility without producing tremendous increases in the heart rate. The net result is an increase in blood pressure without straining the heart by significantly raising its rate. In addition, dopamine is thought to also possibly enhance perfusion to the kidneys and abdominal organs through stimulation of dopaminergic receptors. Because of these properties, dopamine is the most commonly used agent in symptomatic states of hypoperfusion.

Dopamine: Indications

The etiology of hypoperfusion must always be considered prior to treatment. If hypovolemia exists due to fluid depletion, volume replacement should be attempted first in the prehospital environment. If the hypotension exists secondary to bradycardia, the first attempts must address correcting the slow rhythm so as to establish an acceptable rate for a normal cardiac output and blood pressure. If hypoperfusion is the result of decreased myocardial contractility or loss of vascular tone or does not respond to the previous measures, then a dopamine infusion should be started.

In addition, dopamine should be administered for residual hypotension following the return of spontaneous circulation post cardiac arrest.

Dopamine: Side Effects/Precautions

Side effects with dopamine depend on the dose. (See the detailed discussion of dosages below.) At moderate to high dosages, cardiac dysrhythmias or hypertension may occur. The drug should be used cautiously if there are preexisting tachydysrhythmias as well. Dysrhythmias or an excessive acceleration of the heart rate will increase oxygen demand and, with an already-impaired heart, myocardial ischemia becomes an issue. It may be necessary to increase the inspired concentration of oxygen (FiO_2) in this setting.

Since dopamine directly stimulates the sympathetic nervous system, many side effects related to the sympathetic nervous system may become evident. These include:

- ▶ Nervousness
- ▶ Headaches
- ▶ Palpitations
- ▶ Chest pain
- ▶ Dyspnea
- ▶ Nausea/vomiting

Also, because it causes vasoconstriction, dopamine can worsen pulmonary congestion. As the heart is presented with a greater preload and afterload, it may not be able to eject all the blood. Consequently, an increase in hydrostatic pressure in the pulmonary vessels may increase the difficulty in breathing.

Dopamine can cause adverse reactions when administered with some other medications. Dopamine and Dilantin®, when used simultaneously, can cause acute hypertension. When administering dopamine with a monoamine oxidase (MAO) inhibitor, a type of antidepressant, administer one-tenth the normal dose of dopamine. Furthermore, as with norepinephrine, dopamine is chemically inactivated when combined with an alkaline substance such as sodium bicarbonate. When discontinuing a dopamine infusion (as with any vasoactive infusion), gradually taper off the administration so as to avoid acute hypotension.

Dopamine: Contraindications

In symptomatic hypotension, dopamine is always contraindicated before an attempt has been made to correct the underlying abnormality. However, if an attempt has been made and proven ineffective, dopamine should be considered.

Dopamine is relatively contradicted in the presence of symptomatic hypotension with pulmonary congestion. In such situations the fear is that, as mentioned above, dopamine will worsen pulmonary congestion and inhibit the exchange of oxygen and carbon dioxide at the alveolar-capillary interface. However, this must be weighed against the benefits of improved myocardial contractility. As a practical matter, dopamine is often used in patients with pulmonary edema. Carefully think through the effects of dopamine and, if it is applicable, use the drug at the lowest possible dose that proves effective.

Dopamine: Dosages

Dopamine is administered through an IV infusion within the range of 1–20 μg/kg/minute, although more traditionally the prehospital provider will be administering doses within a range of 5–20 μg/kg/minute. As stated earlier, the effects that dopamine produces are considered to be dose-dependent. Simplistically, dopamine dosages can be broken down into the following ranges:

- ▶ *1–5 μg/kg/minute: "Low" Dose*—At this dosage, dopamine was once thought to result in dopaminergic receptor activity in the kidneys and abdomen. Its use for this has been discredited in some literature, and it is currently not used at this range in the prehospital environment.

- ▶ *5–10 μg/kg/minute: "Moderate" or "Cardiac" Dose*—Dopamine administered at this level predominantly interacts with the cardiac beta receptors. The net effects are an observable increase in contractility and increases in the heart rate. Through an increase in cardiac output, blood pressure is also increased. In addition, some stimulation of alpha receptors occurs, causing some vasoconstriction. This action enhances an increase in blood pressure as well.

▶ *10–20 µg/kg/minute: "High" or "Vasopressor" Dose*—At this higher dose of dopamine, alpha receptors are primarily stimulated. In response, there is an overwhelming constriction of the arterial and venous vasculature amounting to an increase in blood pressure.

To prepare an infusion, mix 400–800 mg of dopamine in 250 cc of D_5W. This mixture yields a concentration of 1600 µg/cc or 3200 µg/cc respectively, which should be titrated to the lowest possible dose that achieves the desired effect. At dosages greater than 20 µg/kg/minute, norepinephrine can be added to the dopamine for an increased effect. Like most infusions for advanced cardiac life support, an infusion pump should be used for precise delivery.

Dobutamine

Dobutamine: Mechanism of Action

Dobutamine is another drug used in the treatment of hypotension and low cardiac output, but not routinely in the prehospital environment by the advanced life support provider. Similar to dopamine, dobutamine stimulates the sympathetic nervous system. However, unlike dopamine, dobutamine is a synthetic agent that primarily stimulates the beta 1 receptors located within the myocardium and beta 2 receptors located on the smooth muscle of the bronchioles and peripheral blood vessels.

While dobutamine does stimulate the alpha receptors also found on the myocardium and peripheral blood vessels, this stimulation is insignificant when compared with the beta stimulation that predominates. For this reason, dobutamine produces a greater myocardial contraction with a mild vasodilatory response. Consequently, the heart's work load is eased as increased contractility is balanced by a reduced afterload.

Dobutamine will characteristically induce production of endogenous norepinephrine as the dose increases. When released, the norepinephrine stimulates the sympathetic nervous system in a profound manner. For this reason, at higher dosages, dobutamine may produce an accelerated heart rate *and* increased peripheral resistance. An accelerated response can strain the myocardium and increase its oxygen demands. Therefore, be cognizant of the need for constant monitoring and supplemental oxygen.

Dobutamine: Indications

The ability of dobutamine to increase contractility while dilating the peripheral vascular system makes dobutamine an ideal choice for patients who have pulmonary congestion without significant symptoms of hypoperfusion with a concurrent blood pressure of 70–100 mmHg. In this situation, dobutamine serves to increase the cardiac output while ejecting blood through a lower resistance in the vascular system. Since the dilated vascular system also serves as a reservoir, blood is shifted from the pulmonary vessels into the peripheral vascular system. It is recommended, however, that the endpoints for dobutamine administration be based upon clinical response rather than dose. As such, hemodynamic monitoring is employed to assess the hemodynamic endpoints of enhanced cardiac output and the most advantageous organ system perfusion. This recommended monitoring system, however, eliminates the use of dobutamine as a common medication in the prehospital environment. In the hospital, dobutamine can be considered in the short-term management of patients with congestive heart failure (CHF) or those with left ventricular failure who are unable to tolerate potent vasodilators.

Dobutamine: Side Effects/Precautions

As previously mentioned, dobutamine at higher dosages may produce tachydysrhythmias. A faster heart rate demands more oxygen and, if additional oxygen is not readily available, myocardial ischemia can occur. Additionally, high-dose dobutamine has been known to induce nervousness, hypertension, chest pain, and nausea and vomiting.

Dobutamine: Contraindications

Similar to norepinephrine and dopamine, dobutamine is not indicated in the treatment of symptomatic hypotension until after other treatments have been executed that are geared directly toward correcting the underlying abnormality. And even when volume replacement or correction of a slow heart rate have proven ineffective at increasing cardiac output, dopamine is more reliable and therefore preferred over dobutamine in the stabilization of hypoperfusion.

Dobutamine: Dosage

Dobutamine is not a drug that is administered in the prehospital setting due to the difficulty in achieving optimal dosage (given the inability for central hemodynamic monitoring). It is usually given as an inotropic agent in the hospital for severe left ventricular failure. It may also be considered when the patient is in need of a vasopressor agent but concurrently has pulmonary hypertension (dobutamine does not usually increase pulmonary pressures to the degree that dopamine does).

Part Three: Sympatholytics

The suffix *-lytic,* commonly means to block or inhibit. So when combined with the root word *sympatho-,* the literal meaning is to block the effects of the sympathetic nervous system. Sympatholytics are a unique class of drug that does not exert a specific physiologic action itself; rather it merely inhibits the effects of the catecholamines by occupying the alpha or beta receptor sites of the sympathetic nervous system. This "antagonistic" effect may be exerted on both alpha and beta receptors, on alpha receptors only, or on beta receptors only. The drugs discussed next are known as "beta blockers"; that is, they are sympatholytics that specifically antagonize the beta receptor sites of the sympathetic nervous system.

Beta Blockers

Beta Blockers: Mechanism of Action

Beta blockers antagonize and block the stimulation of the beta receptors. This decreases the heart rate, myocardial contractility, and blood pressure and also decreases the overall workload and oxygen consumption of the myocardium.

Beta blockers also reduce electrical conduction through the AV node and are thus useful in controlling ventricular responses to detrimental atrial rhythms. In addition, since many dysrhythmias occur in response to increased sympathetic activity, beta blockers help prevent the occurrence of such dysrhythmias by blocking the uptake of sympathomimetic catecholamines.

It has been shown through controlled studies that the use of beta blockers in patients experiencing high risk angina, MI, or those who are post-MI all benefit with reductions in the incidences of common complications such as dysrhythmias, reinfarction, or recurrent ischemia.

Beta Blockers: Indications

Beta blockers are used in the control of ventricular tachycardia, PSVT dysrhythmias, and incidences of myocardial ischemia/infarction. In that these disturbances are often related to the circulation of endogenous catecholamines, the blockage of beta receptors can prevent the occurrence of such dysrhythmias. Within the hospital setting, they have also been used in conjunction with fibrinolytic therapy for acute myocardial infarction. Beta blockers are also useful in the long term treatment of a myocardial infarction. As stated above, beta blockers decrease the overall workload and oxygen consumption of the heart. Because an infarction occurs secondary to a mismatch between myocardial oxygen supplies and demands, beta blockers are quite effective in the reduction of mortality following an MI.

In the prehospital setting they are used primarily in the acute management of tachydysrhythmias that present hemodynamically unstable. Commonly, the administration of beta blockers in this clinical situation follows the first line administration of adenosine (or possibly diltiazem). They (specifically labetalol) have also been used in the prehospital setting for the immediate management of a hypertensive crisis.

Beta Blockers: Side Effects/Precautions

Beta blockers can have adverse effects. If the heart rate and contractility are decreased excessively, hypotension and pulmonary congestion can ensue. A patient could also become bradycardic or hypotensive following administration.

Also recall that there are beta receptors on the bronchiole smooth muscle. Inhibiting stimulation of these receptors can precipitate serious bronchospasm. Therefore, you must be aware of any history of asthma, COPD, or congestive heart failure when you contemplate using beta blockers for cardiac situations. As with many other drugs, the effects of beta blockers can be potentiated when combined with drugs of a similar nature, or with drugs that produce a similar clinical response (e.g., calcium channel blockers).

Beta Blockers: Contraindications

Beta blockers are contraindicated in situations where beta receptor stimulation is necessary for normal function. Such situations would include:

▶ Preexisting bradycardia
▶ History of asthma
▶ History of COPD
▶ Congestive heart failure

Blocking the beta receptors may worsen the above situations and cause detrimental complications. Other contraindications include a spontaneous heart rate < 60 bpm, a systolic blood pressure < 100 mmHg, the presence of an atrioventricular conduction defect, or clinically significant hypotension.

Beta Blockers: Dosages

There are several different types of beta blockers commonly used in the prehospital and hospital environments. The route of administration is IV, but dosages vary.

Some of the more common beta blockers, and their dosages, include the following (as always, be familiar with the specific indications for, and the beta blockers used within, your local EMS system):

Esmolol

Esmolol, a rapidly acting beta blocker with a relatively short duration, is administered via an IV infusion.

▶ *IV administration*—initially provide a loading infusion of 500 µg/kg over a 1-minute time frame, followed by a maintenance infusion of 50 µg/kg/min. If the clinical response is inadequate after 4 minutes of maintenance therapy, repeat the loading infusion at 500 µg/kg over 1 minute, and increase the maintenance infusion by 50 µg/kg/min. Repeat with this dosing schedule until either you max out the infusion at 300 µg/kg/min, or resolution of the ectopy or the desired effect occurs.

As an IV infusion, a final concentration of 10 mg/ml is recommended. This is best accomplished by placing 2.5 grams of the drug (one 10-ml ampule), into a 250 ml bag of D_5W.

Atenolol

▶ *IV administration*—5 mg IV push over 5 minutes. If the patient requires it, another 5 mg over 5 minutes can be given 10 minutes later.

Metoprolol

▶ *IV administration*—5 mg IV push over 2–5 minutes. The drug can be readministered twice at 5-minute intervals for a total dose of 15 mg.

Labetalol

▶ *IV administration*—10 mg IV push over 1–2 minutes. The drug can be readministered at the same or doubled dose every 10 minutes to a maximum allowance of 150 mg. Another recommended dosage is to administer a maximum initial dose of 150 mg IV push, and then initiate an infusion at 2–8 µg/min.

Part Four: Antidysrhythmics

Antidysrhythmics is the general classification for those drugs that help to correct disturbances in the heart's electrical activity. First, they may be used to eliminate cardiac conduction disturbances that interfere with the heart's normal rhythm (i.e., rhythm control). Secondly, they may be used to correct some abnormality in the heart's rate if it becomes too fast or too slow (i.e., rate control). Under "Rhythm Control" and "Rate Control," you will find a series of agents that may or may not exert a similar action, but have a common physiologic result.

Rhythm Control

Amiodarone

Amiodarone: Mechanism of Action

Amiodarone is a newer drug available for cardiovascular emergencies that has shown to be very effective with multiple types of dysrhythmias when administered for specific indications. Like many other drugs used in cardiovascular emergencies, amiodarone also exerts its complex actions though mediation of ionic movement. In this situation, the drug affects the actions of sodium, potassium, and calcium across cellular walls during depolarization. These actions enable amiodarone to inhibit abnormal automaticity within the heart, prolong the refractory period of the conduction system, and slow sinus node discharge and junctional node conduction rate. Through added properties of adrenergic blockade of alpha and beta receptors, it acts to depress both atrial and ventricular tachydysrhythmias, and can result in some peripheral vasodilation.

Amiodarone: Indications

Due to amiodarone's extensive range of actions, it has application to many cardiovascular emergencies during prehospital stabilization and transport to the emergency department. These include both atrial and ventricular tachydysrhythmias and cardiac arrest with evidence of ventricular dysrhythmias. Since amiodarone has such a variety of clinical actions, the prehospital provider of advanced cardiac life support must become familiar with their system's utilization of this drug. Specifically, indications for amiodarone can include:

▶ Ventricular fibrillation and pulseless ventricular tachycardia resistant to electrical therapy

▶ Monomorphic and polymorphic ventricular tachycardia with a pulse (stable and unstable)

▶ Wide complex tachycardia of unknown etiology

▶ Supraventricular tachycardias

Amiodarone: Side Effects/Precautions

Side effects become more evident if the drug is administered rapidly in a perfusing patient, so this should be avoided. Also, amiodarone can be *prodysrhythmic* (which means the drug could *cause* dysrhythmias). As such, you will usually administer only one specific agent for rhythm control to avoid the synergistic effect of multiple drugs with similar actions. As an example, it is recommended to exercise caution when administering this drug if another agent which prolongs the QT interval (such as procainamide) is administered. Since amiodarone also has vasodilitory effects, it may induce or exacerbate hypotension. Another way in which amiodarone can contribute to possible hypotension is through its beta antagonistic properties, which can reduce the inotropy of the heart and result in a diminished cardiac output. Finally, amiodarone may increase to toxic levels in the bloodstream should the patient have renal failure, so exercise caution in such cases.

Since amiodarone can induce or worsen hypotension or bradycardia, it is important to know what to do if these outcomes occur. Should either or both occur in your patient following administration of amiodarone, it is recommended first to slow the infusion rate. If hypotension occurs, consider either fluid administration or careful use of vasopressors. If bradycardia is present, that can be countered with an agent to increase the rate (e.g., atropine), or consider transcutaneous pacing.

Amiodarone: Contraindications

An understanding of the contraindications of this drug is simply an extrapolation of its actions. Since this drug slows conduction in the heart, patients with bradycardia induced by sick sinus syndrome, a second-degree AV block (Mobitz I or Mobitz II), or a complete third-degree AV block should *not* be given amiodarone. Likewise, the drug has a negative inotropic action and vasodilatory effects, so its use should be avoided in the patient with clinically significant hypotension. If the patient has a known hypersensitivity to the drug, its use should also be avoided.

Amiodarone: Dosages

As mentioned under "Indications," there are numerous instances when amiodarone can be administered. And the hemodynamic status of the patient may also influence the rate of administration (recall that rapid infusions may precipitate hypotension in susceptible patients). Given the indicated dysrhythmia that is present in the patient, the following identifies three different dosage regimens that could be considered:

> ▶ If the patient is in cardiac arrest (i.g., V-Fib/pulseless V-Tach)
>   – administer 300 mg of the drug via IVP. Repeat at 150 mg via IVP in 3–5 minutes if the dysrhythmias persists.
> ▶ If the patient displays ventricular tachycardia, wide complex tachycardia, or supraventricular tachycardia, and is *hemodynamically stable*
>   – *rapid infusion* is 150 mg administered via IV line over a 10-minute period (which equates to 15 mg/min).
> ▶ If the patient displays ventricular tachycardia, wide complex tachycardia, or supraventricular tachycardia, *and is hemodynamically unstable following cardioversion, OR, if the patient develops bradycardia or hypotension while administering the "rapid infusion" dose*
>   – *slow infusion* of 360 mg of the drug mixed in 5% dextrose and water, and administered over a six-hour period (which equates to 1 mg/min).

The first two above-mentioned doses are considered to be "loading doses" for amiodarone. That is, the administration procedure quickly elevates the blood level of the drug into a therapeutic range so the desired effect is achieved. However, due to degradation of the drug in the body, it is necessary to initiate a "maintenance infusion" to maintain blood levels of the drug in this therapeutic range in order to maintain dysrhythmia suppression once it was achieved. The maintenance infusion for amiodarone is:

> ▶ 1 mg/min via constant IV infusion to a max daily dose (24 hours) of 2.2 grams

It is important to remember that this drug can produce significant side effects or become dangerously toxic if the administration procedure is not strictly adhered to. The use of an infusion pump is strongly recommended. Also, do not initiate a maintenance infusion until the dysrhythmia is abolished by the loading dose. Since a loading dose may be repeated in certain situations, the concurrent administration of both loading doses and maintenance infusions could elevate the serum blood levels to a fatally toxic point.

Lidocaine

Lidocaine: Mechanism of Action

Lidocaine is a drug used by prehospital providers for patients with ventricular irritability, but it is commonly second line to other agents such as amiodarone and procainamide. Ventricular irritability is evident by the frequency and appearance of premature ventricular contractions or independent ventricular rhythms on the ECG tracing.

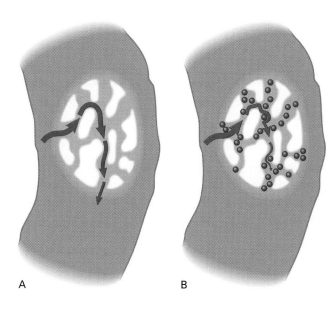

FIGURE 8–3
Conduction through ischemic myocardial tissue. White areas are islands of tissue that are severely depressed and no longer excitable. Gray areas surrounding these islands are also depressed but still excitable. They conduct electrical impulses at reduced velocities. In (A), before lidocaine administration, the electrical impulse, though conducted at reduced velocity, is able to continue through the ischemic area and re-emerge into the normal myocardial tissue, In (B), lidocaine has been administered and has further depressed conduction velocity to the extent that the electrical impulse is blocked and unable to re-emerge into normal myocardial tissue.

A   B

Lidocaine exerts numerous actions to achieve its antidysrhythmic effects. It depresses the conduction velocity through ischemic tissue and depresses the increased automaticity seen with ischemic tissue. These effects can inhibit ventricular rhythms by blocking the conduction wave in areas of ischemia (so it can't re-emerge to excite surrounding tissue) as depicted in Figure 8-3, and it can eliminate ventricular rhythms caused by changes in automaticity of ischemic tissue by depressing phase 4 of spontaneous depolarization as shown in Figure 8-4.

Lidocaine also raises the ventricular fibrillation threshold, thus making it harder for the heart to go into ventricular fibrillation. This is analogous to raising a dam against water flow. As the dam gets higher (raising the threshold), it blocks the water from overflowing; as lidocaine increases the threshold, V-fib is less likely to occur. Finally, lidocaine has little effect on atrial tissue, nor on SA and AV node function, at therapeutic doses. As such, lidocaine does not harm atrial or AV activity when used for ventricular irritability, nor is it useful for atrial dysrhythmias.

Lidocaine: Indications

As mentioned above, lidocaine is one of many drugs that could be used for ventricular irritability in need of suppression, and commonly may not be the first ventricular antidysrhythmic indicated. The following list identifies the uses for lidocaine, but become familiar with your agency's protocol regarding lidocaine usage:

Perfusing Rhythms

▶ Monomorphic ventricular tachycardia (stable and unstable)

▶ Polymorphic ventricular tachycardia (stable and unstable)

— with normal QT interval

— with prolonged QT interval

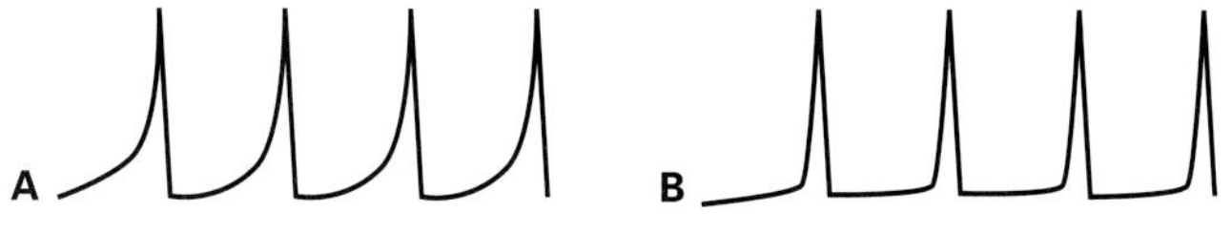

A   B

FIGURE 8–4
Phase 4 cardiac depolarization. (A), before lidocaine administration, shows normal phase 4 depolarization. (B), after lidocaine administration, shows depressed phase 4 depolarization.

▷ Wide complex tachycardia of uncertain type

▷ Occasionally for malignant PVCs

Non-perfusing (Arrest) Rhythms

▷ Ventricular fibrillation

▷ Pulseless ventricular tachycardia

Lidocaine: Side Effects/Precautions

Side effects become more evident as the amount of drug administered increases. At therapeutic doses, lidocaine has minimal side effects of concern. However, at greater dosages lidocaine toxicity manifests itself, primarily in the central nervous system (CNS). The patient may display:

▷ Drowsiness

▷ Irritability

▷ Disorientation

▷ Muscle twitching

▷ Seizures

▷ Bradycardia

▷ Coma (including death)

Precaution should be taken when administering lidocaine to a patient who may have depressed liver function. Regardless of the cause of the dysfunction (e.g., age over 70 years, hepatic disease, hypoperfusion, acute MI), there will be a delay in clearing the lidocaine from the body. This will result in serum levels increasing to toxic levels should the drug be administered continually. In this instance, the maintenance infusion of lidocaine should be reduced by 50%. The loading dose remains the same, since the body still requires that amount of drug to achieve initial therapeutic levels.

Exercise caution as well with the administration of lidocaine concurrently with procainamide, phenytoin, quinidine, and beta blockers.

Lidocaine: Contraindications

Lidocaine is contraindicated in second-degree Type II and third-degree (infra-nodal) heart blocks. Many times there is a ventricular rhythm in conjunction with these conduction blocks. It is important for the prehospital provider to realize that these contractions (albeit abnormally wide) are the only perfusing beat the patient has! If they are abolished by lidocaine or any other ventricular antidysrhythmic considered, the patient may well go into cardiac arrest. This is also true for ventricular escape rhythms.

The same applies for extreme bradycardia with frequent PVCs or other forms of ventricular ectopy. The PVCs may be the body's attempt to maintain cardiac output in the face of the bradycardic rhythm, and abolishing them with lidocaine will worsen the cardiac output. Always remember to treat the rate first with atropine and pacing, then take care of the ventricular rhythms if they persist with a heart rate >60/minute.

Lidocaine: Dosages

As mentioned under "Indications," there are numerous instances when lidocaine can be administered, but almost always it's after another more effective ventricular antidysrhythmic fails. It is important to remember that this drug is initially given and considered for repeat only until the ventricular abnormality is corrected. Only after the abnormality is suppressed should a maintenance infusion be initiated. Since lidocaine undergoes hepatic degradation, a constant infusion is necessary to maintain therapeutic blood levels, but only after the boluses achieve the desired effect. In the research literature, there is a wide variance in dosage recommendations. In light of this inconsistency, the following is only one set of administration guidelines for lidocaine by IV bolus or via tracheal tube installation to a patient with refractory ventricular irritability:

Suppression of Persistent Stable or Unstable Monomorphic Ventricular Tachycardia

▶ Administer 1.0 to 1.5 mg/kg IVP or TT (increase TT dose 2–2.5 times). Repeat every 5–10 minutes at half the initial dose (0.5–0.75 mg/kg). Follow this dosing schedule until 3 mg/kg total cumulative dose has been administered.

Suppression of Persistent Stable or Unstable Polymorphic Ventricular Tachycardia (Normal or Prolonged QT Interval)

▶ Administer 1.0 to 1.5 mg/kg IVP or TT (increase TT dose 2–2.5 times). Repeat every 5–10 minutes at half the initial dose (0.5–0.75 mg/kg). Follow this dosing schedule until 3 mg/kg total cumulative dose has been administered.

Suppression of Persistent Malignant Premature Ventricular Contractions

▶ Administer 1.0 to 1.5 mg/kg IVP or TT (increase TT dose 2–2.5 times). Repeat every 5–10 minutes at half the initial dose (0.5–0.75 mg/kg). Follow this dosing schedule until 3 mg/kg total cumulative dose has been administered.

Conversion of Persistent Ventricular Fibrillation in Cardiac Arrest

▶ Administer 1.5 mg/kg IVP or TT (increase TT dose 2–2.5 times). Repeat every 5 minutes at the same dose. Follow this dosing schedule until 3 mg/kg total cumulative dose has been administered.

Conversion of Persistent Pulseless Ventricular Tachycardia in Cardiac Arrest

▶ Administer 1.5 mg/kg IVP or TT (increase TT dose 2–2.5 times). Repeat every 5 minutes at the same dose. Follow this dosing schedule until 3 mg/kg total cumulative dose has been administered.

As you have probably noticed, lidocaine administration varies, depending on the hemodynamic status of the patient. Allow the following guidelines to help you simplify the administration of lidocaine when appropriate:

▶ **If the patient has a pulse (hence is perfusing)**
— Give 1.0–1.5 mg/kg, and repeat at 0.5–0.75 mg/kg every 5 minutes to maximum of 3 mg/kg.

▶ **If the patient does not have a pulse (hence cardiac arrest)**
— Give 1.5 mg/kg, and repeat once at same dose after 3–5 minutes.

After the IV bolus(es) of lidocaine have achieved the desired effect, and the patient has a relatively stable rhythm and hemodynamic status, it becomes necessary to institute a maintenance infusion of lidocaine to keep the blood serum levels in an acceptable range. You should start by mixing 2 grams of lidocaine into 500 ml of D_5W to yield a 4 mg/ml concentration. Premixed lidocaine is also available, typically packaged as 2 grams in 500 ml of D_5W. This should be administered with a microdrip infusion set or infusion pump at 1–4 mg/min.

Procainamide

Procainamide: Mechanism of Action

Procainamide is yet another ventricular antidysrhythmic drug useful in the suppression of ventricular irritability. Somewhat like lidocaine, it achieves its desired action by depressing phase 4 of the depolarization sequence, which will slow automaticity. In addition, procainamide can depress the slope of phase 0 of cardiac depolarization, which will naturally slow conduction velocity and possibly block an impulse in an already slowed ischemic tissue, which avoids reentry dysrhythmias. As will be discussed shortly, depression of phase 0 may also result in a negative inotropic effect.

In summary, procainamide can reduce ventricular irritability by slowing automaticity and/or conduction velocity. It could also be used for supraventricular tachydysrhythmias due to its ability to reduce automaticity and impulse velocity through the heart's conduction system.

Procainamide: Indications

Procainamide is another drug in the arsenal for combating dysrhythmias that has been used more often over the past several years. However, like other medications, it may precipitate additional undesirable side effects. Also, it is administered as an infusion, so it may take longer to exert an action compared to IV bolus medication. Despite these drawbacks, it has become a preferred agent in terminating dysrhythmic activity. The following list identifies ventricular problems that procainamide may be useful for when lidocaine is unsuccessful:

Perfusing Rhythms

▶ Monomorphic ventricular tachycardia (stable and unstable)
▶ Polymorphic ventricular tachycardia (stable and unstable)
   — with normal QT interval
▶ Wide complex tachycardia of uncertain type
▶ Occasionally for malignant PVCs

Non-perfusing (Arrest) Rhythms

▶ Ventricular fibrillation
▶ Pulseless ventricular tachycardia

Procainamide: Side Effects/Precautions

One of the most significant side effects of procainamide is its negative inotropic effect, which results from depression of phase 0 of depolarization. This slowing of conduction speed has the tendency to also weaken the contraction force, which results in reduced ejection from the ventricles and possibly hypotension. (Hypotension is exacerbated by the fact that procainamide also has a vasodilatory effect.) If hypotension ensues, the procainamide infusion should be eliminated.

Additionally, the depressive effects of procainamide on the cardiac conduction system may result in a widening of the QRS complex. (As phase 0 is flattened, the QRS will be widened and the force of contraction weakened.) Therefore, during procainamide administration, the QRS, P-R, and QT intervals should be monitored for widening. If any interval widens by >50% from its pretreatment width, the procainamide infusion should be stopped.

Procainamide: Contraindications

As with lidocaine, procainamide should not be used if the ventricular dysrhythmia exists with bradycardia. In these instances, the slow rate should be normalized by atropine and pacing first. Additionally, since procainamide has the ability to slow conduction speed, its use in a patient with a conduction disturbance (e.g., second-degree Type II or third-degree block) should be avoided. As well, preexisting hypotension should be a reason to avoid procainamide.

Procainamide: Dosage

Since procainamide is to be administered via infusion, this results in a slow onset of action; effects should be seen in about 5–15 minutes. When treating a patient with the indicated dysrhythmias and other appropriate treatment, a procainamide loading infusion should be initiated at 20–30 mg/min until a maximum dose of 17 mg/kg is achieved. The following outlines a simple approach to procainamide administration:

1. Compute the total amount of drug allowed (multiply the patient's weight in kilograms by 17).
2. Add that amount of drug to a small amount of D_5W (50–100 ml). This places the maximum amount of drug into the D_5W. The benefit is that once the bag is empty you know the maximum dose has been administered.
3. Compute the math for administering the drug at 20–30 mg/min.
4. Stop the loading infusion when one of the following occurs:
   — Ventricular dysrhythmia is abolished.
   — Maximum dose is achieved (17 mg/kg or bag is emptied).
   — QRS, QT, or PR interval widens by 50% of pretreatment width.
   — Hypotension ensues.

If the rhythm is abolished by the procainamide loading dose, stop the loading dose administration and initiate a maintenance infusion to maintain therapeutic blood levels. This is achieved by placing 2 grams of procainamide into 500 ml of D_5W to yield 4 mg/ml. This is then attached to a microdrip administration set (or infusion pump) and infused at 1–4 mg/min (15–60 drops/minute) to maintain suppression of the dysrhythmia. An alternative mixing is 1 gram of procainamide into 500 ml D_5W, to yield 2 mg/ml.

Magnesium Sulfate

Magnesium Sulfate: Mechanism of Action

Magnesium is an important component of numerous biochemical activities within the body. It is integral to the normal functioning of the sodium-potassium pump that, among other things, helps maintain cellular wall stability. Magnesium has also been identified as a "physiological" calcium channel blocker and a blocker of normal neuromuscular nerve transmission. Finally, it plays a role in the movement of potassium across the cellular wall during cellular depolarization.

Magnesium Sulfate: Indications

Research has shown that some patients with a deficiency in magnesium may also suffer from certain cardiac abnormalities. Hypomagnesemia has been associated with life-threatening cardiac emergencies such as ventricular fibrillation, ventricular tachycardia, torsades de pointes, cardiac insufficiency, and sudden cardiac death. As mentioned earlier, these problems have been observed in patients with low levels of magnesium; therefore, its replacement by IV administration may help terminate and/or prevent these occurrences.

Specifically, magnesium sulfate may be warranted for:

- ▶ Persistent or refractory ventricular fibrillation (following lidocaine)
- ▶ Torsades de points without a pulse (polymorphic ventricular tachycardia)
- ▶ Torsades de points with a pulse (polymorphic ventricular tachycardia)
- ▶ Suspected hypomagnesemia (consult first with medical direction)
- ▶ Can be considered for dysrhythmias induced by digitalis toxicity

Magnesium Sulfate: Side Effects/Precautions

Magnesium sulfate in moderate doses has few serious side effects. It has been documented that rapid administration of this drug can result in a drop in the heart rate, diaphoresis, flushing of the skin, and a possible drop in blood pressure. Magnesium should be administered slowly via IV push to minimize these effects. Toxicity associated with higher doses, however, carries with it the more severe side effects of flaccid muscle paralysis (remember that it can block normal neuromuscular transmission), depression of the deep tendon reflexes, respiratory paralysis, and circulatory collapse.

There are some significant drug interactions noted between magnesium and digitalis. Conduction defects may result if magnesium is administered with digitalis. As well, the patient should be continuously reassessed during administration of magnesium. If side effects become severe, or signs of toxicity are present, calcium chloride should be immediately available to administer as an antidote.

Magnesium Sulfate: Contraindications

Magnesium should not be administered to patients in shock or with a heart block, since its physiological "blocking" capability (discussed earlier) may worsen this condition. Magnesium should not be administered to a dialysis patient, or to a patient known to have a lowered calcium level (hypocalcemia).

Magnesium Sulfate: Dosages

The appropriate dose of magnesium sulfate will be defined by the patient's particular ECG rhythm and myocardial status. Alternative dosing regimens are:

Cardiac Arrest (V-Fib/V-Tach or Hypomagnesemia)

- ▶ 1 to 2 grams of the drug should be mixed in 10 ml of D_5W, and administered via IV push over a 1–2 minute period.

Torsades de Pointes (not in cardiac arrest)

- ▶ Loading dose of 1 gram to 2 grams of the drug should be mixed in 50–100 ml bag of D_5W. This should then be administered over a period of 5 to 60 minutes. A maintenance infusion could then be started at 0.5–1.0 grams/hour for up to 24 hours.

Rate Control

Atropine Sulfate

Atropine Sulfate: Mechanism of Action

The heart is innervated by branches of the sympathetic and parasympathetic nervous system. The sympathetic nervous system stimulates the heart; the parasympathetic

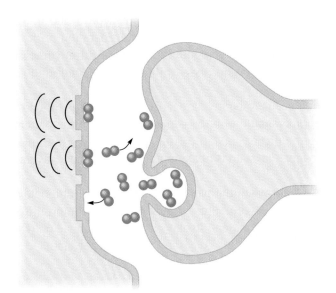

FIGURE 8-5
Activity at nerve synapses of the parasympathetic nervous system. Acetylcholine is released from pre-synaptic nerve endings, travels across the synapse, and stimulates receptors on the post-synaptic nerves. Subsequently, the catecholamines are broken down and the products taken up by the pre-synaptic nerve.

system reduces cardiac activity. The parasympathetic system achieves this by releasing the neurotransmitter acetylcholine (Figure 8-5), which causes a decrease in the heart rate and conduction velocity—without really influencing the strength of ventricular contraction.

Occasionally, you may hear this parasympathetic-mediated reduction in heart rate and conduction velocity referred to as "vagal tone." *Vagal* relates to the vagus nerve, the tenth cranial nerve, which is the primary nerve of the parasympathetic nervous system. Stimulation of the vagus nerve causes the release of acetylcholine and the associated depression of cardiac activity.

Occasionally, excessive vagal tone may be present in a diseased or an ischemic heart. This increase in vagal tone can result in excessive slowing of the heart and/or conduction disturbances. Excessive vagal tone may also be observed secondary to parasympathomimetic overdoses.

Atropine is known to be a *parasympatholytic* drug (*parasympatho-* refers to the parasympathetic branch of the autonomic nervous system, and *-lytic* means to block or stop). Other common names for this drug class include "vagolytic" and "anticholinergic." Atropine exerts its action by blocking the acetylcholine receptors, thereby inhibiting the effect of the neurotransmitter, and diminishing or preventing the influence of vagal tone on the heart. An important distinction is that atropine is not a sympathomimetic drug, as is epinephrine. Atropine increases the heart rate by blocking vagal tone, not by stimulating beta receptor sites as epinephrine would.

Atropine Sulfate: Indications

Since atropine has the ability to counteract vagal tone in the heart, its benefits would be desirable in a patient with cardiovascular compromise from an excessively slow heart rate. Bradycardic rates (< 60/min) may cause instability in the patient because of a drop in cardiac output. This drop, when severe, results in arterial hypotension, organ hypoperfusion, and a decrease in coronary artery perfusion.

Patients who may respond to atropine include those who present with sinus bradycardia and certain conduction blocks of the AV node. Research has shown that individuals with a first-degree AV conduction block or a second-degree Type I AV conduction block may also benefit from atropine. These blocks have more recently been labeled as "nodal" blocks, as the conduction defect is located at or just above level of the AV node. Patients with second-degree Type II and third-degree ("infranodal") heart blocks should be given special consideration prior to atropine administration, as atropine has been reported to be harmful in some of these patients. This consideration will be discussed more under "Contraindications" below.

One important delineation needs to be made regarding the administration of atropine for bradycardia. Atropine should only be administered when the patient has been identified as symptomatic or unstable from the bradydysrhythmia. (Administration of atropine to a patient who is not symptomatic may have adverse consequences.)

"Absolute bradycardia" occurs when the patient displays a heart rate below 60 beats per minute (for example 55) with signs of hemodynamic compromise. "Relative bradycardia" occurs when the patient displays a heart rate above 60 (for example 65), but still has signs and symptoms consistent with hypoperfusion.

Absolute Bradycardia

▶ A spontaneous heart rate < 60 beats/min
    and

▶ Concurrent signs/symptoms of hemodynamic compromise:
— shortness of breath
— chest pain
— altered mental status
— hypotension
— pulmonary edema
— myocardial infarction

Relative Bradycardia

▶ A spontaneous heart rate > 60 beats/min
    and

▶ Concurrent signs of poor cardiac output:
— acute myocardial infarction
— symptomatic hypotension

Atropine has been cited as beneficial in a bradyasystolic heart secondary to excessive vagal tone. Ongoing research results are controversial regarding the appropriateness of atropine in the asystolic heart. However, since the asystolic heart has a poor prognosis for resuscitation, atropine administration is not viewed as harmful. Also, some cases of asystole are thought to result from massive parasympathetic tone. For this reason, asystolic cardiac arrests should routinely receive atropine administration.

Atropine Sulfate: Side Effects/Precautions

Since the effect of atropine is to increase the heart rate, naturally the myocardial oxygen demand will also increase. This is of concern in a patient with an MI or myocardial ischemia, since the imbalance between myocardial oxygen supply and demand may be worsened. This is especially true in a patient with coronary artery disease. Finally, excessive doses of atropine may result in an anticholinergic syndrome characterized by the following symptoms:

Anticholinergic Syndrome

▶ Tachycardia

▶ Blurred vision

▶ Flushed and hot skin

▶ Coma (alterations in mentation)

▶ Muscle incoordination

▶ Dilated pupils

▶ Dry mouth

Atropine Sulfate: Contraindications

As mentioned earlier, atropine should be avoided in patients who are in a symptomatic Type II or third-degree heart block, which are considered "infranodal" (located below the AV node, actually at the level of the ventricle). The reason to avoid atropine in infranodal blocks is logical. There is very little parasympathetic innervation at the level of the ventricles, so in the absence of parasympathetic fibers there cannot be excessive parasympathetic tone, and thus atropine can exert no benefits of increased conduction speed.

Instead, there can be an adverse effect from atropine: If atropine is administered and causes the sinus discharge rate above the conduction block to increase, it may further irritate the conduction defect and worsen the block. A simple analogy would be to take an old wooden covered bridge, only able to support a single lane of traffic, and widen the road that leads to the bridge into a superhighway. As the vehicular traffic increases (i.e., the sinus discharge rate increases), the old bridge will start to break down under the added weight and strain—until it collapses (i.e., the conduction block becomes irritated by the additional electrical traffic from the sinus node until the block is complete).

Since researchers still argue about the exact appropriateness of atropine administration in infranodal blocks, some prehospital protocols may still recommend considering a single atropine bolus. However, if atropine is administered to an infranodal block, watch closely for paradoxical slowing of the ventricular rate. Be prepared to artificially pace the rhythm should the conduction defect worsen.

Atropine Sulfate: Dosages

Atropine is administered via an intravenous line. It can also be administered down the tracheal tube when no IV line is present. When the tracheal route is used, the dose should be 1 to 2 mg diluted with no more than 10 cc of solution. However, when administering more than one dose of atropine, do not rely on the tracheal tube as the sole route, since excessive amounts of fluids will be instilled into the respiratory tree. The following outlines the administration of atropine for the patient suffering from cardiovascular instability:

Hemodynamically Unstable Bradycardia

▶ Initial dose of 0.5–1.0 mg given IVP (or 1–2 mg via TT). Repeat atropine at 0.5 mg–1.0 mg every 3–5 minutes to a maximum dose of 0.03 mg/kg. Up to 0.04 mg/kg has been used in some extreme instances of severe bradycardia.

Cardiac Arrest (Asystole or PEA with Extreme Bradycardia)

▶ Initial and repeat doses are at 1.0 mg every 3–5 minutes until the full vagolytic dose of 0.04 mg/kg is achieved.

As you will notice, the amount you administer is standard (either 0.5 mg or 1.0 mg), but the maximum cumulative dose is based upon the weight of the patient. There is an easy way to determine the maximum dose at 0.04 mg/kg. For every 25 kg of patient weight, administer 1 mg of atropine to achieve the maximum allowance. For example, if the patient weighed 165 pounds, that would convert into 75 kg (divide weight in pounds by 2.2), which results in 3 mg as the maximum amount of drug to be administered. A patient who weighs 100 kg would receive a maximum of 4 mg of atropine.

Also be cautious not to administer less than a 0.5 mg bolus of atropine. At low doses, there has been a documented paradoxical effect worsening the bradycardia, which may possibly lead to V-fib on further hemodynamic instability.

Adenosine

Adenosine: Mechanism of Action

Adenosine is a "purine nucleoside," a naturally occurring body protein. It is a substance found in all body cells. When administered parenterally, it has numerous effects that include slowing of conduction through the AV node and interruption of reentry pathways which may be the underlying etiology of PSVT rhythms.

Adenosine will not convert atrial tachydysrhythmias such as atrial tachycardia, atrial flutter, multifocal atrial tachycardia, or atrial fibrillation into a sinus rhythm. The benefits of adenosine result from its ability to slow conduction through the AV node. In essence, you are creating a form of heart block. For example, if a patient presents with atrial flutter with a 1:1 conduction and a heart rate of 270 prior to adenosine, after adenosine the *atrial* rate may still be 270/minute—but the *ventricular* response may now be 90/minute with a 3:1 conduction block of the atrial flutter. The immediate goal of treating a hemodynamically unstable PSVT is to control the rapid ventricular response. After initial stabilization, the underlying cause of the PSVT can be identified and managed.

Adenosine: Indications

Adenosine is the drug of choice for symptomatic tachydysrhythmias that are supraventricular in nature. Oftentimes with a tachycardic rate, it is impossible to identify the exact cause of the rhythm because the atrial activity and T waves are superimposed on each other. But as noted earlier, this distinction is unnecessary since adenosine will have no effect on atrial tissue; rather it slows AV conduction.

Adenosine is also effective in terminating tachycardias from a reentry pathway. This is probably the most common cause of PSVT. Adenosine is also appropriate for PSVT rhythms associated with Wolff-Parkinson-White (WPW) syndrome. (WPW will be discussed in more detail under "Verapamil and Diltiazem.") Instances when adenosine administration would be appropriate are:

▶ Symptomatic PSVT associated with WPW

▶ Atrial dysrhythmias resulting in a rapid ventricular response

▶ Wide complex tachycardia of unknown etiology

Adenosine: Side Effects/Precautions

Side effects after adenosine administration occur often but, fortunately, are short lived, because its half-life is extremely short, lasting only about 5 seconds. The following list identifies the side effects that the patient should be forewarned about, again remembering that they are of a short, often inconsequential, duration:

▶ Facial flushing

▶ Nausea

▶ Dizziness

▶ Headache

▶ Dysrhythmias

▶ Dyspnea

▶ Chest pain

Adenosine does, however, have important drug interactions that must be given special attention. Methylxanthines (aminophylline) block the receptor sites where adenosine exerts its therapeutic action, so that larger doses may be required for the desired effect. Conversely, dipyridamole (Persantine) blocks the uptake of adenosine and thus potentiates its effects. In this instance, the dose should be decreased. These interactions are extremely important, and the presence or potential use of any of these drugs needs to be determined prior to administration of adenosine.

Adenosine: Contraindications

As with any other drug, an absolute contraindication is known hypersensitivity to the drug. Adenosine should be avoided in patients with a second- or third-degree heart block, since the actions of this drug include delaying AV node conduction. This drug should not be used in patients known to have sick sinus syndrome, especially in the absence of a pacemaker.

Adenosine: Dosage

Successful conversion from the tachydysrhythmia is greatly enhanced if the adenosine administration procedure is strictly followed. Since adenosine has such a short half-life, improper administration could result in the drug being metabolized by the body before it ever reaches the coronary circulation and the myocardium. Adenosine should be administered in the closest medication port to the IV site, preferably in a large antecubital vein, and should be followed by a rapid flush of 20 cc of saline administered immediately after each adenosine bolus. The proper dose and administration procedure are:

Hemodynamically Significant Tachycardia

▶ Initial bolus of 6 mg via rapid IV push over 1–3 seconds. After 1–2 minutes, if the rhythm did not convert, administer 12 mg, then another 12 mg after 1–2 minutes if still unresponsive. The maximum dose of adenosine is 30 mg.

Calcium Channel Blockers: Verapamil and Diltiazem

Verapamil and Diltiazem: Mechanism of Action

Calcium ions are necessary for normal nerve propagation and smooth muscle contraction. Therefore, a drug that alters the normal movement of calcium would also interfere with conduction velocity and smooth muscle contraction.

Verapamil and diltiazem are known as "calcium channel antagonists," or "calcium channel blockers." They act by blocking the movement of calcium across cellular membranes. Although they differ slightly in the degree of effect, verapamil or diltiazem slows conduction velocity through the AV node and relaxes vascular smooth muscle. These benefits would be desirable for patients experiencing a tachydysrhythmia in which the ventricular rate needs to be slowed. Additionally, since these drugs exert negative chronotropic (rate) and inotropic (contractile

TABLE 8–1 Verapamil and Diltiazem: Comparative Actions

	Effect on AV Conduction	Effect on Smooth Muscle Relaxation
Verapamil	Potent negative inotropic and chronotropic effect	Lesser effect on vascular and smooth muscle relaxation
Diltiazem	Mild negative inotropic but potent negative chronotropic effect	Greater effect on vascular and smooth muscle relaxation

force) effects on the heart, they will lessen myocardial oxygen demand. These are desirable anti-ischemic effects. Finally, verapamil and diltiazem result in coronary artery dilation which assists in the treatment of angina.

Although they both are calcium channel blockers, verapamil and diltiazem exert slightly different effects. Table 8-1 identifies the differences in their actions.

Verapamil and Diltiazem: Indications

Because both verapamil and diltiazem slow conduction and prolong refractoriness by interfering with calcium movement across the cellular membrane, it is only logical that they are used in treating tachydysrhythmias. Verapamil was previously the drug of choice in treatment of PSVT rhythms; however, since adenosine can accomplish the same result more reliably with fewer side effects, calcium channel blockers are now used less frequently in the management of symptomatic tachydysrhythmias.

Specifically, verapamil and diltiazem are used when a symptomatic but stable patient has a need for rate control that is unresponsive to adenosine but does not require electrical cardioversion. It is important to remember that the calcium channel blockers should be used with narrow-complex tachydysrhythmias. If used in tachydysrhythmias with a wide QRS (e.g., V-tach, wide complex, with unknown etiology), severe hemodynamic compromise could result, since these drugs have negative inotropic effects. Lastly, IV administration of diltiazem in the patient with known atrial fibrillation or atrial flutter may be more appropriate than verapamil since diltiazem produces less myocardial depression than verapamil.

Verapamil and Diltiazem: Side Effects/Precautions

Precautions associated with the use of calcium channel blockers stem logically from the mechanism of action. Impeding calcium movement exerts a negative inotropic effect. Additionally, vasodilation in peripheral blood vessels occurs. The combination of the side effects may result in the possibility of precipitating hypotension. In fact, the blood pressure must be closely monitored for evidence of hypotension during the administration of calcium channel blockers. For this reason, avoid the use of verapamil, and be cautious about administering diltiazem, in patients with known left ventricular dysfunction. If hemodynamic compromise becomes apparent after the administration of the calcium channel blocker, consider administering calcium intravenously, as this may help restore blood pressure without disturbing the electrical activity of the myocardium.

Significant drug interactions occur with the administration of calcium channel blockers. Typically, you may find that a patient with a PSVT rhythm may already be on certain antidysrhythmic drugs for that problem. If so, your administration of either verapamil or diltiazem may have a synergistic effect, potentiating the seriousness of the side effects. It is not only important to be aware of these possible drug interactions, but you must actively *look for* usage of these drugs while taking the patient's history or by searching the patient's medical records. Table 8-2 identifies these drug interactions.

TABLE 8-2 Calcium Channel Blockers (Verapamil/Diltiazem): Drug Interactions

Calcium channel blockers such as verapamil and diltiazem should not be administered with certain drugs with which they will have negative interactions. These drugs and their interactive effects with calcium channel blockers are listed below.

Drug	Interaction with Calcium Channel Blockers
Digitalis	Conduction disturbance, CHF
Beta blockers	Possible CHF, bradycardia, asystole
Furosemide	Do not simultaneously administer: incompatible

Finally, just as many other drugs do, calcium channel blockers can have some systemic side effects that may be uncomfortable for the patient, but are generally not dangerous.

Minor Side Effects

▶ Nausea

▶ Vomiting

▶ Headache

▶ Dizziness

More Serious (but Less Frequent) Side Effects

▶ Bradycardia

▶ Heart block

▶ Asystole

Verapamil and Diltiazem: Contraindications

A major contraindication to the use of calcium channel blockers is a medical condition known as Wolff-Parkinson-White (WPW) syndrome. This is a condition in which there is an abnormal conduction pathway between the atria and ventricles of the heart. This pathway, when active, allows for a cyclic depolarization wave to move rapidly from the atria to the ventricles and back again. In other words, it allows the impulse to "run in circles" through the upper and lower chambers of the heart. Verapamil or diltiazem administration may actually increase the conduction velocity in the abnormal pathway and allow the rate to increase further. (Fortunately, adenosine does not have this effect and can be used safely in patients with WPW.)

Another contraindication to use of calcium channel blockers results from their ability to slow AV node conduction. Calcium channel blockers should not be administered to someone with a conduction defect (heart block) since it may only worsen the block. Verapamil and diltiazem should be avoided in the patient with severe hypotension and/or cardiogenic shock, because its negative inotropic effects will worsen the cardiac compromise. And finally, remember that these drugs are not indicated for tachydysrhythmias with a wide complex QRS.

Verapamil and Diltiazem: Dosages

Although effective in controlling rapid ventricular rates in patients with PSVT or A-fib/A-flutter, both verapamil and diltiazem are relatively dangerous to administer. It is critical to administer the appropriate dose, at the appropriate rate, at the appropriate timing intervals to avoid disastrous complications. Remember also that, unlike adenosine, verapamil and diltiazem must be administered by slow IV push.

This means: *Administer the medication over at least a 2-minute time period every time it is given, and, in elderly patients, increase this time frame to 3 minutes.*

Verapamil

▶ *For PSVT and A-fib/flutter with rapid ventricular response,* administer 2.5 mg to 5.0 mg initial bolus IVP over 2 minutes, followed by a 5 mg to 10 mg bolus after 15–30 minutes have lapsed. Maximum dose for verapamil under this dosing format is 20 mg.

▶ An alternative dosing is 5 mg of verapamil every 15 minutes till you reach a total cumulative dose of 30 mg.

Diltiazem

▶ *For PSVT* administer an initial dose of 15–20 mg (0.25 mg/kg) as an initial bolus IVP over 2 minutes. After 15 minutes, if the desired effect has not occurred, you can repeat it once at 20–25 mg IVP (0.35 mg/kg).

▶ Upon resolution, you should initiate a maintenance infusion at 5 mg/hour. You can titrate the maintenance infusion to maintain the desired heart rate as long as the infusion does not exceed 15 mg/hour.

Digitalis Glycosides

Digitalis Glycosides: Mechanism of Action

Digitalis glycoside preparations are commonly used in the control of ventricular responses to rapid atrial dysrhythmias. They are not, however, commonly used in the prehospital environment, and as such are mentioned here only for informational purposes.

By inducing vagal tone at the level of the AV node, electrical impulses traveling from the atria to the ventricles are substantially slowed. This slowing action allows for an increased diastolic period in which greater ventricular filling can occur and adequate coronary artery perfusion is achieved. The lengthened diastole also allows for an improvement in left ventricular preload.

Depending upon dose, digitalis also acts as a positive inotrope. By increasing the uptake of cellular calcium, a more forceful contraction is produced. However, the positive inotropic activity of digitalis is negligible compared to that of other inotropic agents, and digitalis is generally not used in situations where positive inotropic activity would be beneficial, e.g., acute CHF. Also, it is not titratable, nor does it have as rapid an onset as other agents.

Digitalis Glycosides: Indications

Digitalis glycosides are useful in two situations: First, digitalis can counteract or correct rhythm disturbances that interfere with ventricular filling. Second, digitalis can have positive hemodynamic effects in the long-term treatment of congestive heart failure.

The first category includes ventricular response to atrial fibrillation or atrial flutter. Generally, a ventricular response of greater than 100 beats per minute is considered uncontrolled. The danger with an uncontrolled ventricular response is that, as it increases, ventricular filling time will be shortened and cardiac output will be reduced. In addition, coronary artery perfusion occurs during diastole, and as diastolic filling decreases, so does the coronary artery perfusion. Therefore, regulation of the ventricular response is paramount in cases of atrial fibrillation, atrial flutter, and PSVT. Digitalis preparations, usually used to achieve long-term control, must be considered for stabilization of PSVT after adenosine, verapamil, and electrical conversion have proven unsuccessful for this purpose.

The second category is long-term treatment of CHF. As stated previously, digitalis glycosides have positive inotropic effects, the ability to bring about a more forceful contraction of the heart. While other medications are more effective in the treatment of *acute* CHF and left ventricular failure, digitalis is useful in the *long-term* treatment of heart failure. The positive inotropic activity is dose dependent and occurs more frequently at lower doses.

Digitalis Glycosides: Side Effects/Precautions

Toxicity is a major potential side effect of digitalis and must be closely monitored. Levels of digitalis that exceed the therapeutic range may produce many different signs and symptoms. These include:

Cardiovascular

- Bradydysrhythmias
- Tachydysrhythmias
- Premature beats
- Hypotension
- Heart blocks
- Cardiac arrest

Non Cardiac

- Anorexia
- Nausea/vomiting
- Abdominal pain
- Yellow vision
- Headache
- Dizziness
- Rash
- Sweating

Patients suffering an acute myocardial infarction or electrolyte disturbances (particularly hypokalemia) are more prone to develop digitalis toxicity. In addition, toxicity can be promulgated through concurrent administration of other medications. For instance, digitalis administered with beta blockers might produce profound bradycardia, or the depletion of potassium by a diuretic can alter the electrolyte balance. Also, quinidine and calcium channel blockers serve to increase overall levels of digitalis.

In any case of toxicity, current levels of administration must be discontinued and the underlying abnormality corrected. In cases of massive toxicity, digoxin antibodies may prove effective in reversal.

Digitalis Glycosides: Contraindications

Digitalis glycosides are commonly used and are only contraindicated in the presence of digitalis toxicity.

Digitalis Glycosides: Dosages

The dosage at which digitalis is administered determines the effect of the medication. Digitalis administered at higher dosages influences the ventricular response, while lower dosages tend to elicit an inotropic response. Digitalis preparations can be administered either orally or via intravenous access.

Other Drugs for Rate Control

As mentioned in the opening to this chapter, some drugs may have more than one application in the treatment of a patient with cardiovascular instability. The drugs listed below are sympathomimetic agents that will increase the heart rate directly by stimulation of the heart or indirectly by stimulation of the sympathetic nervous system. For this reason, they are considered to be drugs that are appropriate for rate control. To understand more fully how these drugs work, review the information about them under "Sympathomimetics" earlier in the chapter.

▶ Dopamine

▶ Epinephrine

▶ Isoproterenol

Part Five: Analgesics and Antianginal Agents

Analgesic agents are used to alleviate pain. The most commonly used analgesics would be morphine (an opiate derivative) or a synthetic narcotic. They are used for pain associated with a myriad of medical or traumatic causes; however, often they are used for the treatment of chest pain from a cardiovascular crisis.

Antianginal agents have similar indications. This drug class includes agents, such as nitroglycerin, that will help alleviate the ischemic chest pain characteristic of a hypoxic heart. Typically, when cardiac pain is not relieved by administered oxygen and nitroglycerin, more potent analgesics are used.

Morphine Sulfate

Morphine Sulfate: Mechanism of Action

Morphine sulfate, a narcotic, is a derivative of the opiates, which are substances that occur naturally in the environment. When administered, morphine interacts with the opiate receptors in the brain where it causes central nervous system effects.

Morphine promotes hemodynamic changes. There is a drop in systemic vascular resistance and an increase in venous capacitance. These hemodynamic changes will lower preload as a result of decreasing venous return and will reduce myocardial afterload (and intramyocardial-wall tension) by dilating the arterial side of the circulation. These changes, in turn, will reduce myocardial workload and oxygen requirements.

Secondly, morphine serves as an analgesic and anxiolytic, thereby diminishing the pain and apprehension associated with an acute MI. This is beneficial since sympathetic nervous system activity is heightened during an MI with an increased demand made on the heart. Morphine will help blunt that effect.

Morphine Sulfate: Indications

The role of morphine sulfate in the management of an MI and other cardiovascular emergencies has been well documented. In general, it is useful whenever there is severe pain (e.g., chest pain) that is compounding the medical emergency, or whenever cardiovascular instability results in acute pulmonary edema (with or without pain). The use of morphine should be considered only after an appropriate physical assessment and patient interview, as long as the vital signs (especially the blood pressure) are within acceptable limits. Typically, you will find yourself considering morphine either after nitroglycerin has failed to relieve the chest pain or as part of the treatment regimen for acute pulmonary edema.

Morphine Sulfate: Side Effects/Precautions

Since it is a narcotic drug with a potential for addiction and abuse, morphine has since been regulated under the 1970 Controlled Substances Act, as a Schedule II drug. This requires care providers using this drug to adhere to specific documentation and security measures.

Morphine acts as a CNS depressant. It can cause profound respiratory depression and possible hypotension. These effects may be pronounced in individuals who already have some type of respiratory impairment or who are receiving CNS-depressant drugs. It is always best to administer morphine in several small incremental doses rather than as large boluses to avoid these complications. Table 8-3 lists potential drug interactions that should be considered prior to morphine use.

As a narcotic drug, morphine can be reversed by naloxone (Narcan®). Undesirable complications of excessive narcosis or respiratory depression can be reversed by administering 0.4 to 2.0 mg of naloxone. Naloxone administration is typically titrated to allow the analgesic and sedative effects to predominate while maintaining a sufficient ventilatory and circulatory status.

Other possible side effects of morphine that should be anticipated include nausea and vomiting, abdominal cramping, blurred vision, altered mental status, constricted pupils, and headaches.

Morphine Sulfate: Contraindications

Morphine should not be administered to anyone with a known hypersensitivity to narcotics (a situation, incidentally, that is rather common). Additionally, because of the hemodynamic effects described earlier, morphine should not be administered to anyone who is hypotensive or thought to be volume-depleted. And due to its vasodilatory effects and depression of the mental status, it should also be avoided in head-injury patients.

Morphine Sulfate: Dosage

Morphine can be administered via the intravascular, intramuscular, and subcutaneous routes. In emergency situations morphine is preferentially given via small intravenous boluses to avoid precipitating excessive respiratory depression and/or cardiovascular collapse.

► *IV administration*—The dose should be started at 2 mg to 4 mg and given slowly via IV push. The dose can be repeated at 5 to 30 minute intervals until the desired effect is achieved.

You should always have the narcotic reversal agent naloxone (Narcan®) readily available when morphine is administered.

TABLE 8-3 | Morphine Interactions

The CNS depressive effects of morphine can be enhanced if administered concurrently with any of the drugs listed below.

- Other sedatives
- Hypnotics
- Antihistamines
- Antiemetics
- Barbiturates
- Alcohol

Nitroglycerin

Nitroglycerin: Mechanism of Action

Nitroglycerin is a nitrate that lowers blood pressure by relaxing vascular smooth muscle. Through its actions, nitroglycerin dilates the vasculature, thereby reducing the pressure against which the heart must eject blood (afterload) and the amount of blood that is returned to the heart for pumping (preload).

The heart constantly requires an adequate oxygen supply. In situations where oxygen supply is depleted—such as a myocardial infarction—myocardial ischemia and subsequent necrosis may result. A reduction in workload results in a reduction in the demand for oxygen. The heart works less because it is pumping against a reduced systemic vascular resistance and has a lower left ventricular filling volume. Nitroglycerin improves the balance between workload and available oxygen. As a result, ischemic pain is alleviated and the possible infarct size limited.

It is also thought that nitroglycerin may dilate coronary arteries and promote collateral circulation to ischemic regions where the normal blood flow is interrupted.

Nitroglycerin: Indications

Ischemic tissue produces pain. If the ischemia can be alleviated, as through the action of nitroglycerin, the pain will most likely resolve. Therefore, nitroglycerin is commonly prescribed for any type of ischemic myocardial pain. This includes pain occurring secondary to angina or as a result of acute myocardial infarction.

Nitroglycerin is also indicated in the emergent treatment of acute congestive heart failure. By increasing capacitance in the venous system, nitroglycerin reduces pressure in the pulmonary vessels and enables a more effective cardiac output, thereby improving respiration and the exchange of gases.

Nitroglycerin: Side Effects/Precautions

Since nitroglycerin can produce a drop in blood pressure, it can also limit the amount of blood available for perfusion of the myocardium. Decreased coronary perfusion worsens myocardial ischemia. For this reason, no more than a 10% reduction in the mean arterial blood pressure is recommended if the patient is normotensive, or 30% if hypertensive. In any situation, however, the blood pressure should not be allowed to drop below 90 mmHg systolic.

Again as a result of the reduction in blood pressure, the patient may experience syncope, dizziness, weakness, and tachycardia. In addition, headache, dry mouth, nausea, and vomiting may occur.

Nitroglycerin should be administered with the patient sitting or lying down due to the potential for a sudden drop in blood pressure. If systemic hypotension does occur, the patient should be immediately placed in the Trendelenburg position (supine, with feet elevated) to facilitate blood flow to the brain and myocardium.

Nitroglycerin: Contraindications

Nitroglycerin should be avoided if preexisting hypotension is present, or if the patient displays hemodynamically significant bradycardia or tachycardia. In addition, nitroglycerin dilates the cerebral veins and can elevate intracranial pressure. Therefore, if increased intracranial pressure exists, nitroglycerin should be used with caution. Finally, anyone with declared sensitivity to nitroglycerin should not be given the drug, nor should a patient who has taken Viagra® within the last 24 hours.

Nitroglycerin: Dosages

Nitroglycerin can be administered through several different routes in varying dosages (either sublingual, transcutaneous with a nitro patch, or by constant intravenous infusion). Since the prehospital provider utilizes the sublingual route almost exclusively during prehospital management, its dosing recommendation is as follows:

▶ *Sublingual spray or tablet*—The sublingual administration of nitroglycerin is a rapid route for administration in the emergent situation. A 0.3 to 0.4 mg starting dose is given and can be repeated at 5-minute intervals, until discomfort is relieved, or a total of 3 tablets or sprays is achieved.

▶ *Intravenous infusion*—Begin at 5 μg/minute and titrate up to 5 μg/minute every 5 to 10 minutes until chest pain is relieved or the hemodynamic response is achieved. Typical response dose is 50 to 200 μg/minute.

Part Six: Diuretics

A diuretic agent is one that will enhance the body's ability to eliminate excess fluid via the renal system. This can be desirable in a patient with congestive heart failure or acute pulmonary edema. These emergencies result from a buildup of fluid caused by failing ventricles. If the fluid backs up as a result of right ventricular failure, peripheral edema, jugular vein distention (JVD), and ascites may be present along with a positive hepatoabdominal reflex. If fluid backs up because of left ventricular failure, the fluid becomes displaced into the alveoli, resulting in diminished diffusion of gases. In either instance, furosemide (Lasix) will reduce the circulating volume by ridding the body of excess fluid. And since the volume is less, there is a drop in preload, which allows the heart to more efficiently pump the remaining fluid.

Furosemide

Furosemide: Mechanism of Action

Furosemide is a potent diuretic that works to reduce vascular volume. In doing so, it removes excess volume from within the lungs, as is seen with acute congestive heart failure or pulmonary edema.

Furosemide exerts its influence in the kidneys where it promotes the excretion of sodium and, ultimately, the water that follows sodium. As volume is removed from the intravascular space, fluid from the extravascular space shifts and is excreted accordingly. This promotes removal of fluid from the lungs, resulting in enhanced gas exchange at the alveolar capillary membrane.

In addition, furosemide exerts a venodilatory effect and increases cardiac output by reducing preload.

Furosemide: Indications

In light of its mechanisms of action, furosemide is applicable in the emergency treatment of pulmonary congestion associated with left ventricular failure (with a systolic pressure above 90 mmHg).

Furosemide: Side Effects/Precautions

As with any diuretic, you must be aware of possible electrolyte disturbances, especially of potassium. Electrolyte disturbances can manifest as electrical dysrhythmias and prove difficult to correct unless the underlying abnormality is targeted. Chronic use of furosemide may precipitate electrolyte disturbances.

Also, severe fluid depletion can result in dehydration and hypotension. Blood pressure and fluid status must be monitored closely during the use of furosemide.

Furosemide: Contraindications

As furosemide is a derivative of sulfamide, it should be withheld from anyone declaring sensitivity to sulfas. Also, preexisting hypotension or dehydration should discount the use of furosemide.

Furosemide: Dosage

In the emergency setting, furosemide should be given intravenously.

▶ *IV administration*—Administer an initial dosage of 20–40 mg or 0.5–1 mg/kg. Delivery should be slow, occurring over 1–2 minutes. If there is failure to respond, furosemide can be repeated at two times the dose, or 2 mg/kg IVP over 1–2 minutes.

Part Seven: Antihypertensives

Another relatively common cardiovascular emergency is hypertension. Well known as the "silent killer," hypertension may also present as an acute emergency requiring immediate reduction in blood pressure. Although the extent and rate at which you should reduce systolic pressure is still disputed by the experts, all agree that if the indicators of a hypertensive crisis are present, reduction of blood pressure should be a priority.

Sodium Nitroprusside

Sodium Nitroprusside: Mechanism of Action

Sodium nitroprusside is a potent and rapid-acting vasodilator that quickly decreases symptomatic hypertension. Sodium nitroprusside dilates the arterial and venous vasculature, thereby dropping blood pressure and reducing myocardial workload.

Sodium Nitroprusside: Indications

Because of its ability to reduce blood pressure rapidly, sodium nitroprusside is useful in a hypertensive crisis. Sodium nitroprusside is titratable and can be used in the management of left ventricular failure or CHF. This drug is most commonly administered in the hospital.

Rarely is it seen in the management of a hypertensive crisis in the prehospital environment by advanced life support providers.

Sodium Nitroprusside: Side Effects/Precautions

Because its vasodilatory effects are so rapid, but overadministering sodium nitroprusside can create a serious state of hypotension. Hepatic and renal dysfunction can slow the clearance of nitroprusside from the body. Since the elderly typically suffer a gradual degradation of hepatic and renal function, the dose of nitroprusside for an elderly patient is commonly reduced.

The effects of sodium nitroprusside can be potentiated by administration with other hypertensive agents. Also, because of the possibility of reduced perfusion, administration of sodium nitroprusside can result in dizziness, hypotension, chest pain, palpitations, nausea, and vomiting. Finally, sodium nitroprusside is susceptible to light and can be rapidly deactivated after exposure.

Sodium Nitroprusside: Contraindications
In the emergency setting, there are no contraindications to the use of sodium nitroprusside.

Other Antihypertensive Drugs
The following drugs may also be considered as alternative agents for reducing the blood pressure. Remember, however, to use more appropriate methods first. A more detailed explanation of these drugs can be found earlier in the chapter.

- ▶ beta blockers (labetalol)
- ▶ nitroglycerin

Part Eight: Fibrinolytics (Thrombolytics) and Other ACS Agents

Acute coronary syndrome (ACS) is a medical emergency in which the blood supply to the heart is incapable of meeting the demands. This blood supply and demand discrepancy is commonly due to chronic changes in the coronary blood flow from such diseases as atherosclerotic or arteriosclerotic heart disease. This is commonly the mechanism behind cardiac angina as discussed previously. A myocardial infarction, however, is actual necrosis of heart muscle from an acute change of (or loss of) blood flow to the heart. Fibrinolytics (thrombolytics) are one of the newer developments for the management of myocardial infarctions that has shown to be a positive factor in decreasing myocardial infarction related deaths. Fibrinolytics (thrombolytics) are agents that facilitate the dissolving of a recently developed blood clot in a coronary vessel, thus allowing reperfusion of blood into that area of the heart (Figure 8-6). If detected early enough, fibrinolysis (thrombolysis) of the clot will prevent cellular death. For this reason, hospitals across the country are instituting protocols within the emergency department to allow the myocardial infarction patient to receive fibrinolytic drug therapy within 30 minutes of arriving at the hospital.

The other ACS agents mentioned in this section are those medications that are used during the initial management of myocardial ischemia and infarction. Many of

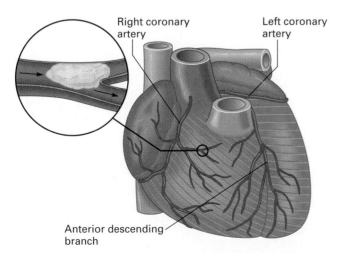

FIGURE 8–6
A clot or embolism forming in a coronary artery prevents oxygenation of a portion of the myocardium, causing ischemia, injury, and infarction. If administered early enough, fibrinolytic drugs dissolve the clot and prevent further myocardial tissue injury.

these agents frequently are used during prehospital, emergency department, and interhospital transport care of suspected myocardial ischemia/infarction emergencies. They are designed to limit the amount of infarction through various mechanisms which affect the thrombus formation until definitive reperfusion therapy can take place.

As a final reminder regarding management of ACS, medications such as oxygen, nitroglycerin, and morphine sulfate are used early in the management of a patient suspected to be experiencing a myocardial emergency. These medications, along with their other uses in advanced cardiac life support, were explained in greater detail in previous sections of this chapter. Additionally, a more complete discussion of acute coronary syndrome can be found in Chapter 9.

Aspirin

Aspirin: Mechanism of Action

Aspirin, when administered early in the management of patients with suspected myocardial ischemia or infarction, has been shown to help reduce the mortality rate. It serves as an antiplatelet agent by way of inhibition of clotting process.

The most common antiplatelet drug in use today, aspirin inhibits cyclooxygenase, a key enzyme in a signaling pathway that leads to platelet activation. While all platelet activation agonists utilize this pathway, most of them can also activate the glycoprotein (GP) IIB/IIIA receptors even if the first pathway is blocked. As a result, aspirin is not a strong platelet antagonist. While extremely cost effective, aspirin shares a common limitation with many other platelet activation antagonists: it targets only one pathway, thus leaving numerous alternate routes for platelet activation available. Other drugs used to inhibit these alternative routes will be discussed later in this chapter.

Aspirin: Indications

Due to its relative safety, ease of administration, and low cost versus benefits, aspirin is considered to be an adjunctive agent to the early management of an acute coronary syndrome. It is most beneficial to those patients who clinically present with ischemic type chest pain.

Aspirin: Side Effects/Precautions

While a relatively safe drug, aspirin has been associated with gastric bleeding in those patients with active ulcer disease, and may be detrimental to individuals with asthma. These precautions, however, are considered to be relative contraindications, and the prehospital advanced life support provider is urged to follow local protocol or medical direction regarding aspirin's use in patients with these specific medical histories.

Aspirin: Contraindications

Specifically, aspirin is contraindicated for those patients having non-cardiac related chest pain, and also in those patients with a known history of hypersensitivity to the drug.

Aspirin: Dosage

Instruct the ACS patient to take 160 mg to 325 mg of chewable (baby) aspirin. This should be administered as early as possible in the treatment algorithm for an acute coronary syndrome. If the patient is unable to chew aspirin, it can be administered by way of rectal suppositories. Medical direction should prevail in the administration of, and route used, for aspirin.

Glycoprotein (GP) IIB/IIIA Antagonists

Glycoprotein IIB/IIIA Antagonists: Mechanism of Action
Upon rupture of plaque in a coronary artery, the clotting cascade begins. This results in the adhesion of platelets that, ultimately, causes coronary artery occlusion and subsequent infarction of tissue distal to the thrombus site. What is considered the "final common pathway" of this platelet adhesion and thrombus formation is the utilization of IIB/IIIA receptors in the platelets' membranes. During this clotting process, if these receptor sites in the platelets are blocked (antagonized), the continued thrombus formation from platelet aggregation can be stopped. As such, the administration of a GP IIB/IIIA medication can reduce the ischemic complications from the plaque rupture.

Glycoprotein IIB/IIIA Antagonists: Indications
Generally, medications in this category are used during in-hospital management and during interhospital transport situations. Although the specific indications and dosing for available GP IIB/IIIA medications vary somewhat (and are beyond the scope of this text), they include patients who have:

> ▶ Patients with non-ST segment elevation MIs

Glycoprotein IIB/IIIA Antagonists: Side Effects/Precautions
Because these medications interfere with the body's ability to clot, any bleeding disorders become a concern in a patient who is under consideration to receive these drugs. For example, it has been noted that bleeding may occur at the site of any catheter insertion. As such, caution should be exercised with any known history of bleeding disorders, traumatic injuries, or medical (surgical) procedures.

Glycoprotein IIB/IIIA Antagonists: Contraindications
The following are contraindications to the use of glycoprotein IIB/IIIA antagonists:

> ▶ Systemic hypertension
> ▶ Active internal hemorrhage,
> ▶ Recent (within 30 days) major trauma or surgery procedures
> ▶ History of intracranial hemorrhages
> ▶ Low platelet count
> ▶ Concurrent use of another IIB/IIIA antagonist
> ▶ Known hypersensitivity to the drug

Angiotensin Converting Enzyme (ACE) Inhibitors

ACE Inhibitors: Mechanism of Action
ACE inhibitors have been shown to serve as useful adjunctive therapy to patients experiencing myocardial infarctions with diminished left ventricular function. Angiotensin I is a physiologically inactive substance in the bloodstream that, when combined with the angiotensin-converting-enzyme, becomes angiotensin II. Angiotensin II is a powerful vasopressor that contributes to the workload on the heart by increasing systemic vascular resistance. This naturally places greater workload on the heart that is already failing. ACE inhibitors work by blocking the conversion of angiotensin I into angiotensin II, thus promoting vascular relaxation, a drop in systemic vascular resistance, and eventual diminishment of myocardial workload due to the drop in left ventricular afterload. This improved left ventricular

function enhances cardiac output, limits infarction size, slows the progression of heart failure, and decreases sudden death and the recurrence of infarctions.

ACE Inhibitors: Indications

ACE inhibition therapy is usually given within the first 12–24 hours of the progressing acute coronary event. Although this therapy is not administered in the prehospital environment, it may be encountered by the provider during interhospital transports. It commonly follows the standard initial management and stabilization interventions common to MI patients after reperfusion measures have been taken and the patient is hemodynamically stable. These drugs are usually indicated in the following situations:

- ▶ Suspected infarctions with ST-segment elevations to ≥ 2 anterior leads
- ▶ Poor left ventricular ejection fraction (< 40%)
- ▶ Heart failure in the absence of systolic hypotension unresponsive to traditional therapies (diuretics and/or digitalis preparations)
- ▶ Systemic hypertension

The medications are usually given orally, starting with a low dose, and increased to the full therapeutic dose over the next 24 to 48 hours.

ACE Inhibitors: Side Effects/Precautions

Since these drugs promote a drop in systemic vascular resistance through inhibition of angiotensin II formation, detrimental hypotension could result. Monitor the patient's hemodynamic status diligently to avoid this. Also remember that these drugs are adjuncts to other AMI patient management, and should not be administered within the first 6 hours of infarction, nor prior to the administration of reperfusion therapy.

ACE Inhibitors: Contraindications

There are very specific situations in which ACE inhibitor administration should be avoided. Patients with a systolic pressure < 100 mmHg, renal failure (or known renal stenosis), angioedema, or who are pregnant should not receive this medication. Per usual, patient hypersensitivity to any of the ACE inhibitors should preclude their use.

Heparin

Heparin: Mechanism of Action

Heparin is another drug used to help decrease the size of the infarction. It does this by inhibiting a series of reactions that lead to the clotting of blood and the formation of fibrin clots. Heparin inhibits the conversion of prothrombin to thrombin, thrombin being necessary to the conversion of fibrinogen to fibrin. Once thrombosis has developed, heparin can prevent coagulation by inactivating the thrombin that is already present. In this way, although heparin does not break up existing clots, it does act to halt the development of further clots.

Heparin: Indications

While its use is still controversial in specific clinical situations, heparin can still be considered as adjunctive treatment to fibrinolytic therapy early in the management of a myocardial infarction. Numerous generations of heparin are available, some of which have advantages such as ease of administration, or having been shown to be more beneficial given the clinical presentation of the patient. For example, unfractionated heparin (UFH), works well in patients with a large anterior MI, atrial fibrillation, previous embolus, or undergoing direct or adjunct percutaneous coronary intervention (PCI). However, it carries with it problems such as having numerous contraindications (discussed later) and the need to obtain certain laboratory blood values prior to its administration, mainly PTT (partial thromboplastin time). These concerns may delay or prohibit the drug's administration.

A newer generation of heparin, known as low molecular weight heparin (LMWH), is also available and has been shown to be beneficial when administered early. This type of heparin preparation is used in a patient who is strongly suspected to be experiencing an MI, but who does not show pathologic Q wave development on the ECG or who clinically presents with unstable angina. Additionally, this type of heparin has fewer side effects, a lower number of contraindications, does not necessitate a PPT determination before its administration, and has the added benefit of being administered subcutaneously.

If heparin is to be administered in the prehospital setting, it will most likely be an LMWH preparation such as enoxaparin (Lovenox) that can be given subcutaneously. This allows the MI patient to receive the benefits of heparin actively without the risks associated with unfractionated heparin or the need to obtain laboratory studies.

Generally, after insuring that the patient is being oxygenated, has received a 12-lead ECG, has had venous access established, and is receiving nitroglycerin, aspirin, and morphine therapy as needed, interventions such as antithrombin therapy with heparin and administration of glycoprotein IIB/IIIA antagonists may be considered (Refer to Chapter 9 on myocardial infarctions for additional details).

Heparin: Side Effects/Precautions
Since it acts as an anticoagulant, heparin could result in intracranial hemorrhage or hemorrhage elsewhere in the body. Because there are different heparin preparations (unfractionated versus LMWH), the prescribing physician must use these agents with caution and perform ongoing assessment for complications, to include heparin-induced thrombocytopenia.

▶ Use enoxaparin with extreme caution (if at all) in patients with heparin-induced thrombocytopenia.

Heparin: Contraindications
Heparin has the same contraindications as fibrinolytic therapy. These include:

▶ Known hypersensitivity (e.g., pork products)
▶ Severe hypertension
▶ Bleeding disorders or history of gastrointestinal bleeding
▶ Recent major surgery or major trauma
▶ Recent history of intracranial hemorrhaging

Heparin: Dosage
Enoxaparin (Lovenox) and dalteparin (Fragmin) are both LMWH preparations that can safely be administered by prehospital professionals under the guidance of medical direction. Enoxaparin is given with much greater frequency than dalteparin.

The dose for enoxaparin and dalteparin is the same, and should be administered in conjunction with aspirin.

▶ Initial dose is 1 mg/kg, to be given subcutaneously. It is to be given BID (twice daily), so realistically the prehospital provider will only be giving the first dose.

Fibrinolytic (Thrombolytic) Therapy

Fibrinolytic Therapy: Mechanism of Action

Fibrinolytic therapy (also known as thrombolytic therapy) has revolutionized the treatment of and decreased the mortality rate from acute myocardial infarction. Through a chemical conversion, fibrinolytics activate enzymes that proceed to dissolve the thrombus or clot that is occluding the coronary artery. When this occurs, a reperfusion of the oxygen-starved myocardium takes place. Consequently, the process of infarction can be halted and areas of ischemic myocardium salvaged.

Fibrinolytic Therapy: Indications

Fibrinolytics should be initiated as soon as possible to anyone who is under 75 years of age, satisfies predetermined criteria, and does not exhibit any contraindications to the therapy. The age limit can be higher than 75 years, but the therapy's benefit is diminished. Predetermined criteria include a history and clinical presentation compatible with a myocardial infarction, ST segment elevation that suggests infarction, and/or a presumably new left bundle branch block. Fibrinolytics should be administered within the first 12 hours of onset of symptoms to achieve the greatest benefit.

Research shows that a significant decrease in mortality was *not* realized with prehospital administration versus early emergency department (< 30 minutes) administration of the drug. Therefore, given the risk of potential complications, the use of fibrinolytic drugs in the prehospital environment is uncommon. The authors recommend that readers keep abreast of continued research on these drugs.

Fibrinolytic Therapy: Side Effects/Precautions

As fibrinolytics promote the dissolution of blood clots, bleeding is a serious complication of fibrinolytic therapy. This is a major concern if trauma is induced by CPR, there are excessive venipuncture attempts, or the patient has a propensity toward intracranial hemorrhage. In addition, caution must be exercised when fibrinolytics are administered to anyone with a history of GI bleeding or cardiovascular problems that may result in internal hemorrhage. Generally, if any of the above has been reported within 2 to 4 weeks preceding the cardiac event, care should be exercised.

Care should also be exercised if a patient presents with hypertension, has a history of chronic hypertension, is pregnant, or is receiving anticoagulant therapy. Since certain fibrinolytics can cause hypotension, if this occurs, the infusion should be reduced and the blood pressure carefully monitored. Allergic reactions have been known to occur and should be treated with appropriate medications such as steroids and diphenhydramine.

It must be noted that the process of thrombus formation is an ongoing process. After a clot is dissolved, it may start to reform. Therefore, adjunctive therapy, such as heparin, is often used in conjunction with fibrinolytic agents.

Furthermore, as clots are dissolved, residual pieces can break free and travel throughout the body as emboli. The emboli can then create other occlusive problems such as pulmonary embolism or cerebrovascular accident. Therefore, vigilant patient monitoring for such complications is a must.

Fibrinolytic Therapy: Contraindications
In the administration of fibrinolytics, many absolute contraindications and relative contraindications are based on the danger of promoting deadly hemorrhage.

Absolute Contraindications

▶ Active internal hemorrhage within the past 21 days

▶ Suspected aortic aneurysm

▶ Recent head trauma or known intracranial tumor

▶ Surgery within past 14 days

▶ History of stroke in the past 12 months

▶ Known bleeding disorders

Relative Contraindications

▶ Recent trauma or surgery within the past 2 months

▶ Initial blood pressure of > 180 mmHg systolic and/or > 110 mmHg diastolic pressure that is controlled by medical treatment

▶ Active bleeding ulcers

▶ History of stroke, tumor, injury, or brain surgery

▶ Known bleeding disorder or use of warfarin (Coumadin)

▶ Significant kidney or liver dysfunction

▶ Previous use of the thrombolytic agents streptokinase or anistreplase within the past 12 months

▶ Known cancer with possible thoracic, abdominal, or intracranial abnormalities

▶ Prolonged CPR efforts

Part Nine: Other Cardiovascular Drugs

The remaining two drugs, used in specific cardiovascular emergency situations, do not readily fit into any of the aforementioned categories. As such, they have been placed here at the end of the chapter under a general heading. But be aware that this placement is not meant to imply that these drugs are unimportant or ineffective. It is actually quite the opposite: When these drugs are called for, they are often the only option you have to correct the abnormality.

Sodium Bicarbonate

Sodium Bicarbonate: Mechanism of Action
Cardiac arrest produces a lack of adequate perfusion and oxygenation at the cellular level. The body rapidly uses up all the residual oxygen in the blood while allowing the accumulation of waste products. After all the oxygen has been depleted in the cells, and in an attempt to maintain normal activity, the metabolism will change from aerobic to anaerobic. Anaerobic metabolism, however, creates important waste products, mainly hydrogen ions (H+) and carbon dioxide (CO_2), which accumulate in the body to toxic levels. This profound acidosis has a nega-

tive impact on cellular function, myocardial activity, and survivability from cardiac arrest.

Normally, the body can handle the acid production by combining the "strong" hydrogen acid waste product with a base (alkaline) substance. This in turn yields a "weak" acid, carbonic acid, which in turn dissociates into carbon dioxide and water (see below). The carbon dioxide is eliminated through the respiratory system, while the water is eliminated by the kidneys.

hydrogen ion [plus] bicarbonate ion [equals] carbonic acid
[which yields] carbon dioxide and water

Or, as a chemical formula:

$$H^+ + HCO_3^- \rightleftarrows H_2CO_3 \rightleftarrows H_2O + CO_2$$

This process is known as "blood buffering" of hydrogen ions, the process by which the body maintains acid-base balance. Unfortunately the body's compensatory mechanism, the buffering process, is overwhelmed in cardiac arrest because excessive amounts of hydrogen and carbon dioxide are produced. This propels the process in the opposite direction to produce hydrogen ions and increased acidosis. Sodium bicarbonate may be useful when this occurs.

Sodium bicarbonate is nothing more than a "salt," which will dissociate into sodium (Na^+) and the bicarbonate ion (HCO_3^-). The bicarbonate ion liberated during this process is then available to bind the excess hydrogen waste products, which will help lower the acidity of the blood. Integral to the success of this process, however, is adequate pulmonary blood flow and ventilation to eliminate CO_2 produced at the end of the reaction.

Sodium Bicarbonate: Indications

Years ago, sodium bicarbonate was one of the cornerstone medications used in cardiac arrest. The theory was that profound metabolic acidosis accompanies cardiac arrest, and sodium bicarbonate administration would correct that abnormality. Subsequent studies have not supported the routine use of sodium bicarbonate in cardiac arrest.

The poor tissue perfusion that accompanies CPR does not allow for sufficient elimination of the CO_2 that is produced by the bicarbonate buffering process. The produced CO_2 accumulates, pushing the buffering reaction in the reverse direction to re-produce hydrogen ions. Since carbon dioxide diffuses easily into the cells, there is a resultant worsening of intracellular acidosis. This finding has been associated with many adverse reactions.

As a result, sodium bicarbonate has a less important role in the management of cardiac arrest. Effective ventilations and chest compressions have been shown to adequately limit the accumulation of acid in cardiac arrests of short duration. This is because most acidosis in early cardiac arrest states is caused by respiratory insufficiency. Thus, in the early phases of CPR, a buffering agent is unnecessary.

Under certain circumstances, sodium bicarbonate may still play a role in cardiac arrest management. For example, if there is confirmed preexisting metabolic acidosis or hyperkalemia, sodium bicarbonate administration may be beneficial. During routine cardiac arrest management, however, bicarbonate administration should be considered only after the other interventions—CPR, defibrillation, intubation, ventilation, and epinephrine administration—have failed to produce successful results. Sodium bicarbonate is also indicated in known, pre-existing hyperkalemia and tricyclic antidepressant overdose.

Sodium Bicarbonate: Side Effects/Precautions

As alluded to earlier, a major concern with sodium bicarbonate administration is the worsening of intracellular acidosis when carbon dioxide is rapidly produced from buffering hydrogen ions. This high level of CO_2 is actually more immediately damaging to the myocardium than the accumulation of the hydrogen ions, since they do not pass through the cellular walls as rapidly as CO_2 does. This serves as the first precaution when using sodium bicarbonate.

Also, since the bicarbonate is attached to a sodium ion that is liberated upon administration, hypernatremia and hyperosmolarity are also concerns when larger quantities of sodium bicarbonate are used. Excessive metabolic alkalosis caused by bicarbonate overutilization also impedes the release of oxygen from hemoglobin at the tissue level.

Lastly, as a general rule, do not administer sodium bicarbonate when sympathomimetic drugs are being given. Sympathomimetics (e.g., epinephrine, dopamine) can be deactivated in an alkaline environment. If you are administering sodium bicarbonate and other drugs through the same IV line, be sure to properly flush out the line after each medication administration.

Sodium Bicarbonate: Contraindications

Actually, there are no absolute contraindications to the use of sodium bicarbonate as long as the precautions identified above are understood and followed. But again, remember that sodium bicarbonate is not a first line agent in the treatment of metabolic acidosis in cardiac arrest. It should only be administered after the interventions described above have been completed.

Sodium Bicarbonate: Dosage

When sodium bicarbonate is to be used, it should not be administered for the first 10–20 minutes of cardiac arrest management unless hyperkalemia or pre-existing acidosis is present. Administer sodium bicarbonate only after other interventions have been proven unsuccessful.

▶ *IV administration*—Administer 1 milliequivalent per kilogram (1 mEq/kg) IV bolus. The dose can be repeated at half its initial amount (0.5 mEq/kg) every 10 minutes thereafter.

Preferentially, use arterial blood gas analysis to guide the administration of sodium bicarbonate.

Calcium Chloride

Calcium Chloride: Mechanism of Action

Calcium, like magnesium, is an elemental ion that is necessary for numerous physiological activities of the body. Calcium chloride replaces calcium in cases of hypocalcemia. Its main role in the management of cardiovascular emergencies, is its influence on muscle contraction. Calcium ions increase the force of myocardial contractions. They do this by entering the portion of the cell where actin and myosin filaments interact. Here, calcium can initiate and strengthen the myofibril shortening. Calcium may also aid in peripheral vasoconstriction, which will allow for a rise in blood pressure when coupled with its myocardial effects.

Calcium Chloride: Indications

Although it is well established that calcium plays a critical role in myocardial performance, studies have so far not shown administration of calcium chloride in cardiac arrest to be beneficial. This may be due to the excessively high levels of calcium that develop with its administration. Therefore, it has a limited (albeit important) role in the management of the patient experiencing a cardiovascular emergency.

Listed below are specific conditions in which calcium administration would be desirable.

▶ Acute hyperkalemia (elevated potassium)

▶ Acute hypocalcemia (decreased calcium)

▶ As prophylactic therapy preceding the use of calcium channel blockers

▶ Calcium channel blocker toxicity

In these instances, the main role of calcium is to prevent the negative effects of the initial disturbance (e.g., changes in potassium or calcium levels). Remember to try to guide the administration of calcium chloride by documented abnormalities in blood lab values.

Calcium Chloride: Side Effects/Precautions

One of the most important considerations when administering calcium chloride is to first ascertain if the patient is on digitalis. Calcium can cause digitalis toxicity and ventricular irritability. Additionally, be sure to administer calcium through a secure IV line, since extravasation of this drug can result in local tissue necrosis. Also important are the precautions pertaining to drug interactions for calcium chloride. If calcium chloride and sodium bicarbonate are simultaneously administered into an IV line, mixing the two will result in the formation of a precipitate.

Be sure to also administer the drug dose over the appropriate amount of time. Administering calcium chloride too quickly has been associated with a slowing of the cardiac rate. Other side effects relating to the drug itself include:

▶ Nausea

▶ Vomiting

▶ Syncope

▶ Bradycardias

▶ Dysrhythmias

▶ Cardiac arrest

Calcium Chloride: Contraindications

Since the complications that result from promoting digitalis toxicity are so severe, the use of calcium should be avoided in those patients concurrently receiving a digitalis preparation.

Calcium Chloride: Dosages

Of the different preparations available, it is best to use the 10% calcium chloride solution, since this has been shown to be the most effective in increasing plasma levels of calcium. Based upon the need for the calcium administration, the dosage may vary.

Prophylaxis when Administering Calcium Channel Blockers

▶ Using the 10% solution of calcium chloride, administer 2 mg/kg to 4 mg/kg via slow IV push. If the desired effects are not seen, you can repeat the drug administration at the same dose after 10 minutes.

Hyperkalemia and Calcium Channel Blocker Overdose

▶ In these instances, the dose of calcium needs to be increased in order to receive the desired benefit. As such, administer 8 mg/kg to 16 mg/kg via slow IV push. If, however, there is no clinical response after 10 minutes, you can repeat administration at the same dose.

CASE STUDY FOLLOW-UP

On your favorite Tuesday night TV show, *Code Blue, Stat!*, a patient named Mr. Hedger has called EMS for severe chest pain, diaphoresis, and dizziness. You are especially interested in this episode, because you had a patient just like Mr. Hedger only a few hours ago while at work. You settle back to match wits with the fictional prehospital providers, and to second-guess the assessment and care the script-writers have thought up for this patient.

Assessment

From the assessment performed by the TV actors, you believe that the patient is most likely experiencing either myocardial ischemia or infarction complicated by bradycardia. In this instance, just like the one you saw at work, the goals of treatment are to decrease anxiety, ensure oxygenation, normalize the rate, and limit or reverse the myocardial ischemic process. Before getting too involved in the way the TV team is managing this patient, however, there are certain assessment parameters that you would like to know about.

Your mind drifts back to the assessment you performed on your patient, including a full set of vitals, airway and breathing patency, lung sounds, 12-lead ECG, skin characteristics, and associated signs and symptoms.

The patient provides some history in how he was feeling as the TV emergency providers continue the assessment: the pain is described as substernal, radiating into the left arm, started 2 hours ago, lungs clear, abdomen benign, no peripheral edema, skin cool and diaphoretic, 12-lead shows early ischemia in the inferior leads, vitals are BP 122/76 mmHg, HR 42/minute, RR 26/minute.

Treatment

You are pleased by the appropriateness of the TV show demonstrating that these assessment findings were completed prior to the main treatment. However, the TV actors seem to be having some trouble deciding what to administer to the patient. One provider hesitates as the cardiac monitors and gadgets flash and blink and fill the air with a chorus of hums, clicks, beeps, and rings. You talk to the TV as if the EMS crew can hear you. "OK, pal, you already have the patient oxygenated and an IV initiated. Let's get the ball rolling so this guy doesn't go farther down the tubes. Give some aspirin to stop the clotting."

You decide to give the TV crew some more advice. You remind them that certain drugs, like oxygen, nitroglycerin, and morphine, have the ability to decrease the workload on the heart, which is appropriate to help reduce ischemia. As well, Mr. Hedger is bradycardic, and for this you advise starting with atropine at 1 milligram IV push, since it is a parasympatholytic that will increase the heart rate with only a small increase in the workload. If this doesn't work, you point out, transcutaneous pacing is always an option.

The TV actors? Well, they mumble out something about giving nitroglycerin sublingual at 0.3 mg. "Good boy," you say. "That may help reduce the ischemic pain and decrease the ischemic area." Next they mention dopamine. "What???" you yell to the TV. "How about finishing out the administration of atropine or use TCP before using such a strong sympathomimetic?!" Well, the TV actors don't seem to be listening to you. They continue with 10 μg/kg/min intravenously. "No, no!" you groan. "Start at 5 μg per kilogram per minute with an infusion, then work your way up!"

While packaging the patient for transport, one provider chimes in that the blood pressure is starting to drop. The other provider increases the dopamine to 20 micrograms per kilogram per minute, and you yell, "Fluid bolus, fluid bolus!!"—recalling that careful administration of a fluid bolus can increase preload and

continued on next page

myocardial stretch, which enhances contractility. "By the way," you ask the TV team, "has the chest pain resolved? If not," you urge, "try some morphine—cautiously—perhaps 2 mg IV push. That will help, as long as the systolic blood pressure isn't too low." This time, fortunately, the crew seems to have heard you. One provider consults with medical direction and he orders the morphine after the patient continues to complain of chest pain.

Suddenly you're pulled away from the TV show because your telephone is ringing. It's your friend Dawn. You and she got off work at the same time tonight. She says, "Hey, switch to Channel 3. *Code Blue, Stat!* is on and they are really botching up this MI. "I know," you tell her. "I'm watching it. . . . I'm just glad we didn't treat our MI patient like that today. We would probably both be mopping the station floor if we did!"

▓ SUMMARY

Pharmacological therapy is an integral component of successful cardiac arrest management. The health care provider must become completely familiar with the most common drugs used. There are no short cuts. You must learn and stay abreast of current medications. For each drug, you must learn the mechanisms of action, indications, side effects and precautions, contraindications, and dosages. You must not rely on pocket references and charts. In the heat of an emergency, there is no time to look things up and, unless you already have a thorough understanding of *how each drug works,* mistakes are easy to make.

REVIEW QUESTIONS

1. While treating a patient experiencing a cardiovascular emergency, which of the following drugs is most likely to be initially administered?
   a. atropine
   b. nitroglycerin
   c. oxygen
   d. 0.45% sodium chloride

2. Why is atropine beneficial in the management of a patient with sinus bradycardia?
   a. Atropine mimics the effects of enhanced parasympathetic stimulation.
   b. Atropine blocks the effects of enhanced parasympathetic stimulation.
   c. Atropine mimics the effects of sympathetic stimulation.
   d. Atropine blocks the effects of sympathetic stimulation.

3. Epinephrine administered via IV push during cardiac arrest increases coronary and cerebral perfusion by
   a. dilating coronary and cerebral blood vessels.
   b. constricting coronary and cerebral blood vessels.
   c. reducing systemic vascular resistance.
   d. increasing systemic vascular resistance.

4. What type of adrenergic stimulation accounts for the changes in coronary and cerebral perfusion identified in Question 3?
   a. alpha
   b. beta
   c. dopaminergic
   d. synaptic

5. Which one of the following drugs could alter the pupillary findings in a patient?
   a. atropine
   b. lidocaine
   c. oxygen
   d. nitroglycerin

6. ACE inhibitors are beneficial to the MI patient because
   a. they drop systemic vascular resistance.
   b. they help keep the size of the infarction from enlarging.
   c. they inhibit calcium ion movement across the cellular membrane to decrease SVR.
   d. a and b are correct

7. Which of the following rhythm(s) could procainamide be used for?
   a. PSVT uncontrolled refractory to traditional dosages of adenosine
   b. stable wide complex tachycardia of unknown etiology
   c. ventricular fibrillation refractory to amiodarone and lidocaine
   d. all of the above

8. Verapamil and diltiazem share what common mechanism of action?
   a. Both are calcium channel blockers.
   b. Both are sympathomimetics.
   c. Both are diuretics.
   d. Both are vasoconstrictors.

9. Based on their mechanism of action, what is the major indication shared by verapamil and diltiazem?
   a. Both may be used to treat tachydysrhythmias.
   b. Both may be used to treat bradycardia.
   c. Both may be used to treat pulmonary edema.
   d. Both may be used to treat hypotension.

10. Procainamide's mechanism of action is most similar to the action of
    a. atropine.
    b. adenosine.
    c. lidocaine.
    d. verapamil.

11. Which of the following drugs would be most appropriate for a patient with symptomatic tachycardia and a history of Wolff-Parkinson-White (WPW) syndrome?
    a. verapamil
    b. diltiazem
    c. morphine
    d. adenosine

12. Of the following drugs, which is most dissimilar to the other three?
    a. magnesium sulfate
    b. lidocaine
    c. procainamide
    d. diltiazem

13. When appropriate, the same drug may be applicable in numerous situations. Epinephrine, for example, can be used for both
    a. bradycardia and hypertension.
    b. chest pain and ventricular irritability.
    c. cardiac arrest and bradycardia.
    d. b and c are correct

14. What is the major indication for sodium bicarbonate?
    a. symptomatic hypotension
    b. systemic hypokalemia
    c. respiratory acidosis
    d. metabolic acidosis

15. An increase in venous capacitance and a reduction in systemic vascular resistance is characteristic of which one of the following drugs?
    a. dopamine
    b. procainamide
    c. morphine
    d. nitrous oxide

16. Which of the following drugs will have a depressive effect on the pumping action of the heart?
    a. atropine
    b. calcium chloride
    c. diltiazem
    d. epinephrine

17. Which of the following will **not** depress the pumping action of the heart at therapeutic doses?
    a. lidocaine
    b. diltiazem
    c. propranolol
    d. atenolol

18. Which of the following drugs is **primarily** an alpha receptor stimulator?
    a. epinephrine
    b. norepinephrine
    c. dopamine
    d. All of the above equally stimulate alpha receptor sites.

19. If you are treating a patient with diminished systemic vascular resistance, which of the following drug(s) could help restore the vascular tone?
    a. epinephrine
    b. norepinephrine
    c. dopamine
    d. All of the above could help restore vascular tone.

20. Which of the following drugs would be the most similar in action to dopamine when used to raise blood pressure?
    a. atropine
    b. dobutamine
    c. isoproterenol
    d. metoprolol

21. Esmolol exerts its action by
    a. inhibiting alpha adrenergic receptor sites.
    b. inhibiting calcium ion movement.
    c. increasing systemic vascular resistance.
    d. blocking beta adrenergic receptor sites.

22. Based on its actions as addressed in Question 21, esmolol may be indicated for treatment of which of the following conditions?
    a. stable angina
    b. a slow heart rate
    c. hypotension
    d. b and c are correct

23. All of the following drugs can result in peripheral vasodilation except for
    a. nitroglycerin.
    b. morphine.
    c. digitalis.
    d. nitroprusside.

24. Which of the following is **not** a mechanism of action for the class of drugs known as "beta blockers"?
    a. depress contractility
    b. diminish oxygen requirements to the heart
    c. decrease the heart rate
    d. increase the blood pressure

25. You are treating a patient suffering from severe congestive heart failure (CHF). Based on the mechanisms of action of the following drugs, which would you most likely **avoid?**
    a. nitroglycerin
    b. lasix
    c. morphine
    d. verapamil

26. The initial dose of 2.5 mg IV push is appropriate for which of the following medications?
    a. oxygen
    b. verapamil
    c. adenosine
    d. diltiazem

27. **Initial** therapy for a patient with chest pain, dyspnea, and symptomatic bradycardia should include which of the following?
    a. atropine at 2.5 mg/kg
    b. oxygen via nonrebreather at 15 lpm
    c. external pacing
    d. dopamine at 2.5 µg/kg/min

28. Epinephrine is traditionally repeated at
    a. 1 mg.
    b. 3 mg.
    c. 5 mg.
    d. none of the above

29. What drug, when administered for hemodynamically unstable bradycardia, has the **maximum** dosage of 0.04 mg/kg?
    a. epinephrine
    b. isoproterenol
    c. dopamine
    d. none of the above

30. What drug has the initial dose of 1–1.5 mg/kg?
    a. lidocaine
    b. amiodarone
    c. procainamide
    d. magnesium sulfate

31. Which of the following drugs does **not** have an initial dose of 1 mg?
    a. epinephrine
    b. atropine
    c. sodium bicarbonate
    d. none of the above

32. The repeat dose of amiodarone for ventricular fibrillation is
    a. 150 mg/kg.
    b. 300 mg/kg.
    c. 150 mg.
    d. 300 mg.

33. What drug, used for symptomatic paroxysmal supraventricular tachycardia (PSVT), may be administered at 6 mg IVP as an initial dose?
    a. verapamil
    b. adenosine
    c. diltiazem
    d. none of the above

34. What drug used for symptomatic PSVT is administered at 10 mg IVP as an initial dose?
    a. adenosine
    b. verapamil
    c. diltiazem
    d. none of the above

35. How much magnesium sulfate should be mixed with 10 ml of D_5W for administration in ventricular fibrillation?
    a. 1 mg
    b. 1 gram
    c. 1 mg/kg
    d. none of the above

36. Which of the following drugs is **not** usually administered in milligrams per kilograms for the initial bolus?
    a. sodium bicarbonate
    b. lidocaine
    c. diltiazem
    d. none of the above

37. What is the appropriate dose for the correct answer in Question 36?
    a. 1 mEq/kg
    b. 10 mEq/kg
    c. 5 mEq/kg
    d. none of the above

38. Morphine is administered at
    a. 2–10 mg slow IVP.
    b. 1 mg/kg slow IVP.
    c. 0.5 mg to 1.0 mg slow IVP.
    d. none of the above

39. Which of the following is an appropriate dose of calcium chloride in a patient with known hyperkalemia, or calcium channel overdose?
    a. 3 mg/kg
    b. 6 mg/kg
    c. 8 mg/kg
    d. none of the above

40. What sympathomimetic infusion can be administered initially at 2 µg/min?
    a. procainamide
    b. epinephrine
    c. dopamine
    d. none of the above

41. To allow for stimulation of beta adrenergic receptor sites in the heart, dopamine should be run at
    a. 10 μg/kg/min.
    b. 2 μg/kg/min.
    c. 20 μg/kg/min.
    d. none of the above

42. To allow primarily for stimulation of alpha adrenergic receptors sites in the vasculature, **dopamine** should be run at
    a. 2 μg/kg/min.
    b. 5 μg/kg/min.
    c. 10 μg/kg/min.
    d. 20 μg/kg/min.

43. Which of the following infusions for bradycardia does **not** have a maximum infusion rate of 10 μg/min?
    a. epinephrine
    b. isoproterenol
    c. dopamine
    d. none of the above

44. A correct initial dose of amiodarone for ventricular fibrillation would be
    a. 300 mg.
    b. 7.5 mg/kg.
    c. 150 mg.
    d. 300 mg/kg.

45. What drug is usually administered at 20–30 mg/min?
    a. atropine
    b. dopamine
    c. procainamide
    d. none of the above

46. When administering 0.4 mg doses of nitroglycerin sublingually for chest pain, the maximum dosage should be
    a. 1 mg.
    b. 1.2 mg.
    c. 3 mg.
    d. none of the above

47. What would be an appropriate starting dose for a lidocaine maintenance infusion?
    a. 5 μg/min
    b. 2 mg/min
    c. 3 mg/kg/min
    d. none of the above

48. Vasopressin is administered for what purpose?
    a. to decrease myocardial workload in an MI
    b. to enhance conduction velocity in an infranodal block
    c. to reduce afterload during a hypertensive crisis
    d. none of the above

49. What would be an acceptable loading dose of furosemide for a 55 kg patient?
    a. 55 mg
    b. 10 mg
    c. 22.5 μg
    d. none of the above

50. Fibrinolytics have what mechanism of action?
    a. They dissolve plaque fissures.
    b. They dissolve calcium deposits in coronary vessels.
    c. They dissolve newly formed embolic clots.
    d. They dissolve fibrous scar tissue found in ventricular walls following an MI.

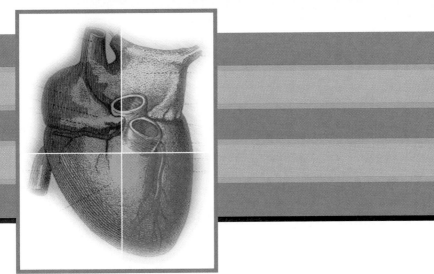

Acute Coronary Syndromes

Annually, over 1,000,000 people experience an acute myocardial infarction (AMI or MI), with nearly 500,000 of these lives being claimed. Furthermore, the majority of these deaths, about 250,000 annually, take place outside of a medical facility, with many occurring before any medical attention is ever sought. Remarkably, this figure does not account for the millions of people permanently disabled by an acute MI. From this perspective, health care professionals must develop a great appreciation of the devastating impact that the acute myocardial infarction has, not only on the individual but on society as a whole.

Topics in this chapter are:

- The Heart as a Pump
- Pathophysiology of an AMI
- Assessment of the Ischemic Chest Pain/AMI Patient
- Management of Ischemic Chest Pain/AMI: Prehospital, ED, and Hospital Considerations
- Management of Specific AMI Presentations

NOTE: The guidelines for management of patients with ischemic chest pain and acute MI discussed in this chapter have been published by the American Heart Association in collaboration with the International Liaison Committee on Resuscitation. "Guidelines 2000 for Cardiopulmonary Resuscitation and Emergency Cardiovascular Care: International Consensus on Science, Part 3: Adult Basic Life Support." Circulation. 2000; 102 (suppl I): I-22–I-59.

CASE STUDY

You are called to a residence for a male patient complaining of chest discomfort. Upon arrival, you find Steve, a 48-year-old male, who is pale, disoriented, diaphoretic, and complaining of constant chest pain that radiates to his upper back.

With much difficulty and confusion, Steve tells you that he has had this chest pain for the past day and a half. He continues on to state that he has had several episodes of "blacking out" and difficulty in breathing. In addition, you discover that Steve has a history of previous heart attacks and hypertension.

Quickly, you obtain a set of vitals which include a pulse of 52 beats per minute, respirations at 32 per minute with noted effort, and blood pressure of 78 by palpation. You inquire whether Steve has taken any medications for his present condition. Instead of replying, Steve turns slightly combative and noncompliant.

How would you proceed to assess and care for this patient? This chapter will describe the assessment and management of a patient suffering ischemic chest pain, acute MI, or acute coronary syndrome. Later, we will return to the case and apply the procedures learned.

INTRODUCTION

Frequently, an acute MI occurs secondary to coronary artery disease. The magnitude of the threat of acute MI becomes quite evident when we consider the estimates that well over 6 million Americans have significant coronary artery disease! Regrettably, an acute MI and subsequent disability and/or death are often the first, and sometimes the last, sign of decades of coronary artery disease.

Advances in medicine have produced interventions that can successfully counter the adverse effects of the myocardial infarction and have made surviving an acute MI a realistic possibility. However, the process of reperfusing myocardial muscle by use of fibrinolytics or procedures such as angioplasty is extremely time dependent and may vary dramatically in response to the variety of infarct presentations. Therefore, to appropriately manage an acute MI or other coronary syndrome, you must have a strong working knowledge of the heart and its relation to the rest of the human body.

This chapter will provide a framework and basic knowledge required for effective management of the acute myocardial infarction.

THE HEART AS A PUMP

The heart functions as a pump. Through the circulatory system, the heart pumps blood to every organ, tissue, and cell in the human body. Each living cell depends upon the continual circulation of blood for the delivery of oxygen and elimination of wastes. *Without sufficient circulation, the organs, tissues, cells, and subsequently the human organism will die.* Therefore, the effective pumping action of the heart is critical to the maintenance of life. Any problem with the muscular pump can result in serious disability and even death.

The effective circulation of oxygenated blood relies on two distinct pumping actions, one on the right side of the heart and one on the left side (Figure 9-1). Consequently, the heart must be viewed as two distinct pumps that function simultaneously.

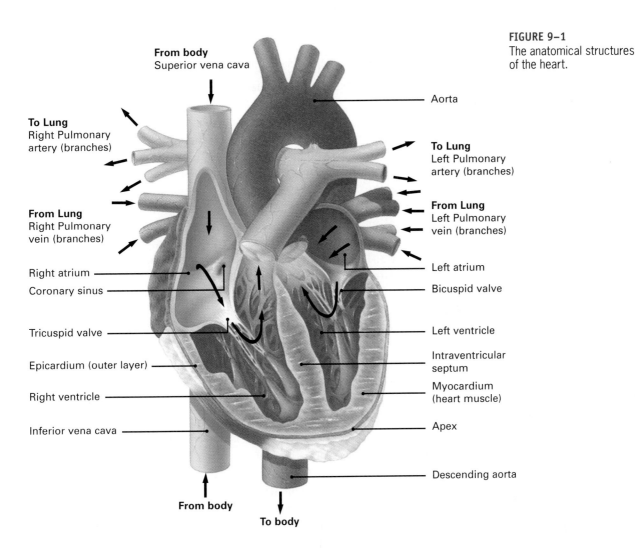

FIGURE 9–1
The anatomical structures
of the heart.

From body
Superior vena cava

Aorta

To Lung
Right Pulmonary
artery (branches)

To Lung
Left Pulmonary
artery (branches)

From Lung
Right Pulmonary
vein (branches)

From Lung
Left Pulmonary
vein (branches)

Right atrium

Left atrium

Coronary sinus

Bicuspid valve

Tricuspid valve

Left ventricle

Epicardium (outer layer)

Intraventricular
septum

Right ventricle

Myocardium
(heart muscle)

Inferior vena cava

Apex

Descending aorta

From body

To body

The Right-Side Pump

The right atrium and right ventricle compose the right-side pump. The function of
the right side of the heart is to eject the unoxygenated blood that has been returned
to the heart by the venous system into the capillaries of the lungs for reoxygenation. This delivery is very dependent on the effective contraction of the right ventricle. *Any compromise in right ventricular contraction can cause blood to back up
into the venous system, thus resulting in a reduction of blood sent to the lungs for
oxygenation and, subsequently, a shortage of blood available to be distributed
through the left side of the heart to the tissues and cells of the body.*

The Left-Side Pump

Similar to the right side, the left-side pump consists of the left atrium and the
thick-walled left ventricle. The left-side pump works to deliver the freshly oxygenated blood that has been returned to the heart from the lungs to every cell in the
human body. As the powerful left ventricle contracts, blood is ejected into the arterial system. *Any compromise in left ventricular contraction can reduce the amount
of blood ejected into the arterial system and cause an increase in pulmonary vessel hydrostatic pressure, leading to a reduction in the amount of oxygenated blood
for distribution to the tissues and cells of the body.*

The Cardiac Output

With each contraction of the heart, blood is ejected into the circulatory system. The quantity of blood that the heart ejects with each contraction is commonly referred to as *stroke volume*. The stroke volume is very dependent on *preload* (blood available from the right side of the heart), *afterload* (pressure against which the heart must eject the blood), and *contractility* (the muscular contraction of the ventricles). If preload is inadequate, the stroke volume will decrease. Similarly, a significantly elevated afterload will also decrease stroke volume in that it is more difficult for the heart to eject blood against high pressure.

Contractility depends on preload to fill and stretch the ventricular muscle fibers. Myocardial muscle fibers are elastic, and after incoming preload sufficiently stretches them, a mechanical stimulus causes the muscle fibers to "snap" back to original size. This is the action that provides the mechanism of contraction. The principle of this action is referred to as *Starling's Law* which states that the greater the stretching of the myocardium (to a certain point) the more forceful the subsequent contraction will be. With this in mind, it is easy to understand how an inadequate preload, and resulting inadequate stretching of the myocardial fibers, can cause a significant decrease in stroke volume.

The amount of blood pumped in one minute is referred to as the *cardiac output*. Cardiac output is dependent on both stroke volume and heart rate. In equation form:

$$\text{Cardiac Output} = \text{Stroke Volume} \times \text{Heart Rate}$$

Heart rate and stroke volume can interact in a variety of ways to determine cardiac output. If the stroke volume remains constant while the heart rate increases, the overall cardiac output will rise. However, if the stroke volume is compromised, an increase in heart rate will not result in increased cardiac output. This is a danger with paroxysmal supraventricular tachycardia (PSVT). Conversely, a bradycardic rhythm with no increase in stroke volume will result in a decreased cardiac output. And, even if the stroke volume increases, the slow heart rate will prevent it from effecting an optimal cardiac output. The interplay between stroke volume, heart rate, and cardiac output is summarized below.

Stroke Volume/Heart Rate Changes	Cardiac Output Result
Increased stroke volume with an increased or unchanged heart rate	Increased
Increased heart rate with an increased or unchanged stroke volume	Increased
Increased stroke volume with a decreased heart rate	Unchanged
Decreased stroke volume with an increased heart rate	Unchanged
Decreased stroke volume with a decreased or unchanged heart rate	Decreased
Decreased heart rate with a decreased or unchanged stroke volume	Decreased

Unacceptable cardiac output must be examined in terms of the heart rate plus preload, contractility, and afterload (the latter three being the factors that affect stroke volume). If you know which factor or factors are at fault, you can determine which interventions are most likely to restore an adequate cardiac output.

The nervous system varies cardiac output to meet the ever-changing demands of the body. With all parameters functioning normally, the heart is able to supply a cardiac output that is in balance with the needs of every tissue and cell. If a greater amount of blood is needed to provide oxygen and waste removal, the stroke volume and heart rate can be increased so as to increase the cardiac output. The reverse happens during times of rest when the cells do not require much oxygen and waste removal.

Optimal cardiac output is essential for the perfusion of the myocardium. If the cardiac output falls to dangerously low levels, the availability of oxygenated blood to the myocardial cells themselves also decreases. This represents a serious situation, in that the heart must sustain a certain level of arterial perfusion in order to continue to function as a pump.

It is important to emphasize that *myocardial workload and oxygen requirements are directly proportional to the status of the preload, contractility, afterload, and heart rate.* As these factors increase, so do the myocardial workload and oxygen demand. Conversely, the diminishment of these variables results in a heart that consumes less oxygen because it is working less.

As you might assume, *alteration in the heart's ability to pump blood is a distinct possibility in the setting of an acute MI.* Because intervention varies in relation to the presentation of the infarct, it is critical that the clinician have a commanding knowledge of the heart's role as a pumping mechanism and the many variables that affect cardiac output.

PATHOPHYSIOLOGY OF AN AMI

A myocardial infarction must be viewed as a *continuing process* that starts when the heart cells are deprived of oxygen. In order to power the electrical and mechanical actions that permit the heart to pump blood, the myocardial cells must receive an uninterrupted supply of oxygenated blood. In the absence of oxygen, the affected heart cells will become *ischemic* and eventually undergo detrimental changes that promote cellular *injury.* If the provision of oxygen is still not resumed, the injured cells will eventually die and be replaced by nonfunctional scar tissue. This cellular death is termed *infarction.*

The damage inflicted by the acute MI typically arranges into three distinct regions (Figure 9-2). From the center to the outside, these regions are:

- ▷ Infarcted tissue
- ▷ Injured tissue
- ▷ Ischemic tissue

The center of the infarct consists of the actually infarcted (dead) tissue. Since this tissue is nonfunctional, *electrical conduction and active depolarization do not occur.* If the infarct is of significant size, the decrease in active wall motion can seriously impair the ability of the heart to effectively pump blood.

Encircling the infarcted tissue is a ring of injured (but not yet dead) heart cells, which is immediately surrounded by a ring of ischemic heart cells (oxygen-deprived, but not yet injured). The ischemic and injured cells have the potential to *aberrantly conduct electrical impulses.* Electrical aberrancy can result in the production of *lethal* and *nonlethal dysrhythmias.* Additionally, *myocardial ischemia produces pain.* This explains the retrosternal chest pain that is frequently experi-

FIGURE 9–2
A myocardial infarction
typically has three distinct
regions.

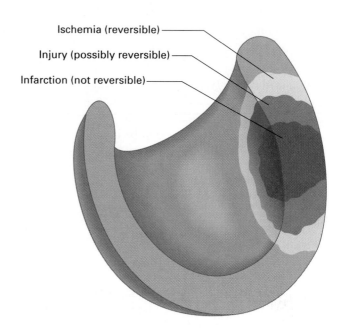

Ischemia (reversible) —————

Injury (possibly reversible) —————

Infarction (not reversible)—————

enced during an acute myocardial infarction. Restoring oxygen to the ischemic cells can reverse ischemia and effectively alleviate the discomfort.

Myocardial ischemia is reversible! This is a critical concept to remember when managing the acute MI. Quick restoration of oxygen to the ischemic heart cells can halt the process of injury and infarction, thus not only alleviating ischemic pain but also preventing further damage and improving patient outcome.

With injured cardiac cells, reversal of the detrimental changes is extremely time dependent. If addressed in a timely fashion, the injury process can effectively be stopped and possibly even reversed. If a significant delay in reoxygenation occurs, the injury will become permanent and possibly result in cellular infarction.

Unfortunately, once the heart cells infarct, their function cannot be restored.

Myocardial infarction occurs secondary to an *insufficient supply of oxygenated blood* for the demanding myocardial cells. Most frequently, this inadequacy is precipitated by coronary artery disease. As the deposition of atherosclerotic plaque narrows the lumen of the coronary arteries, the amount of blood that can pass through the arteries is diminished. In addition, the atherosclerotic surface is covered with plaque, which is rough and prone to the formation of a blood clot, or *thrombus,* that can cause total occlusion with subsequent infarction.

Total occlusion can also occur secondary to a sudden rupture of the plaque, which creates a raw surface upon which a thrombus can form. Again, if the preexisting narrowing is sufficient, the thrombus can generate a total occlusion that deprives any distal cell of necessary oxygen. From this point on, the process of myocardial infarction begins.

In addition to atherosclerosis, an acute MI can be precipitated by a sudden spasm of a coronary artery. Such spasm is often an effect of cocaine or unstable angina. Other causes of infarction include microemboli, severe hypotension, and hypoxemia from acute respiratory failure.

The size and location of an infarct are directly related to the specific coronary artery that has been affected. Recall that the left side of the heart is supplied by the left coronary artery, left circumflex artery, and left anterior descending coronary artery (Figure 9-3). If one of these arteries becomes occluded, an infarct

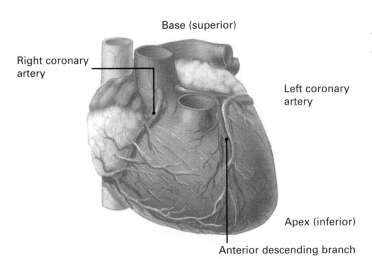

Base (superior)

Right coronary artery

Left coronary artery

Apex (inferior)

Anterior descending branch

FIGURE 9–3
The coronary vessels of the heart.

is likely to occur somewhere in the left ventricle. The more proximal the occlusion, the greater the potential damage, in that more cells beyond the occlusion are now deprived of oxygen. Because pumping blood throughout the body is harder work than pumping blood to the lungs, the left ventricle is larger and more muscular than the right ventricle. Due to its size and workload, the left ventricle is frequently the site for an acute MI.

Similarly, the right coronary artery perfuses the right side of the heart—including the inferior and posterior regions of the myocardium. If the right coronary artery or one of its branches becomes occluded, an infarct must be suspected within the right ventricular region, possibly including the inferior wall of the left myocardium. The right ventricle is affected less often than the left ventricle (Figure 9-3).

An unchecked myocardial infarction can inflict varying degrees of damage to the myocardium. This damage can extend through the entire thickness of the heart wall (*transmural*) or only affect a partial depth of muscle (*subendocardial*). Usually the innermost portion of the heart is affected first. The two types of infarct can be readily differentiated through examination of the ECG tracing. The more serious transmural infarction is identifiable by changes in the normal Q wave. If no changes in the Q wave are observed, but existence of an acute MI is otherwise confirmed, a subendocardial infarction is likely (Figures 9-4A and 9-4B).

Myocardial infarction is a devastating event that can produce two basic complications:

▶ **Abnormal electrical conduction.** *Abnormal electrical conduction arising from the ischemic and injured myocardial tissues can produce lethal and nonlethal dysrhythmias.* This electrical aberrancy indicates serious underlying problems with the myocardium. *Most deaths associated with an acute MI occur secondary to electrical instability.*

During the early hours of infarction, *ventricular fibrillation* is the most common life-threatening dysrhythmia. Other rhythms, such as bradycardia or PVCs, warn of underlying abnormalities that may lead to an immediate life threat if not addressed. Death from electrical dysrhythmias, when it occurs within 1 hour of the onset of cardiac symptoms, is termed sudden death.

▶ **Mechanical pumping failure.** *Mechanical pumping failure secondary to the loss of effective depolarization and contractility is another danger that*

Transmural infarction
after 2-3 days

Subendocardial infarction
after several days

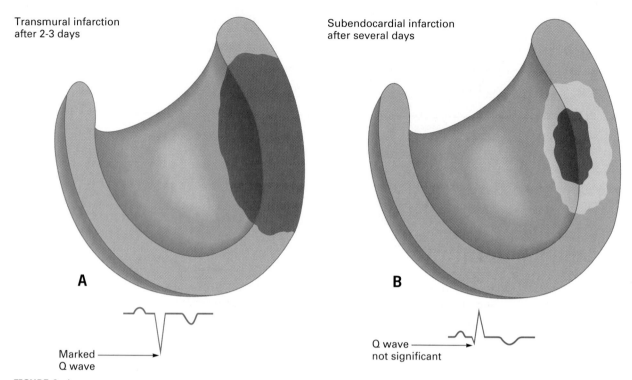

A

B

Marked
Q wave

Q wave
not significant

FIGURE 9–4
(A) A transmural infarction and typical ECG tracing. (B) A subendocardial infarction and typical ECG tracing.

accompanies the acute MI. Extensive infarction can result in significant myocardial wall damage. Infarcted tissue is nonfunctional and does not actively participate in contraction, thus decreasing overall pumping effectiveness and cardiac output. Also, infarcted tissue is weak and has the potential for the formation of aneurysms. If conditions are right, these aneurysms contain the inherent risk of ventricular wall rupture.

All in all, dysrhythmias and the loss of effective contraction can compromise the heart's ability to provide an adequate cardiac output that satisfies the needs of all tissues and cells within the body. If severe, the net result can be disability and even death.

Who Is at Risk?

Many risk factors greatly enhance one's chance of incurring a heart attack. As previously suggested, coronary artery disease is a frontline contributor to the increased incidence of myocardial infarction. While everyone has the potential for coronary artery disease, some individuals are more prone than others to the development of atherosclerotic arteries.

Many risk factors are unchangeable. These include genetics, age, and gender. Conversely, many factors are changeable and, when modified, can significantly reduce the risk of myocardial infarction. When combined with coronary heart disease, these factors place an increased workload on the heart—a workload for which it is not built! These modifiable risks include physical inactivity, obesity, and diets high in fat and cholesterol.

Awareness of nonmodifiable and modifiable risk factors, with relevant and appropriate life-style modification, remains the best way of preventing an acute myocardial infarction.

General Presentation of an Acute Myocardial Infarction

An acute MI can manifest itself with a variety of signs and symptoms. The specific signs and symptoms depend on the *size* and *location* of the infarct and the response of the body to ischemic pain, dysrhythmias, and possible compromise in ventricular pumping ability.

Chest Pain

Chest pain, the most common complaint in the acute myocardial infarction, can occur at rest, or with physical exertion, or as a result of emotional stress. As discussed earlier, chest pain originates from ischemic tissues. Frequently, this pain is described as "oppressive" or "crushing" and is typically located behind the lower half of the sternum. Often, chest pain from an acute MI crescendos in intensity and can radiate to the shoulders, jaw, neck, arms, or back. However, radiation is not a constant. An MI can occur without this pain pattern. Also, myocardial ischemic pain will sometimes locate in the epigastric region, often with the unfortunate result of being dismissed as indigestion. As discussed later in this chapter, some acute MIs are painless or exhibit other symptoms.

Respirations

There are dramatic variations in respiratory presentation relating to factors such as pain, anxiety, electrical dysrhythmias, and pump problems. While a small infarct may result in no respiratory deficit, a large infarct of the left ventricle may cause signs of hypoxia and labored breathing as blood backs up behind the left ventricle, engorges the pulmonary capillaries, and impairs the diffusion of oxygen at the alveolar-capillary membrane.

Edema

If there is a major pump problem, the retention of blood and disturbance of lymphatic fluid drainage may be observable in different regions of the body. Severe right-side pump failure will cause the backup of blood from the right ventricle into the body itself. Engorged neck veins, distended abdomen, enlarged liver, pedal edema, and edema to the lower back of bed-confined patients are all indications of inadequate right-ventricle pumping. These signs may also be evident with a left ventricular failure that has caused right ventricular impairment through the massive backup of blood through the lungs into the right ventricle itself.

Skin Characteristics

Any patient who has cool, clammy skin and is complaining of chest pain must be thoroughly examined! In the presence of an acute MI, skin of either presentation (cool or clammy or both) suggests *hypoperfusion* and activation of the *sympathetic nervous system*. The sympathetic nervous system brings about an increase in heart rate and blood pressure which forces a weak heart to work harder. Therefore, the sympathetic influence upon an infarcting heart is detrimental.

Other Signs and Symptoms

A variety of other complaints may be noted when evaluating a patient with an acute MI. Such complaints can include anxiety, weakness, general malaise, nausea, vomiting, and syncope.

It must be reiterated that an acute myocardial infarction can present with a variety of signs and symptoms. Generally, the presentation is determined by the size and location of the infarct. *Ironically, some individuals suffering an acute MI may complain only of shortness of breath or a vague uneasiness without accompanying pain!* Diabetics, women, and the elderly are more prone to this unique presentation because of nerve degeneration and a lowered ability to perceive pain. *In addition, some patients may have no complaints and suffer what is termed a "silent" MI.* Totally asymptomatic, a silent MI can only be diagnosed by observing delayed ECG changes or characteristic cardiac enzyme elevations.

Regardless of the severity or mildness of outward appearances, it must be recognized that all myocardial infarctions destroy valuable heart tissue and can produce immediate or delayed compromises in normal heart activity. Therefore, anyone with a suspected acute MI or chest pain of probable cardiac origin must be promptly examined and a definitive diagnosis made. This includes any individual with a history of angina who experiences chest pain that is unrelieved by rest and nitroglycerin or who experiences a sudden change in the pattern or duration or severity of the episodes of anginal chest pain.

 # ASSESSMENT OF THE ISCHEMIC CHEST PAIN/AMI PATIENT

Physical examination of the patient with ischemic chest pain focuses on the heart and its ability to pump blood. Recall that during a myocardial infarction the heart is prone to serious electrical dysrhythmias and contractile failure—both of which can adversely affect cardiac output. While not every acute MI will produce a dysrhythmia or pumping failure, the potential does exist and must be taken seriously. In consequence, a targeted assessment of the heart's electrical and hemodynamic capabilities must be rapidly initiated and completed within 7 to 10 minutes.

General Presentation

Initial evaluation focuses on the *general presentation* of the patient. Through rapid observation, an impression of the patient's current problem and level of distress can be quickly developed. Patients suffering an acute MI rarely thrash about but choose to remain still. However, keep in mind that cerebral hypoxia secondary to an inadequate cardiac output can result in a combative, confused patient. Also, pump failure tends to force patients into a sitting position, since the supine position enhances blood return to the heart and forces the strained myocardium to work harder to pump this blood.

The ABCs

Following a quick observation, *the airway, respiratory, and circulatory status* of the cardiac patient must be evaluated.

Airway
If the airway appears obstructed, rapid correction of the obstruction is necessary. Correction can occur, as indicated, through positioning, suctioning, placement of an oropharyngeal airway, or placement of a tracheal tube. Because an infarct occurs secondary to myocardial hypoxia, it is paramount that the airway provide an unobstructed conduit for delivery of oxygen into the lungs.

Breathing
A rapid but thorough evaluation of the respiratory status is crucial. In addition to observing rate and effort, it is necessary to perform a comprehensive auscultation

of all lung fields. As stated earlier, a left ventricular pump problem and consequent inability to eject blood from the ventricle, will cause an increase in the hydrostatic pressure in the pulmonary capillaries, which will result in rales and/or wheezing.

Clear lung sounds could indicate a myocardial infarction without pumping complications, or may suggest only right ventricular involvement. (Recall that right ventricular compromise will promote the accumulation of blood in the venous system, not in the lungs.) A pulse oximeter will be useful in determining the status of oxygen delivery to the tissues.

Circulation

The pumping ability of the heart can quickly be determined by palpating peripheral pulses. In states of low cardiac output, the radial and pedal pulses may be weak or not present at all. Strong distal pulses indicate a heart that is pumping and circulating blood well. Electrical dysrhythmias may cause the pulse to be irregular, fast, or slow. Finally, heart tones and the auscultation of carotid bruits can contribute valuable information as to the current status of the myocardium.

If a pump problem is suspected, *effective management is dependent upon identifying and treating the cause.* If inadequate cardiac output and hypoperfusion result from ventricular failure without dysrhythmias, the ventricle at fault must be identified.

Left Ventricular Failure

As previously discussed, a failing left ventricle can cause unejected blood to pool in the pulmonary capillaries. Depending on the severity of the left ventricular dysfunction, respiratory distress with rales and wheezing may be noted upon auscultation. In addition to dyspnea, severe failure of the left ventricle can bring about a profound decrease in cardiac output.

Right Ventricular Failure

A decrease in the efficiency of the right ventricle causes the backup of blood in the dependent areas of the body, accompanied by relatively clear lung sounds. Again, depending on the severity, failure of the right ventricle to deliver blood through the lungs to the left ventricle can also precipitate a dramatic decrease in cardiac output.

Occasionally, left ventricular failure can provoke right ventricular failure. As blood backs up through the pulmonary circulation and into the right ventricle, there will be signs of right-side failure along with pulmonary congestion.

Vital Signs

Vital signs are not reliable in the diagnosis of an acute myocardial infarction. Depending on the infarct location and severity and the nervous system response, the presenting vital signs can vary tremendously. A sympathetic response can result in a rapid heart rate, but if the parasympathetic response predominates, the result can be a bradycardic rate. Also, dysrhythmias may cause an irregular heart rate.

Blood pressure measurements can also vary. Hypotension in the presence of an acute MI is an ominous sign, suggesting that a significant decrease in cardiac output or profound parasympathetic tone now exists.

In spite of the wide variations in vital signs that can accompany an acute MI, it is important that the examiner monitor the vital signs and view them as valuable clues that can aid in determining the location of damage and the appropriate treatment.

ECG Tracings

In the acute myocardial infarction, electrical dysrhythmias originating from ischemic and injured tissues are a common complication. These dysrhythmias can prove unstable and life threatening. Of particular concern is ventricular fibrillation, which is an immediate life threat and the primary cause of cardiac arrest in the infarcting patient. *Ventricular fibrillation may occur suddenly, with no warning whatsoever.* If treated immediately with defibrillatory shocks, ventricular fibrillation is a correctable rhythm.

While not immediately life threatening, other dysrhythmias such as PVCs and bradycardia may be a warning of underlying abnormalities. Such warning dysrhythmias must be heeded and the underlying abnormality identified and corrected. *If underlying disturbances are ignored, warning dysrhythmias can swiftly degenerate into lethal dysrhythmias with rapidly ensuing death!*

In the setting of an acute MI, electrical monitoring of the heart is paramount. Effective pumping is dependent on solid electrical conduction. Electrical monitoring of the heart is accomplished with an electrocardiograph monitoring device.

While the 3-lead ECG machine adequately illustrates the heart's rate and rhythm, the 12-lead ECG monitor provides a more comprehensive picture of the myocardium during an acute infarction. The 12-lead machine reveals 12 distinct views of the myocardium and can isolate areas of ischemia, injury, and actual infarction (Figure 9-5).

On the 12-lead ECG tracing, ischemia is illustrated by *symmetrically inverted T waves and/or ST segment depression.* Cells incurring injury exhibit an *elevation of the ST segment of more than 1 mm in height.* As stated earlier, infarcted tissue is exhibited by the presence of a *pathologic Q wave* (Figure 9-6). For a relative diagnosis, these changes must be viewed in two or more contiguous leads. This is a general description, and exceptions do apply to certain leads.

It must be remembered that ischemic and injured myocardial cells show the above-mentioned changes immediately, while the pathologic Q waves that define infarction take hours to days for development. Up to 20% of initial ECGs are normal on patients later found to have acute MI. *Therefore, the emergency health care provider must suspect an acute MI on the basis of a compatible history and ECG changes indicative of ischemia and injury.* If the clinician were to remain passive and attempt to discount an MI by the absence of the pathologic Q waves, a fatal mistake could be made.

Table 9-1 correlates the site of infarction and coronary artery with the leads that view them.

Often, the acute MI knows no boundaries. In such cases, infarcts are not exclusive to the anterior wall or lateral wall. Rather, infarcts can cover multiple areas such as the anterolateral or anteroseptal.

History

In addition to the physical exam, a targeted history should be rapidly attained. While suspicion of an acute infarction is based on the patient's symptoms and ECG tracings, a targeted cardiac history can reinforce this suspicion and provide a further guide for specific management.

A cardiac history should focus on the onset, nature, and duration of symptoms associated with the current emergency as well as previous cardiac history. Any symptoms that may potentially pertain to the physiological actions of the heart should be discussed. Questions should address the presence and location of

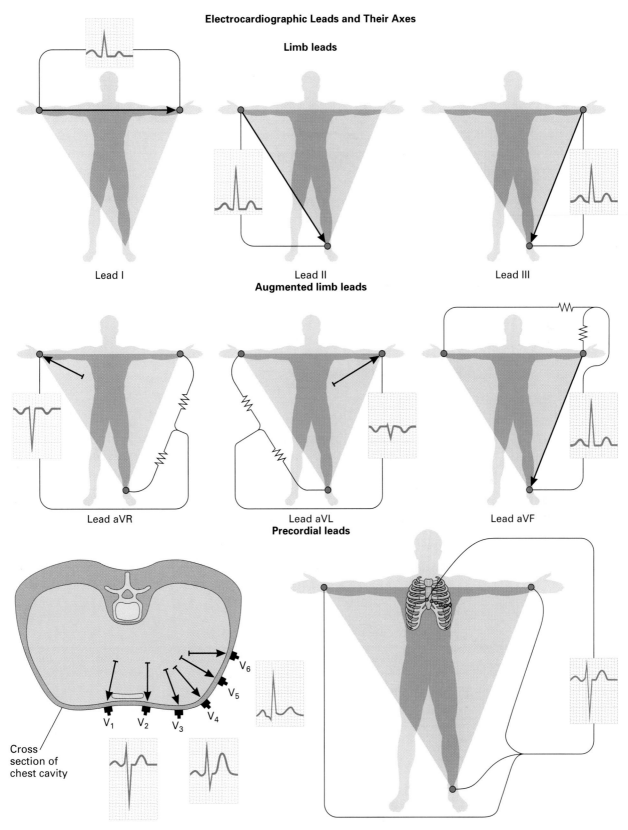

When current flows toward arrowheads (axes), upward deflection occurs in ECG
When current flows away from arrowheads (axes), downward deflection occurs in ECG
When current flows perpendicular to arrows (axes), no deflection occurs

FIGURE 9–5
12-lead placement and views of the heart.

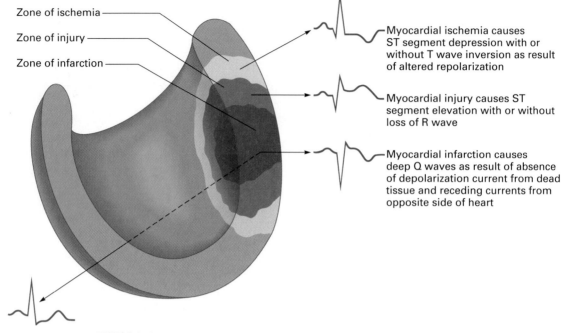

Zone of ischemia

Zone of injury

Zone of infarction

Myocardial ischemia causes ST segment depression with or without T wave inversion as result of altered repolarization

Myocardial injury causes ST segment elevation with or without loss of R wave

Myocardial infarction causes deep Q waves as result of absence of depolarization current from dead tissue and receding currents from opposite side of heart

FIGURE 9–6
ECG changes reflecting ischemia, injury, and infarction.

chest pain, radiation of pain, shortness of breath, orthopnea (difficulty breathing if not in an upright position), diaphoresis, syncope, weakness, and so forth. The examiner should also establish the patient's actions at the time of onset, past medical history, and a list of all medications used within the last 6 months.

If the history reinforces suspicion of an acute MI, the interviewer should attempt to determine the patient's eligibility for fibrinolytic therapy. This information centers on:

▶ History of trauma, surgery, or bleeding

▶ History of stroke within the last 6 months

▶ Pregnancy

▶ Any bleeding problems

See the discussion of indications and contraindications to fibrinolytic therapy later in this chapter under "Management of the Uncomplicated AMI," subsection "Fibrinolytic Therapy."

TABLE 9–1   Correlation of Infarction Sites and Leads

Site	Leads	Coronary Artery Affected
1. Anterior wall	V_1 to V_4	Left coronary artery or left anterior descending artery
2. Inferior wall	II, III, aVF	Right coronary artery
3. Right ventricle	II, III, aVF, right precordial V_{4R}	Right coronary artery
4. Lateral wall	I, aVL, V_5, V_6	Left circumflex artery

Conclusions

Suspicion of an acute myocardial infarction is based on a compilation of the information obtained through the patient presentation, clinical evaluation, and supportive history. The definitive diagnosis of an acute myocardial infarction is made upon serum enzyme changes and the development of pathologic Q wave changes. In that pathologic Q waves are not immediate, presumption is further reinforced through the characteristic changes noted with ischemia and injury. *However, let the clinician beware: Even if all aspects of the physical and electrical exam appear unremarkable, an individual still may be actively infarcting!*

MANAGEMENT OF ISCHEMIC CHEST PAIN/AMI: PREHOSPITAL, ED, AND HOSPITAL CONSIDERATIONS

The location and size of an acute myocardial infarction will determine the manner in which it outwardly presents. The acute MI can present with a variety of signs and symptoms indicating complications such as (but not limited to) dysrhythmias, pump failure, or absolutely no complications other than chest pain.

For instance, an infarct of the anterior left ventricle will present differently than an infarct of the posterior right ventricle. Along the same lines, an occlusion high in the left coronary artery will affect the heart differently than an occlusion low in the left anterior descending artery. Regardless of size and location, any infarct represents a serious situation in which early and aggressive intervention must be deployed.

The following discussion outlines the management essentials for an acute MI, followed by additional information identifying specific steps and interventions that should be taken by health care providers as the patient moves from the prehospital environment to the hospital's cardiac care unit.

Halting the process of infarction is the overriding goal in the emergency management of the acute MI. This can be achieved through several different interventions that must be tailored to the particular presentation. Essentially, these interventions work toward the following goals:

- ▷ Alleviation of pain and apprehension
- ▷ Prevention and management of dysrhythmias
- ▷ Limitation of the infarct size
- ▷ Initiation of fibrinolytic therapy or percutaneous coronary intervention (PCI)

All of these serve to reduce the cardiac workload and myocardial oxygen consumption, ward off electrical or mechanical complications, and protect the healthy myocardium from greater infarct. The underlying purpose of all these interventions is to protect and preserve as much of the heart as is possible, thus enabling it to continue functioning to the best of its ability.

Alleviation of Pain and Apprehension

Pain and apprehension stimulate sympathetic nervous innervation. Sympathetic innervation results in high production of *catecholamines* which increase the preload, contractility, afterload, and heart rate. *Consequently, the heart works harder to pump blood and increases its demand for oxygen, which is already in short supply.* The alleviation of pain and apprehension serve to decrease the level of circulating catecholamines and their detrimental effects on the ailing myocardium. Through a decrease in preload, contractility, afterload, and heart rate, the workload and oxygen consumption of the heart decrease, thus reducing potential ischemic damage and irreversible infarct.

Prevention and Management of Dysrhythmias

Electrical dysrhythmias must be evaluated and addressed. Warning dysrhythmias must be rectified before they degenerate into harder-to-manage potentially lethal dysrhythmias. Dysrhythmias represent aberrant conduction and abnormal stimulation of the heart that can promote an inadequate cardiac output.

Limitation of the Infarct Size

Remember, rapid management of ischemic and injured tissue can halt the progression of a myocardial infarction. If successful, this prevents greater heart involvement and reduces the chances of detrimental complication. The concept of myocardial salvaging can significantly decrease morbidity and mortality.

Initiation of Fibrinolytic Therapy or Percutaneous Coronary Intervention (PCI)

Fibrinolytics have revolutionized the treatment of the acute MI. They dissolve blood clots and thus serve to reopen occluded arteries and reoxygenate the ischemic and injured tissue. As the injured myocardium is repertused, there is an improvement in left ventricular function resulting in higher perfusion pressures. As coronary perfusion is improved, the overall size of the infarct is limited and the remaining myocardium protected. *Early initiation is paramount to the overall success of the treatment, as fibrinolysis is extremely time dependent.*

Percutaneous coronary intervention (PCI), such as direct coronary angioplasty and stent placement, has recently been found in clinical trials to yield potentially superior results to those of fibrinolytics. In most clinical trials, PCI has been shown to provide better coronary artery flow rates, lower rates of reocclusion and post-infarction ischemia, and fewer complications than fibrinolytics. One of the difficulties with PCI, however, is that the hospital must have an on-site coronary catheterrization facility and experienced interventional cardiology capabilities for optimal outcomes. Current recommendations are to triage certain types of high risk patients to facilities with PCI capabilities. These patients include those with contraindications to fibrinolytic therapy, as well as those suffering from LV dysfunction, such as when presenting with signs of shock, pulmonary congestion, tachycardia, and/or hypotension.

MANAGEMENT OF SPECIFIC AMI PRESENTATIONS

Because the myocardial infarction can present in a variety of ways, treatment of the ischemic chest pain/acute MI is quite variable. Therefore, management will be discussed in terms of the following presentations:

- ▶ The ischemic chest pain/acute MI patient without complication
- ▶ The acute MI with dysrhythmias
- ▶ The acute MI with hemodynamic alteration

The following guidelines are recommended for advanced prehospital care providers who care for patients presenting with an actual or suspected myocardial infarction. The guidelines have been developed by a consortium of professional entities that include the American College of Cardiology and the American Heart Association, based on the best currently available medical information, research, and technology. The recommendations are incorporated into the discussion in this chapter. They are briefly summarized in Table 9-2.

The management of the ischemic chest pain/acute MI patient begins with a brief, targeted history and thorough assessment that is geared toward the cardiovascular and associated systems. If an MI is suspected, management must be decisive and expedient. The ischemic chest pain algorithm (Figure 9-7) outlines the treatment of the uncomplicated myocardial infarction and represents a basis on which all other presentations of a heart attack are managed. Keep in mind that not every intervention in the algorithm may be applicable to the particular MI at hand; therefore, each AMI must be considered individually.

Management of the Uncomplicated AMI

An uncomplicated AMI is one that presents without any electrical dysrhythmias or hemodynamic alteration. The following section discusses components of the AHA guidelines for management of the acute myocardial infarction as outlined in the ischemic chest pain algorithm (Figure 9-7).

TABLE 9–2 **Summary of Recommended Guidelines for the Management of Myocardial Infarction**

Prehospital Issues

Class I	1. 911 access
	2. EMS service education on identifying, triaging, and initiating treatment for ischemic chest pain patients
	3. Prehospital 12-Lead ECGs
	4. First responder defibrillation
Class IIa	1. Community education on MI recognition, EMS access, and medications
	2. Prehospital fibrinolytic therapy with > 60 minute transport time or on-scene physician

Emergency Department Management

Class I	1. MI protocol designed to identify the MI patient and obtain a 12-lead ECG within 10 minutes of arrival and deliver fibrinolytics within 30 minutes of arrival if applicable
	2. Routine measures to include: oxygen, intravenous nitroglycerin, fibrinolytic therapy, eligibility for primary PTCA, and specific pharmacological management of concurrent dysrhythmias

Hospital Management

Class I	1. Continual ECG monitoring for reocclusion
	2. Management of recurrent chest discomfort
	3. Avoidance of Valsalva, bed rest
	4. Hemodynamic monitoring as appropriate
	5. Intra-aortic balloon counterpulsation as needed
	6. Continued management of concurrent rhythm disturbances
	7. Consideration for surgical interventions
Class IIb	1. Routine use of anxiolytics
Class III	1. Prolonged bed rest in uncomplicated MI patients

This summary is from recommendations of the American College of Cardiology and the American Heart Association.

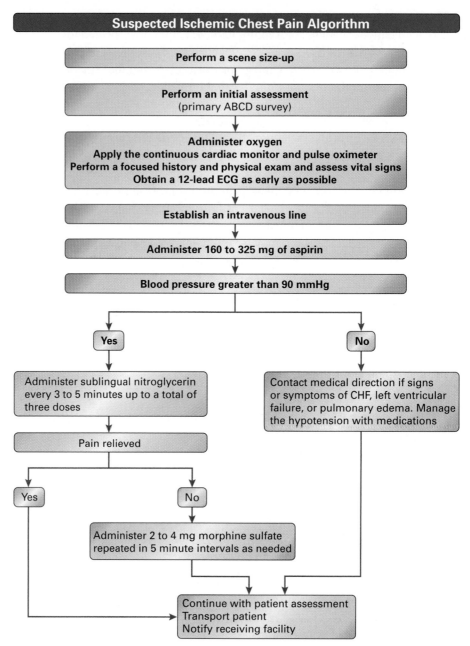

FIGURE 9–7
Algorithm for ischemic chest pain.

Immediate Assessment

The initial care of the ischemic chest pain patient must begin with an immediate assessment to determine the patient's status. The immediate assessment must include measurement of vitals signs, determination of oxygenation status, IV access, 12-lead ECG, targeted history and physical exam, chest x-ray, and various laboratory studies. There are some special considerations related to performing certain portions of this assessment.

Intravenous Access   Due to the potential need for pharmacologic and fluid therapy, intravenous access in the myocardial infarction patient must be promptly established. Optimally, a large bore catheter should be placed in an arm/vein.

Emergency Care Protocol: Suspected Ischemic Chest Pain

1. Ensure scene is clear of safety hazards. Call for additional resources if necessary.

2. Perform an initial assessment. Establish an airway if necessary. Assess breathing. If inadequate breathing, begin positive pressure ventilation with supplemental oxygen connected to the ventilation device. If breathing is adequate, administer oxygen.

3. Apply ECG monitor and pulse oximeter; establish an intravenous line.

4. Perform a focused history and physical exam. Assess vital signs.

5. Administer 160–325 mg of aspirin.

6. If blood pressure is greater than 90 mmHg, administer nitroglycerin sublingually by tablet or spray.

7. If patient has no relief from nitroglycerin and blood pressure remains above 90 mmHg, administer 2–4 mg of morphine sulfate. Continue with 2 mg of morphine at 5-minute intervals as needed to control pain.

8. Obtain a 12-lead ECG.

9. Transport. Notify receiving facility.

Concerning IV access in the AMI patient, several points are worthy of discussion. First, intravenous cannulation is painful and can promote anxiety and the release of catecholamines. Recall that catecholamines can induce a heart to work harder, thus encouraging the process of infarction. This is exactly the process that you are trying to prevent! So IV access must be established quickly and without multiple attempts.

Because of the anticoagulatory effects of drugs such as aspirin, heparin, and fibrinolytics, any injury to the vein, which can cause hematoma or infiltration, must be avoided. Along the same lines, central access into noncompressible veins such as the subclavian is frowned on due to the potential complication of vascular bleeding and difficulty in controlling possible hemorrhage in this area.

While obtaining IV access, it is prudent to obtain blood samples for electrolyte, enzyme, and coagulation studies.

Electrocardiograph Monitoring   Since most early deaths associated with an acute myocardial infarction occur secondary to electrical disturbance, rapid application of the cardiac monitor is necessary. Dysrhythmias can present at any time and must be promptly evaluated. Even if they are not immediately life threatening, remember that such electrical disturbances can quickly degenerate into lethal dysrhythmias. Additionally, keep in mind that an individual suffering an acute MI is most prone to ventricular fibrillation during the first hour following the onset of cardiac symptoms. Successful conversion of ventricular fibrillation into a viable rhythm is time dependent. If the cardiac monitor/defibrillator is already in place, delays in identification and defibrillation are avoided. So as IV initiation is considered standard treatment, so is ECG monitoring. It should be initiated early in the prehospital environment (if possible) and continued during the patient's movement through the emergency department and subsequent CCU and step down units.

As discussed earlier, a 12-lead cardiac monitor is optimal for the identification and location of ischemia, injury, and infarct. If a 12-lead machine is unavailable, a 3-lead monitor can supply the basic rate and rhythm information. *Remember, however, that a normal ECG tracing by itself does not preclude the presence of an AMI!* 12-lead ECG monitoring is recommended as a Class I intervention in the out-of-hospital environment, and is an absolute necessity in the emergency department. Acquisition of a 12-lead ECG is of paramount importance in the process of identifying the MI patient with acute ischemic-type chest pain.

Immediate General Treatment

Following the immediate assessment, the ischemic chest pain patient requires standard immediate general treatment. The non-sequential mnemonic "MONA," referring to oxygen, nitroglycerin, aspirin, and morphine, can be utilized as a memory tool to remind you of the different components of immediate treatment. Keep in mind that this mnemonic serves as a device only for remembering the components of the immediate general treatment, not the sequence. Typically, oxygen is administered first, followed by nitroglycerin and aspirin, only to be followed by morphine if pain still persists.

Oxygen   *Oxygen is the most important and most effective drug in the treatment of the acute myocardial infarction!* As such, it is considered to be a Class I intervention for symptomatic chest pain, and IIa with an uncomplicated MI during the first 2 to 3 hours. Because the infarcting myocardium is starving for oxygen, the administration of supplemental oxygen helps to relieve the discomfort of ischemic pain and limit the progression of the infarction.

Simply stated, oxygen must be given to any patient in whom an AMI is suspected. Even in the absence of dysrhythmias or other complications, supplemental oxygen must be provided.

Oxygen is administered in enough quantity to maintain an arterial saturation of >97%. This may be possible via a low-flow volume of 4–6 liters per minute through a nasal cannula, or by way of a nonrebreathing face mask utilizing a volume of 10–15 liters per minute. Any existing hypoxemia must be reversed. In the setting of an AMI, there are no immediate dangers in the utilization of oxygen. A pulse oximeter provides invaluable feedback on the effectiveness of oxygen therapy and avoids arterial puncture, which may be contraindicated with the use of fibrinolytics.

Aspirin   Aspirin has become a prominent agent in emergent and long-term management of the acute myocardial infarction and is considered a recommended therapeutic intervention for known acute MI or suspected ischemic-type chest pain. Studies indicate the administration of aspirin in the setting of an AMI has achieved significant reduction in mortality comparable to some fibrinolytic agents. Economically, aspirin is the most cost-effective therapy available.

Through a complex series of actions, aspirin functions as an antiplatelet factor that decreases the coagulation potential of the blood. This makes thrombus formation less likely in arteries with pre-existing occlusion. Even though the arteries are compromised, delivery of oxygenated blood to the myocardium can continue and help to limit ischemic pain and infarct size.

Aspirin should be given as soon as possible! Any patient with a presentation suggestive of an acute MI should receive aspirin, barring a declared hypersensitivity. Relative contraindications to the application of aspirin are actively bleeding ulcers or asthmatic conditions.

Aspirin should be given by mouth at a suggested dosage range of 160–325 mg. As always, avoid any oral tablet administration in the patient with a severely decreased level of consciousness to prevent possible airway occlusion and/or aspiration.

Platelet inhibition can lead to bleeding complications. As discussed earlier, carefully weigh the potential benefits against potential complications of administering aspirin to a patient with actively bleeding ulcers or a history of asthma.

Nitroglycerin Nitroglycerin is an effective drug in the management of an acute myocardial infarction. Nitroglycerin works to promote *venous dilation.* As a result, the veins retain a greater volume of blood and decrease preload. The decrease in arterial wall tension also lowers afterload. *These outcomes effectively decrease the myocardial workload and oxygen utilization.* Additionally, nitroglycerin may dilate coronary arteries and promote collateral circulation. This action allows for *the flow of blood into regions of the heart originally deprived of oxygen.* In accomplishing all this, *nitroglycerin assists in the alleviation of ischemic pain, stabilization of an electrically unstable myocardium, and limitation of infarct extension.*

Nitroglycerin is a Class I intervention for any patient with AMI complicated by CHF, hypotension, persistent or recurring ischemia, or anterior involvement. It is considered Class IIb, acceptable but only possibly helpful, for AMI not complicated by any of these factors. Caution should be exercised when considering nitroglycerin for a patient with a systolic pressure under 90 mmHg or a heart rate less than 50 or greater than 100 beats per minute. Nitroglycerin can be administered through a variety of routes in a variety of dosages, as outlined in Table 9-3.

Because it causes vasodilation, nitroglycerin must be used with extreme caution in any patient who actively exhibits hypotension. In this situation, a single tablet of nitroglycerin may be tried with caution if IV access for judicious fluid administration has been established. Since right ventricular infarcts typically present with hypotension, the administration of nitroglycerin must be used with extreme caution, if at all, in the presence of suspected right ventricular infarction. (Suspect right ventricular infarction in patients with ECG changes consistent with inferior wall MI and hypotension unexplained by the heart rate.) Nitroglycerin administration should be avoided if the patient declares sensitivity to the drug.

As stated, nitroglycerin can significantly lower the overall blood pressure. While in many cases this is beneficial, it must be emphasized that too drastic a pressure decrease can be detrimental. A sudden drop in blood pressure can induce syncope, bradycardia, reflex tachycardia, or even cardiac arrest as coronary artery perfusion bottoms out in relation to a decreasing diastolic pressure. IV infusion allows for the most control of the drug. An IV line should be initiated prior to oral administration, ready for prompt measures to counteract side effects.

If any of the above occurs, volume expansion should accompany the normal ACLS procedures for any dysrhythmia. Furthermore, the patient must be placed supine with the legs elevated to enhance blood return to the heart and increase coronary artery perfusion. Pressor therapy (which acts to relieve the symptom of hypotension) should be avoided unless and until fluid volume expansion (which addresses the underlying problem) proves ineffective.

TABLE 9–3 Nitroglycerin Administration

Routes	Dosages
Sublingual pill	0.3–0.4 mg every 5 minutes
Sublingual spray	1 spray every 5 minutes
IV infusion	10–20 µg per minute. Increase 5–10 µg per minute every 5–10 minutes

For the above reasons, remember that nitroglycerin should be used with extreme caution in the hypotensive patient. Additionally, after the blood pressure of a normotensive patient has sustained a mean drop of 10%, or a hypertensive patient has sustained a mean drop of 30%, continued administration should be carefully scrutinized.

Morphine Sulfate   Morphine sulfate is another agent that can be used in the management of the acute myocardial infarction. Similar to nitroglycerin, morphine sulfate decreases preload and afterload through the *dilation of the venous and arterial systems,* thus decreasing myocardial workload, alleviating ischemic chest pain, and limiting the overall progression of the infarct. In addition to the hemodynamic alterations, morphine also acts on the brain to produce an *analgesic effect.* Pain perception is decreased, in turn reducing the stress and anxiety that promote the release of harmful endogenous catecholamines.

Like nitroglycerin, morphine can be considered for the anxious acute MI patient complaining of continuing chest pain unresponsive to nitrates. Morphine should be discontinued if hypotension ensues and the systolic blood pressure drops below 90 mmHg. If hypersensitivity exists, morphine should be avoided.

Morphine is administered via IV in dosage increments of 2–4 mg. These dosages can be repeated as often as every 5 minutes until total pain alleviation has been accomplished. The total dosage of morphine must be evaluated in reference to a stable blood pressure.

Additionally, since morphine can depress the respiratory center in the medulla, the patient's breathing must be monitored continuously.

A drastic reduction in preload and afterload can precipitate a decrease in cardiac output and dangerous hypotension, as with nitroglycerin. Again, the provider must be observant for a sudden drop in blood pressure and the dangerous manifestations of this drop. Should such a decrease bring about syncope, shock, bradycardia, reflex tachycardia, or cardiac arrest, judicious fluid therapy should accompany the normal ACLS protocol for the presenting dysrhythmias. The supine position with elevated legs should be implemented. Pressor agents should be avoided until it is obvious that the fluid challenge is ineffective.

If the administration of morphine sulfate results in dangerous hypoventilation, positive pressure ventilation is necessary. In severe cases of respiratory depression, naloxone (Narcan) can be given at 0.4–2.0 mg.

It is important to remember that morphine sulfate should not be used by itself, but in conjunction with nitroglycerin, oxygen, and other appropriate interventions in the acute myocardial infarction.

Adjunctive Treatments

Following completion of the immediate general treatment, adjunctive treatments may be initiated. Specific therapy decisions should be derived utilizing information obtained in the initial assessment, 12-lead ECG findings, and by completing a process of risk stratification which will be described later. The adjunctive treatments discussed below can all be found in the ischemic chest pain algorithm (Figure 9-7).

Fibrinolytic Therapy   Fibrinolytic therapy has revolutionized the effective treatment of acute myocardial infarction occurring secondary to a thrombus-blocked artery.

Fibrinolytic agents act to quickly dissolve an occluding blood clot and reopen a pathway through which the myocardium can receive vitally needed oxygenated blood. Subsequent reperfusion delivers oxygen to ischemic tissues and halts the infarction process. As a result, the overall size of the infarction can be limited and portions of the susceptible myocardium salvaged.

Fibrinolytic eligibility determination and administration should occur as soon as possible! As "time is muscle," the maximum fibrinolytic benefit appears to be achieved if the fibrinolytic is administered within 3 hours of onset of symptoms (optimally within 30–60 minutes), although definite benefit is still seen in patients who receive the therapy within the first 12 hours of infarction. Fibrinolysis is now known to be beneficial to most patients, irrespective of the individual's age, past medical history, or gender. However, some increased risks (e.g., intracranial hemorrhage) have been identified in those patients who are over 75 years of age or display hypertension (SBP > 180 mmHg or DBP > 110 mmHg).

Fibrinolytics may be administered to a patient with objective evidence that indicates infarction, especially those suffering a transmural MI. Definitive diagnosis of an AMI is dependent on characteristic enzyme changes and the development of pathologic Q waves. As discussed earlier, the development of pathologic Q waves can lag hours to days behind the actual death of cardiac tissue. Additionally, ascertainment of laboratory results may require time. The progression of infarction is not considerate of such delays and continues right along at a rapid pace. Therefore, *fibrinolytics may be administered on the presumption of infarction.* This presumption can be made upon ECG changes indicating injury (ST elevation) with a compatible history. The presumption of an MI can also be made if the patient displays evidence of a new left bundle branch block (common to left anterior descending arterial occlusion) with a compatible history.

Several contraindications exist to the administration of fibrinolytics. These contraindications all revolve around the potential for serious hemorrhage, as the human body's compensatory clotting mechanism is temporarily disabled by the fibrinolytic. As listed by the AHA, absolute contraindications to fibrinolytic therapy are:

▶ Previous hemorrhagic stroke

▶ Other stroke or cerebrovascular event within 1 year

▶ Active internal bleeding (menses excluded)

▶ Suspected aortic dissection

Relative contraindications, in which the practitioner must use extreme discretion in the administration of fibrinolytics, are:

▶ Severe uncontrolled hypertension on presentation:
  –systolic >180 mmHg
  –diastolic >110 mmHg

▶ History of severe chronic hypertension

▶ Current use of anticoagulants; known bleeding disorder

▶ Recent trauma (within 2 to 4 weeks), including head and traumatic CPR or major surgery (< 3 weeks)

▶ Recent (2 to 4 weeks) internal bleeding; active peptic ulcer disease

▶ Pregnancy

▶ For streptokinase: allergy or prior exposure (especially 5 days to 2 years)

Currently, several fibrinolytic agents exist and are given intravenously. These agents and their dosage regimens are listed in Table 9-4.

It is important to remember that ventricular fibrillation can occur during the administration of fibrinolytics! Refer to Chapter 8 for a detailed discussion of fibrinolytics.

TABLE 9–4 Fibrinolytics Administration

Fibrinolytic Agent	Regimen
anistreplase	30 U IV over 2–5 minutes
alteplase	100 mg IV (60 mg in first hour—6–10 mg IV push initially—then 20 mg/hour over the next 2 hours) Accelerated regimen: • Give 15 mg IV bolus • Then 0.75 mg/kg over next 30 minutes (not to exceed 50 mg) • Then 0.50 mg/kg over next 60 minutes (not to exceed 35 mg)
reteplase	10 U IV bolus over 2 minutes (30 minutes later give second 10 U bolus over 2 minutes)
streptokinase	1.5 million U in a 1-hour infusion
tenecteplase	30–50 mg IV bolus

Reperfusion Therapy: Percutaneous Coronary Intervention (PCI)   PCI refers to methods of clearing an atherosclerotic-narrowed artery by mechanical means. The most common form of PCI used today is PTCA (percutaneous transluminal coronary angioplasty). In PTCA, a long catheter is inserted through a peripheral artery (usually brachial or femoral) and threaded through the aorta into the involved coronary artery. A balloon at the distal end of the catheter is inflated and deflated many times to flatten the atherosclerotic accumulation against the vessel wall. The net result is an opened coronary artery and reperfusion of an oxygen-deprived myocardial region. Frequently, a stent (a cylindrical wire mesh support) is also placed inside the artery lumen during the angioplasty procedure to aid improving patency rates and preventing arterial reocclusion. Other forms of PCI include several types of atherectomy, procedures in which the arterial plaque is either cut or ground away.

PCI addresses the underlying cause of the myocardial infarction, the atherosclerotic-narrowed coronary artery. Where fibrinolytics will rectify a thrombogenic occlusion by dissolving the clot, PCI opens the occluded artery by mechanically widening the lumen.

Individuals suffering an AMI for which fibrinolytic therapy is contraindicated, or who don't respond to fibrinolytic agents, are candidates for PCI. Also, PCI has shown positive results for those afflicted with cardiogenic shock or acute pump failure. Further, PCI is indicated for those with occluded vein grafts from coronary artery bypass graft surgery.

PCI must be performed by a specialist in the catheterization laboratory and, just like fibrinolytic therapy, is considered a Class I intervention. It assumes a class IIa rating when a patient is a candidate for reperfusion but has a risk of bleeding. In most clinical trials, PCI has been shown to provide better coronary artery flow rates, lower rates of reocclusion and post-infarction ischemia, and fewer complications than fibrinolytics.

Heparin   Heparin is an anticoagulant that has no lytic effect on existing clots. Often heparin is used in conjunction with certain fibrinolytic agents or by itself after fibrinolysis has occurred.

Even after fibrinolytics effectively dissolve an occlusive clot, a rough atherosclerotic surface remains. This surface provides an opportunity for the reformation of a thrombus with subsequent reocclusion. Through its anticoagulant properties, heparin works to prevent the recurrence of thrombus formation and provides for the maintenance of a patent coronary artery.

Also, in the setting of post-fibrinolytic therapy, pieces of the thrombus may break off and be transported by the blood, only to lodge (as emboli) elsewhere in the body. Consequently, complications such as stroke and/or further infarct can arise. Heparin appears to decrease the incidence of such complications.

Among clinicians, there appears to be some controversy concerning the administration of heparin. However, heparin is considered a Class I indication for patients undergoing percutaneous or surgical revascularization, and a Class IIa intervention when administered with fibrinolytics. Finally, it is a Class III intervention for routine IV use within 6 hours to patients receiving a nonselective fibrinolytic agent, who are not at a high risk for systemic embolism.

In the presence of active bleeding, severe hypotension, recent intracranial surgery, or bleeding tendencies, heparin is contraindicated for the same reasons as are fibrinolytics. The administration and dosing regimen for heparin are summarized in Table 9-5.

Beta Blockers   Beta blockers inhibit the uptake of catecholamines at the myocardial beta receptors. As a consequence, circulating catecholamines are prevented from increasing the heart's rate, contractility, and electrical excitability, in turn preventing adverse effects on workload and myocardial consumption of oxygen, ischemic pain, and ultimately infarct size. For these reasons, the administration of beta blockers can be considered a Class I intervention for the management of recurrent chest discomfort unresponsive to initial therapy.

Despite fibrinolytic therapy, ischemic and injured tissues can continue to degenerate into dead tissue because of ongoing myocardial work. The administration of long-term beta blockers attempts to stop this process by chronically inhibiting the workload of the heart. In the presence of an MI, beta blockers also appear to decrease the incidence and mortality of ventricular fibrillation.

Beta blockers should be considered for any patient suffering an acute MI with excessive adrenergic activity. This activity includes an elevated heart rate or hypertension.

Because of their ability to reduce the activity of the heart, beta blockers are contraindicated in hypotension, congestive heart failure, and bradycardia. Recall that the bronchi and bronchioles are susceptible to beta stimulation and rely on this influence for relaxation. For this reason, beta blockers are contraindicated with any asthmatic or bronchospasmodic disposition.

Although many approaches are acceptable, the regimens of beta blockers commonly used are summarized in Table 9-6.

The administration of beta blockers in the setting of an AMI can be dangerous and must be used with judicious caution. By nature, beta blockers induce

TABLE 9–5 | Heparin Administration

AHA-Recommended Options	Dosing Regimen
Option 1: Administer heparin simultaneously with the fibrinolytic agent.	Bolus IV: 60 IU/kg (maximum 4000 IU)
Option 2: Administer heparin on completion of a fibrinolytic infusion.	Continue: 12 IU/kg/hr (maximum 1000 U/hour for patients > 70 kg).
Option 3: Administer heparin empirically in patients with large anterior AMIs without fibrinolytics.	

TABLE 9-6 | Beta Blockers Administration

Beta Blocker	Regimen
metoprolol	5 mg IV infusion every 5 minutes to a total of 15 mg
atenolol	5 mg infusion over 5 minutes. Wait 10 minutes and give second dose of 5 mg over the course of 5 minutes.
propranolol	0.1 mg / kg by slow IV push divided into 3 equal doses at 2 to 3 minute intervals
esmolol	50 μg/kg/min over 1 minute followed by a continuous infusion at 500 μg/kg
labetolol	10 mg IV push over 1 to 2 minutes. May be repeated at 10 or 20 mg every 10 minutes to max dose of 150 mg

myocardial depression and therefore require constant observation. Always monitor for symptomatic bradycardic dysrhythmias.

The reduction in electrical excitability, heart rate, and contractility can adversely affect the stroke volume and cardiac output. Consequently, a balance between decreased cardiac workload and optimal cardiac output must be found. Beta blockers are often continued 1 to 2 years after infarct.

Emerging Therapies: Glycoprotein (GP) IIB/IIIA Antagonists and Low Molecular Weight Heparin (LMWII)   Patients suffering from MI without ST elevation or high risk unstable angina may be candidates for Glycoprotein (GP) IIB/IIIA antagonists, such as abciximab (Reopro®), eptifibitide (Integrilin®), and tirofiban (Aggrastat®). Through a complex chemical mechanism, these substances serve to inhibit platelet aggregation, thereby inhibiting clot formation. Clinical trials have shown the GP IIB/IIIA antagonists to reduce death, MI, and the need for revascularization procedures in unstable angina and non-ST segment elevation MI patients.

Low molecular weight heparin (LWMH) serves much the same function as the GP IIB/IIIA antagonists. Additional clinical trails are being conducted to establish the role of LMWH in the same sub-set of acute coronary syndrome patients. LMWH is already considered an equivalent alternative to standard heparin (see below) in patients with non-ST-segment elevation MI or unstable angina, and the combination of LMWH with GP IIB/IIIA antagonists looks very promising for the future.

Angiotensin Converting Enzyme Inhibitors (ACEI)   ACE inhibitors (ACEI) have been used for many years as oral anti-hypertensive agents. Over the past several years, they have also been studied as potential adjunctive agents for use following acute MI. Initiation of ACEIs within 12–24 hours of symptom onset has been shown to decrease mortality and CHF associated with MI. Typically, ACEI therapy is started after the patient has stabilized and after initial therapy with fibrinolytics, beta blockers, and nitrates has been initiated.

Risk Stratification with the First 12-lead ECG
Making a decision as to how to treat patients suspected of having ischemia chest pain or AMI requires additional diagnostic measures and subsequent risk stratification. This is imperative to finding the correct tract to follow in the ACLS ischemic chest pain algorithm (review Figure 9-7). At the center of this risk stratification process lies the initial 12-lead ECG. This ECG is used to triage patients into one of three different categories:

> ST-Segment Elevation—suspicious of myocardial injury

> ST-Segment Depression (≥ 1 mm)—suspicious of myocardial ischemia

> Nondiagnostic or normal ECG

As a general rule, patients presenting with ST elevation are assumed to be suffering from an AMI, while those with ST-segment depression are considered to be at high risk for both non-ST-elevation MI or unstable angina.

The ACLS ischemic chest pain algorithm stands as a general outline of interventions that should be considered in the emergent management of ischemic chest pain and acute myocardial infarction. Keep in mind, however, that consideration for the listed items should be done on an individual basis, with application tailored to the individual suffering the chest pain or acute myocardial infarction. It is imperative that the care provider be familiar with both the details of the algorithm and the specifics of each of the therapies discussed previously.

Management of AMI Complicated by Dysrhythmia

Short of unstable dysrhythmias or cardiac arrest, the algorithm for ischemic chest pain, as described above, also finds application to the acute myocardial infarction complicated by electrical dysrhythmia. Often, an electrical disturbance secondary to an acute MI serves to warn of extensive ischemia or serious underlying abnormalities such as acid-base imbalance, hypocalcemia, hypokalemia, or hypomagnesemia. Hence, these dysrhythmias are termed *warning dysrhythmias* and warrant immediate attention.

Frequently, warning dysrhythmias are rectified through application of the guidelines as described earlier. Among others, this includes the administration of MONA (oxygen, nitroglycerin, aspirin, morphine), fibrinolytics, and beta blockers. Therefore, prior to pharmacologic therapy specific to the dysrhythmia, these and other standard AMI treatment measures should be attempted with their effectiveness constantly evaluated. If the dysrhythmias persist despite these measures, standard therapy specific to the dysrhythmia should be considered.

An unstable rhythm or cardiac arrest requires immediate intervention—*regardless of the presence of an acute myocardial infarction.* The following section contains information that pertains to the management of the common dysrhythmias that occur secondary to an acute MI. As always, *treat the patient, not the monitor!*

The ACLS standard treatment algorithms for all of the dysrhythmias discussed below will be examined in detail in Chapter 10.

AMI and PVCs

When PVCs occur during an active infarction, it is essential to determine the cause. Often, PVCs in the setting of an acute MI occur secondary to an underlying abnormality. Underlying causes may include poor oxygenation, hypotension, electrolyte abnormalities, acid-base imbalances, high state of catecholamine stimulation, and others. It is up to the clinician to identify the cause and correct it, which should correct the PVCs as well.

In the presence of PVCs, examine the status of adequate oxygenation, efforts at pain relief, and the administration of nitroglycerin, morphine, and beta blockers. If PVCs are associated with a bradycardic rhythm, it is likely that the premature ventricular beats are escape beats and can be corrected by addressing the bradycardic rhythm itself.

Treatment with lidocaine (see Chapter 8 for the dosing regimen) can be considered if the PVCs persist despite the above measures and if they satisfy one or more of the following criteria:

▶ Six or more PVCs per minute

▶ PVCs that are closely coupled

▶ PVCs that fall on the preceding T wave (R-on-T phenomenon)

▶ PVCs that occur in couplets or runs of three

▶ PVCs that are multiform

AMI and Ventricular Dysrhythmias

Ventricular fibrillation must be promptly defibrillated. If ventricular fibrillation occurs in the presence of an acute MI, defibrillation should be conducted immediately. The incidence of ventricular fibrillation is highest during the first hour following the onset of myocardial infarction and continues over the next 48 hours. Ventricular fibrillation can be described as one of two types:

▶ *Primary ventricular fibrillation* occurs as a result of a problem with the heart itself. An example is aberrant conduction related to the ischemic and injured myocardial tissues.

▶ *Secondary ventricular fibrillation* typically occurs because of a problem elsewhere in the body. Among others, hypovolemia and pH disturbances are possible causes of secondary ventricular fibrillation. Because the underlying cause is external to the heart, secondary ventricular fibrillation is more difficult to correct. Successful treatment often relies on addressing the underlying abnormality.

Ventricular fibrillation is a potentially convertable rhythm, and prompt defibrillation carries a high incidence of conversion. Ventricular tachycardia often deteriorates into ventricular fibrillation and, therefore, must also be treated promptly. The clinician must first determine whether the patient with ventricular tachycardia is stable, unstable, or pulseless and manage it accordingly.

AMI and Bradycardia

Bradycardia commonly accompanies an acute MI and is quite prevalent during the first hour of infarct. This slow rhythm often occurs in response to an increased parasympathetic influence and is frequently associated with an inferior- or posterior-wall MI. Bradycardia can present with a variety of underlying rhythms, including sinus bradycardia, junctional escape rhythms, and an assortment of different heart blocks.

Management of sinus bradycardia in the presence of an AMI represents a tricky issue. A slow rate can cause a decrease in cardiac output and produce insufficient peripheral and coronary artery perfusion. Consequently, the infarct can be worsened and cardiac arrest may result.

Conversely, a slow heart rate may exert a protective effect by slowing down the heart. From this perspective, the heart is intrinsically limiting ischemia and injury through a self-initiated decrease in workload and oxygen demand.

Any bradycardia that occurs secondary to an AMI should not be treated with pharmacologic therapy unless the patient is symptomatic and produces signs of hypoperfusion. As always, the provider should assure adequate oxygenation and pain relief in the attempt to limit the infarct progression.

AMI and Tachycardia

An acute MI with associated tachycardia is a signal that something else is occurring! Often, tachycardia is the physiologic response to stress, anxiety, heart failure, or hypovolemia. Tachycardia is a dangerous rhythm that must be immediately addressed, for the accelerated rhythm stands to worsen an overall infarct by *increasing the myocardial workload and overall oxygen consumption, leading to extensive myocardial damage.* Additionally, it is thought that excessive tachycardia lowers the threshold for the occurrence of ventricular fibrillation. As with PVCs, the key lies in the identification and treatment of the causal mechanism.

If sinus tachycardia, atrial flutter, atrial fibrillation, or atrial tachycardia is present, the clinician must ensure that effective oxygenation, pain control, and all other appropriate interventions of the ischemic chest pain algorithm have been correctly and adequately initiated. The use of beta blockers and morphine sulfate have special application with tachycardia.

Excessive tachycardia can lead to unstable conditions such as shortness of breath, pulmonary congestion, hypotension, increased chest pain, and shock. Tachycardias of this nature must be terminated immediately and are managed with synchronized electrical shock therapy and medications.

AMI and Conduction Blocks

An acute MI can present with a variety of conduction blocks. While some of these blocks require no more than careful observation, others are an ominous sign of extensive damage and require immediate and extensive intervention.

First-Degree Conduction Block A first-degree conduction block requires little more than observation. The concern with a first-degree block is the progression to a more serious block. If a first-degree block is encountered, careful observation is necessary.

Second-Degree Conduction Blocks There are two types of second-degree blocks. Second-degree Type I block usually signifies an AV node block that is frequently caused by an enhanced vagal discharge. In the absence of symptomatic bradycardia and other symptoms, this block only requires *observation* for progression to a more serious block. If *symptomatic,* this block can be treated using the symptomatic bradycardia algorithm in Chapter 10.

Second-degree Type II block represents a very serious situation. This block signifies ischemia and damage to the myocardial conduction system. *With this block, there is significant risk for the transformation into a full heart block.* If encountered, a transvenous or transcutaneous pacemaker must be applied in anticipation of the progression to a third-degree block.

Third-Degree Conduction Block A third-degree heart block in an acute MI indicates extensive damage from the infarction. The only means of cardiac output comes from the ventricular escape rhythm. *Because this pacemaker is very unstable, a temporary pacemaker must be implemented as soon as possible.*

Intraventricular Block If the intraventricular block is clinically significant and the patient is unstable, pacing and therapeutic management should be aggressively initiated. Pacing is a must in a right bundle branch block; however, authorities are unsure of its effectiveness in a left bundle branch block. If the patient is stable, there is no specific prehospital treatment.

Management of AMI with Hemodynamic Alteration

Depending on the nervous system response or the contractile damage to the heart as a pump, variable hemodynamic states can accompany the acute myocardial infarction. The following section discusses the acute MI with hypertension and the acute MI with hypotension. As emphasized earlier, all interventions listed in the algorithm need to be evaluated for implementation on a one-by-one basis.

Keep in mind that hemodynamic alteration can occur in response to mechanisms that are not related to the MI. Such causes include massive pulmonary embolism, hypovolemic shock, septic shock, cardiac tamponade, and a dissecting aortic aneurysm.

AMI and Hypertension

During the process of myocardial infarction, a patient may present with hypertension, which can be typical for the patient or may signify an increased circulation of catecholamines secondary to pain and anxiety. *Regardless of its origin, hypertension (systolic > 140 mmHg and/or diastolic > 90 mmHg) in the setting of an acute MI needs to be addressed.*

Because the heart must work harder to eject blood against an increased afterload, hypertension can produce an *increase in myocardial oxygen demand and result in an extension of the infarct.* For the same reasons, persistent hypertension can also harm the recovery of a weak heart. Further, hypertension in the setting of an acute infarction can precipitate wall rupture as the weakened tissue is subject to heightened stress from an increased effort to eject blood.

Many times, hypertension is transient; rest and reassurance along with the administration of supplemental oxygen, nitroglycerin, and morphine are enough to alleviate the release of catecholamines. If these measures prove ineffective in reducing the hypertension, or if the hypertension is severe, IV nitroglycerin (10–20 µg/min) and beta blockers may be effective. If all of these measures fail, nitroprusside (0.1–5.0 µg/kg/min) can be administered.

AMI and Hypotension

Symptomatic hypotension in the presence of an acute myocardial infarction is an ominous sign. Hypotension indicates a decrease in cardiac output due to a decrease in stroke volume or a heart rate that is too slow or too rapid to permit adequate ventricular filling. *Symptomatic hypotension can result in hypoperfusion of the body tissues, including the heart itself. Without intervention, further damage or cardiac arrest can ensue.*

Hypotension associated with an acute MI can be of several origins, as discussed below. The etiology must be identified and corrected as is appropriate.

Bradycardia   As the heart rate is slow, the cardiac output has fallen. See the earlier section of this chapter, "AMI and Bradycardia," for the proper management of this condition.

Tachycardia   As the heart rate is too rapid, adequate ventricular filling is discouraged. Consequently the cardiac output falls. See the earlier section of this chapter, "AMI and Tachycardia," for the proper management of this condition.

Left Ventricular Pump Failure   Left ventricular pump failure occurs when a significant-sized infarct decreases the effective wall motion necessary for contraction. Through this complication, the heart is unable to eject an acceptable stroke volume. When left ventricular pump failure occurs, a decrease in cardiac output and/or pulmonary congestion ensue. Even though the patient is hypotensive, the cardiac output may still be able to meet the immediate demands of the body; but be aware of the potential for deterioration into cardiogenic shock, as discussed below.

Initial treatment of left ventricular failure focuses on aggressive airway control and oxygenation. If the heart rate is not the cause, treatment should center on enhancing systemic vascular resistance to increase the blood pressure. The suggested guidelines are outlined in Table 9-7. These approaches are dictated by blood pressure readings. The possible use of vasodilators and beta blockers must be carefully weighed in light of the patient's hypotensive state.

Cardiogenic Shock   *When cardiac output is no longer adequate to perfuse the tissues of the body and the heart, cardiogenic shock must be suspected.* Cardiogenic shock will manifest itself with systemic hypotension and pulmonary edema. Cardiogenic shock results when more than 35% of the left ventricle has been destroyed by an infarct. The majority of patients do not survive.

Treatment originates with aggressive airway management and oxygenation. The treatment of cardiogenic shock is similar to the treatment of left ventricular failure. Dopamine and/or norepinephrine at the lowest effective dose is advised. Pulmonary edema secondary to cardiogenic shock should be treated as described under "AMI and Pulmonary Edema," below. Cardiogenic shock is an indication for advanced procedures such as PTCA and intra-aortic balloon pump counterpulsation.

Right Ventricular Pump Failure   In right ventricular failure, the right ventricle cannot eject blood into the pulmonary circulation. This results in a decreased volume available for the left ventricle to pump to the remainder of the body. Consequently, profound hypotension ensues with the associated danger of decreased systemic and coronary artery perfusion.

The key to treatment lies in the administration of fluids. Under *Starling's Law* of contractility, the more the ventricle is stretched, the more forceful the contraction will be. Therefore, if a greater preload is available to the right ventricle, the ventricle will eject more volume into the lungs, thus delivering a greater amount of blood to the left ventricle for systemic disbursement. Vasodilators should be strictly avoided, in that these will only serve to decrease preload and worsen the entire situation.

AMI and Pulmonary Edema
If the pumping ability of the left ventricle has been seriously impaired and blood backs up into the pulmonary vessels, as described earlier, the pressure increase can force serum and other fluids from within these vessels into the interstitial spaces

TABLE 9–7	Treatment for AMI with Hypotension (Pump or Volume Problem)

Initial treatment for symptomatic hypotension in the presence of an AMI focuses on aggressive airway control and oxygenation. If there is a pump or volume problem (if heart rate is not the causal mechanism), treatment should center on vasoconstriction to increase the blood pressure, as follows:

Systolic Blood Pressure	Agent/Dosage
< 70 mmHg with signs of shock	Norepinephrine 0.5–30 µg/min
70–100 mmHg with signs of shock	Dopamine 5–15 µg/kg/min Add norepinephrine if > 20 µg/kg/min

and even into the alveoli. This series of events not only compromises cardiac output but also impairs the ability of the lungs to adequately oxygenate blood for delivery to the entire body.

In pulmonary edema, respiratory distress is accompanied by adventitious lung sounds (rales). Depending on how seriously the left ventricle has been damaged, and the degree to which the adrenergic nervous system has been stimulated, the clinician may note profound hypotension or adrenergically induced hypertension as the body attempts to compensate for this deficit. In severe cases, blood and other frothy material from the lungs can be seen at the patient's mouth and/or nose.

Emergency treatment of acute pulmonary edema revolves around decreasing the amount of blood that the impaired left ventricle must eject and the resistance against which it must pump. This will reduce the buildup in the pulmonary vessels and, in turn, reduce the pressure that forces the blood from the pulmonary vessels into the interstitial spaces and/or alveoli.

After sitting the patient upright and administering high-flow oxygen, nitroglycerin is useful in increasing the venous capacitance and decreasing the amount of preload presented to the heart for pumping. Because of its similar action, morphine sulfate may also find application in this situation. Finally, if an increase in venous capacitance does not rectify the situation, the diuretic furosemide (Lasix) can be given at a dosage of 0.5–1.0 mg/kg via IV bolus to reduce pressure by stimulating the kidneys to excrete water. IV nitroglycerin, nitroprusside, or dopamine can be administered if the blood pressure is greater than 100 mmHg.

If the patient is hypotensive and vasodilators are not applicable, dopamine can be utilized in an attempt to raise the overall blood pressure. Dobutamine administered at a dosage of 2–20 μg/kg/minute functions to increase the contractility of the heart with reflex decreases in systemic vascular resistance.

As always, remember that ventilatory effort may need assistance with positive pressure ventilation so as to force fluid from the alveoli and increase the delivery of oxygen into the pulmonary fields.

■ SUMMARY

Acute coronary syndromes, mainly acute myocardial infarctions, are devastating events that claim many lives each year. Many of these deaths are unnecessary because both preventive practices and rapid treatment have led to improved patient outcomes.

Successful management of the acute MI hinges on an application of procedures tailored to the particular presentation of the infarction. Consequently, a strong working knowledge of the heart as a pump and the overall cardiovascular system is a must.

The fact that treatments exist for the acute MI is only half the battle. Individuals suffering an acute MI tend to wait 2 to 4 hours before seeking medical attention. "Time is muscle," and the success of many management techniques is extremely time dependent. These delays result in unnecessary disability and death.

It is the responsibility of the community at large to become educated in the prevention and recognition of infarction symptoms. General awareness and avoidance of modifiable risk factors, recognition of a heart attack, and training in CPR are just a few examples of how the myocardial infarction can be challenged in the community. Most important of all may be an understanding of the need to seek help promptly. Here the phrase *"dial first, dial fast, dial 911"* finds poignant application.

CASE STUDY FOLLOW-UP

You respond to the scene and find Steve who has been suffering chest pain for more than 24 hours and, as you talk with him, is becoming somewhat combative.

Assessment

Your initial assessment of Steve reveals a lethargic male patient with a cardiac history experiencing a possible myocardial infarction. Upon further investigation, you note obvious distention of the jugular veins accompanied by edema to the abdomen and feet. While the lung sounds are clear, you obtain a pulse oximetry reading of only 68%. Knowing that decisive action must be taken quickly, you prepare to treat the patient for ischemic chest pain.

Treatment

Because of the important role oxygen plays in the treatment of chest pain, you quickly place Steve on a non-rebreather at 15 lpm. While applying the cardiac monitor, you instruct your partner to initiate an IV of normal saline.

Once Steve is on the 12-lead cardiac monitor, you note a bradycardic rhythm at a rate of 48 beats per minute that includes unifocal PVCs at a rate of 12 per minute. The 12-lead ECG reveals ST-segment elevation and Q wave changes to the right precordial lead.

Your partner asks if you want him to administer nitroglycerin for the chest pain or lidocaine hydrochloride for the PVCs. You instruct him not to, as the patient is already hypotensive and the PVCs are most likely escape beats resulting from the slow rhythm. Rather, you order a complete set of lab tests and a fluid bolus of 500 cc of normal saline in an attempt to increase cardiac output by raising the left ventricular filling pressure.

Additionally, you administer 1 mg of atropine and apply the transcutaneous cardiac pacer as a precaution. Within a minute, Steve's heart rate increases to 68 beats per minute with a blood pressure reading of 88/50 mmHg. There is also a concomitant increase in his level of orientation and ability to respond.

You administer 325 mg of aspirin and complete a checklist for fibrinolytic therapy. Steve appears eligible for fibrinolytic therapy, and you include this information when you notify the receiving hospital. You quickly transport Steve to the awaiting facility.

The next evening, you get a call from Steve's wife informing you that he successfully underwent fibrinolytic therapy for a thrombus in the right coronary artery. She tells you that Steve is now on heparin and will be in the ICU for the next two weeks. The cardiologist has told them both that he expects Steve to make a full recovery but that he will have to modify his lifestyle if he is going to live to see his grandchildren get married!

Knowing that your actions were integral to Steve's successful outcome, you proceed into the break room with a large grin on your face. You are about to eat a large jelly-filled donut when it occurs to you that this may be part of the lifestyle that landed Steve in the hospital. You decide on an unbuttered bagel instead—and are just about to take the first bite when you get a call for a multiple gunshot wound victim.

Your work is never done. . .

REVIEW QUESTIONS

1. Of the following situations, which would serve most to diminish the cardiac output?
   a. increase in afterload with a decrease in preload
   b. increase in heart rate while stroke volume remains the same
   c. decrease in heart rate with an increase in stroke volume
   d. decrease in stroke volume with an increase in heart rate

2. A patient suffering an acute MI presents with systemic hypotension and lung sounds that are clear of any adventitious noises. Which of the following should be suspected by the health care professional?
   a. possible left ventricular failure
   b. possible right ventricular failure
   c. a left ventricular MI with right ventricular involvement
   d. an acute MI with no ventricular involvement

3. In which of the following situations will the myocardial oxygen demand be decreased the most?
   a. increase in afterload
   b. increase in preload
   c. decrease in afterload
   d. increase in contractility

4. You are administering oxygen to a patient with an acute MI. Which of the following is most likely to occur as a result?
   a. increase of activity in the infarct region
   b. restoration of function to all injured cells
   c. increase in myocardial workload
   d. improvement of function to ischemic tissue

5. Of the following patients, which could be said to be suffering the greatest infarct in terms of size?
   a. patient with occlusion in the left coronary artery
   b. patient with occlusion in the left descending coronary artery
   c. patient with blockage in the left circumflex artery
   d. patient with blockage of the left subclavian artery

6. In the acute MI, which of the following pathophysiological processes is responsible for the majority of deaths?
   a. myocardial wall rupture
   b. electrical instability in the infarcted tissue
   c. aberrant conduction through ischemic and injured tissue
   d. the formation of aneurysms on the left ventricle

7. When assessing a patient with a possible acute myocardial infarction, which of the following would most support the evaluation that an acute MI is occurring?
   a. the presence of chest pain
   b. ST elevation in leads V_4 and V_5
   c. a blood pressure of 90/66
   d. ST elevation in leads V_2 and V_5

8. A 53-year-old female patient has the chief complaint of shortness of breath. Upon questioning, she denies the presence of chest pain. On the cardiac monitor, you note a sinus rhythm of 88 beats per minute with ST elevation in leads V_3 and V_4. You would suspect
   a. the patient has COPD.
   b. the patient has an occlusion of the right coronary artery.
   c. no infarction is occurring because of the absence of chest pain.
   d. a possible anterior-wall infarction is occurring.

9. Of the following choices, which **definitively** indicates an acute myocardial infarction?
   a. patient with serum enzyme changes and pathologic Q waves
   b. patient with ST elevation in leads V_3 and V_5
   c. patient with shortness of breath and chest pain
   d. patient with symmetrically inverted T waves in leads V_5 and V_6

10. A 67-year-old male presents with crushing chest pain and is diaphoretic. Upon inspection, you note sinus bradycardia with ST elevation in lead V_{4R}, blood pressure of 94/70, and engorgement of the neck veins. Which of the following represents the **best** course of treatment for this patient?
    a. oxygen
    b. oxygen with nitroglycerin and morphine
    c. oxygen with a bolus of normal saline
    d. oxygen with nitroglycerin and beta blockers

11. A physician orders a bolus of heparin to a patient after fibrinolytic therapy has been completed. The rationale for such a move is to
    a. keep opened artery patent.
    b. lower the returning preload.
    c. decrease myocardial workload.
    d. prevent active bleeding elsewhere in the body.

12. Which of the following choices represents the most prudent order of treatment for a hemodynamically stable MI patient presenting with 10 multifocal PVCs per minute?
    a. lidocaine, oxygen, beta blockers
    b. oxygen, lidocaine, nitroglycerin
    c. lidocaine, oxygen, morphine
    d. oxygen, nitroglycerin, lidocaine if needed

13. A COPD patient is incurring a left ventricular infarction. The patient is confused, diaphoretic, and displays a pulse oximeter reading of 87%. Which of the following treatments would be most beneficial for the patient?
    a. high-flow oxygen delivered by a nonrebreather
    b. oxygen at 4 liters per minute delivered through a simple face mask
    c. low-flow oxygen delivered through a nasal cannula
    d. withhold oxygen so as not to depress respiratory drive

14. After administering nitroglycerin to a chest pain patient, the patient's blood pressure drops drastically, and she goes into pulseless electrical activity (PEA). Your best course of action would be to
    a. place the patient supine with legs elevated and defibrillate.
    b. give large amounts of fluid while administering CPR.
    c. administer dopamine at 10 µg/kg/min.
    d. administer CPR only.

15. Of the following patients, which would be most eligible for fibrinolytic therapy?
    a. male with transmural infarct and BP 150/120
    b. female with transmural infarct and stroke 11 months ago
    c. male involved in car crash with right ventricular infarct and head injury
    d. female with left ventricular infarction and pregnant

16. Which of the following electrical disturbances represents the greatest life threat to occur within the first hour post infarct?
    a. PEA
    b. ventricular tachycardia
    c. asystole
    d. ventricular fibrillation

17. You are treating a severely lethargic patient in cardiogenic shock from a massive left ventricular MI. Which of the following regimens best describes the appropriate treatment of this patient?
    a. oxygen, dopamine, norepinephrine
    b. intubation, oxygen, nitroglycerin, dopamine
    c. oxygen, IV, cardiac monitor, nitroglycerin
    d. intubation, oxygen, dopamine, norepinephrine

18. Of the following cardiac drugs, which is the most important in the management of the acute myocardial infarction?
    a. nitroglycerin
    b. oxygen
    c. morphine sulfate
    d. beta blockers

19. You are treating a patient who complains of chest pain and exhibits respiratory distress with adventitious lung sounds heard on auscultation. As you examine the patient, you note a pink froth beginning to appear at the corners of her mouth. You note a systolic blood pressure of 140 mmHg. Which of the following represents the **best** choice for the initial treatment of this patient?
    a. oxygen at 15 lpm
    b. IV nitroglycerin
    c. furosemide
    d. nitroglycerin given by mouth

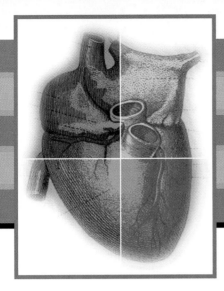

Prehospital Algorithms and Emergency Cardiac Care Protocols

An algorithm is a simplified visual method to illustrate a systematic approach to prehospital emergency cardiac care. An emergency cardiac care protocol, which may be presented in an algorithm format, also serves as a guideline to providing prehospital care. Prior to employing any treatment protocol, it must be approved by the emergency medical services medical director. The series of steps recommended in this chapter should be used as a guideline to stimulate thought and clinical action and should not be used as a legal standard of care. These algorithms and emergency cardiac care protocols are based on the scientific evidence and recommendations found in the American Heart Association's "Guidelines 2000 for Cardiopulmonary Resuscitation and Emergency Cardiovascular Care" or on standard practice. They are identified as a recommended course of treatment for the various types of cardiac arrest and cardiovascular and cardiopulmonary conditions.

Topics in this chapter are:

- Key Considerations in the Algorithm Approach to Emergency Cardiac Care
- Prehospital Algorithms and Emergency Cardiac Care Protocols for Patients in Cardiac Arrest
- Postresuscitation Patient Management in the Prehospital Setting
- Prehospital Algorithms for Patients Not in Cardiac Arrest

You respond to the scene for an unknown problem. As you approach the residence and walk up onto the front porch of the house, the door suddenly flies open and an older man comes running frantically out the door. He is out of breath and screaming, "My wife, my wife! Please help her!" He runs back into the house and runs up the stairs. You cautiously proceed after him while watching for any evidence of scene hazards. You find an elderly woman who is supine on the floor. She is ashen gray and motionless. You tell your partner to contact dispatch to send a backup unit for a nonbreather.

How would you proceed to assess and care for this patient? This chapter will describe the systematic algorithm approach to managing a patient in cardiac arrest or one who is suffering from a cardiovascular or cardiopulmonary compromise. Later we will return to the case and apply the procedures learned

INTRODUCTION

The algorithm approach to managing a patient in cardiac arrest or one who is suffering from cardiovascular or cardiopulmonary compromise is an oversimplified guideline that is used mainly as an educational tool to illustrate and summarize important emergency care steps. The prehospital emergency cardiac care protocols are also designed as a guideline for providing care to patients in the prehospital environment who are suffering a cardiac crisis. These are not rigid and inflexible steps that set a legal standard of care; instead, they are designed to provide a systematic approach to consider when managing these types of patients. The steps should stimulate thought that is based on clinical understanding. When proceeding through the various steps, a key element to remember is to treat the whole patient and not just the rhythm. If the underlying condition causing the rhythm is not detected or managed, the rhythm will not improve and will likely deteriorate and lead to death. Thus, use your assessment skills including a scene size-up and a history and physical examination in an attempt to determine any potential underlying cause for the presenting cardiac rhythm whether the patient is in cardiac arrest or not.

KEY CONSIDERATIONS IN THE ALGORITHM APPROACH TO EMERGENCY CARDIAC CARE

When applying the algorithms and emergency cardiac care protocols to patient management, it is necessary to consider the following clinical recommendations:

▶ Treat the patient, not a rhythm. It is necessary to consider the etiology of a rhythm when providing care. Likewise, you must attempt to determine the reason why a patient may be in a persistent rhythm. This is accomplished by managing the "whole" patient and not developing tunnel vision while performing specific skills. Be sure to consider characteristics found in the scene size-up that may provide clues to the potential underlying cause. For example, drug paraphernalia is found at the scene near the patient. You may suspect the cardiac arrest rhythm is a result of an overdose or illicit drug reaction. Also, be sure to collect as much of a history from the patient's immediate family, relatives, or friends to include events and complaints prior to the cardiac arrest or episode. For example, you determine the patient's atenolol prescription that was filled yesterday is now empty. When performing your assessment, be sure to look for possible clues as to an underlying cause. As an example, a patient in pulseless electrical activity has subcutaneous emphysema present to his neck and upper chest and has absent breath sounds to the right hemithorax.

▶ Proceed through the algorithm until the rhythm is changed or the patient is no longer in cardiac arrest.

▶ Continue CPR throughout the algorithm as long as the patient remains in cardiac arrest.

▶ Consider using the termination of resuscitation in the field protocol in patients who has been in asystole for ten minutes or greater.

▶ Perform alternative interventions when the appropriate indications exist.

▶ Only perform those interventions and administer those medications that are approved by your medical director and allowed by your local protocol.

▶ Airway management, effective ventilation, oxygenation, chest compressions, and defibrillation are key basic components in patient management. These interventions take precedence over more advanced care such as intravenous therapy and medication administration.

▶ Lidocaine, atropine, and epinephrine can be administered down the tracheal tube at 2 to 2.5 times the intravenous dose.

▶ Intravenous medications should be administered by a rapid bolus, with a few exceptions. Follow the administration with a 20 to 30 ml bolus of intravenous fluid. This expedites delivery of the medication to the core circulation, which may take 1 to 2 minutes.

▶ The sequence of shock–drug–shock should be used in ventricular fibrillation and pulseless ventricular tachycardia.

▶ Vasopressin is an alternative drug used only in the initial treatment of ventricular fibrillation and pulseless ventricular tachycardia.

▶ Transcutaneous pacing must be done as early as possible in the treatment of asystole to be a potentially useful intervention.

PREHOSPITAL ALGORITHMS AND EMERGENCY CARDIAC CARE PROTOCOLS FOR PATIENTS IN CARDIAC ARREST

General Approach to the Cardiac Patient

Any resuscitation efforts must begin with a general approach to cardiac care in the prehospital environment (Figure 10-1). Often, the first arriving EMS crew has limited personnel that is responsible for initiating and continuing the emergency care and resuscitation effort. Often, a second or backup EMS crew will arrive on the scene to assist with the patient management. Thus, it is necessary to assess the resources available upon arrival at the scene, make decisions as to what interventions will be performed immediately, and who will be responsible for performing those interventions. As additional backup personnel arrive on the scene, the responsibility of the team members may change.

The general approach to cardiac care algorithm follows the primary ABCD survey and secondary ABCD survey that was covered in Chapter 2, Systematic

Approach to Emergency Cardiac Care: The Primary and Secondary Survey. It is a systematic approach that allows you to make a quick initial assessment and develop a management plan based on the presenting rhythm, precipitating events that led to the cardiac arrest, and any other information that is pertinent to the differential diagnosis of the patient.

Key Points

▶ Perform a scene-size up to ensure the scene is clear of safety hazards. Also, be aware of potential safety hazards at the scene when performing defibrillation. Call for additional resources upon determination that the patient is in cardiac arrest.

▶ Performing the primary ABCD survey is no different than the standard initial assessment that you perform on all patients: perform a general impression, assess responsiveness, establish an open airway, assess breathing and provide positive pressure ventilation if necessary, assess circulation, and immediately assess the cardiac rhythm if the patient is pulseless and apneic.

▶ Early recognition and defibrillation of ventricular fibrillation or pulseless ventricular tachycardia is imperative to successful resuscitation.

▶ Open the airway and assess for breathing. If the patient is breathing, assess for adequacy and the need for ventilation. Place the patient in the recovery position if there is no suspicion of a spinal injury. Provide positive pressure ventilation if necessary, initiate oxygen therapy, initiate intravenous therapy, and assess vital signs. If necessary, intubate the patient. Gather a history, perform a physical examination, and attach a continuous ECG monitor. Acquire a 12-lead ECG if necessary.

▶ If no breathing is present, administer two slow breaths and check for a pulse. Assess for a carotid pulse. If the patient is pulseless, begin chest compressions and ventilation.

▶ Defibrillation is the most important intervention that can be performed. As soon as the defibrillator is available and ventricular fibrillation or pulseless ventricular tachycardia is verified, defibrillate the patient.

▶ If defibrillation is not indicated, proceed to the secondary ABCD survey. Continue CPR, intubate the patient, confirm tube placement, assess effective ventilation, initiate an intravenous line, attempt to determine the etiology of the cardiac arrest and rhythm, and administer the first line resuscitation drugs.

▶ If the patient is pulseless and electrical activity is present, with the exception of ventricular fibrillation and ventricular tachycardia, proceed to the pulseless electrical activity (PEA) algorithm.

▶ If the patient is pulseless and no electrical activity is noted on the oscilloscope, proceed to the asystole algorithm. Consider the following possibilities when confronted with a flat line on the monitor:

– The leads are loose.

– The leads are not connected to the patient.

– The leads are not connected to the monitor/defibrillator

– The power to the monitor/defibrillator is not turned on.

– The ECG gain is set too low.

– Isoelectric VF/VT or true asystole exist.

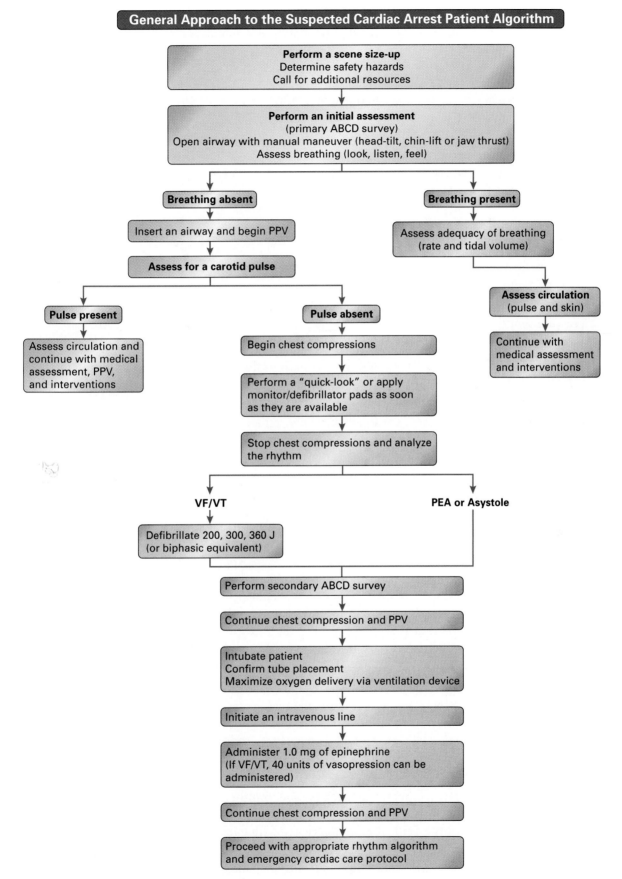

FIGURE 10-1
Algorithm for general approach to the suspected cardiac arrest patient.

Emergency Cardiac Care Protocol: General Approach to the Suspected Cardiac Arrest Patient

1. Ensure the scene is clear of safety hazards. Call for additional resources if cardiac arrest is suspected or confirmed upon your entry into the scene.

2. Perform an initial assessment and determine or confirm that the patient is unresponsive, apneic, and pulseless.

3. If a defibrillator is available, immediately perform a "quick look" with the defibrillator paddles or attach the "hands off" defibrillator pads and analyze the patient's rhythm. If the defibrillator is not immediately available, begin chest compressions and positive pressure ventilation. Defibrillation is the primary critical intervention that must be done as soon as possible. Do not delay analysis of the rhythm or defibrillation for any other intervention.

4. If the rhythm is ventricular fibrillation or pulseless ventricular tachycardia, immediately deliver three defibrillations at 200, 300, and 360 joules or the biphasic equivalent.

5. If the rhythm is pulseless electrical activity, immediately resume chest compressions and positive pressure ventilation.

6. If the rhythm is asystole, confirm it in another lead, and resume chest compressions and positive pressure ventilation.

7. Intubate the patient, confirm the tracheal tube placement, and establish an intravenous line.

8. Administer 1 mg of epinephrine via intravenous push. If the rhythm is ventricular fibrillation or pulseless ventricular tachycardia, a one-time dose of 40 units of vasopressin can be administered via intravenous push.

9. Continue with the appropriate cardiac arrest rhythm protocol while attempting to establish the underlying cause of the cardiac arrest.

Ventricular Fibrillation/Pulseless Ventricular Tachycardia (VF/Pulseless VT) Algorithm

Ventricular fibrillation or pulseless ventricular tachycardia is the most viable cardiac arrest rhythm that a patient can be in. Approximately 80% to 90% of patients in nontraumatic sudden cardiac arrest initially present with VF or VT. Within minutes, the rhythm will deteriorate into a nonviable rhythm. The earlier defibrillation is done, the better the chance of converting the patient's rhythm into a perfusing rhythm. That is why early defibrillation is imperative in increasing the survival rate of patients in out-of-hospital cardiac arrest (Figure 10-2).

Key Points

▶ Ventricular fibrillation is the most common rhythm that patients will be in immediately following collapse from cardiac arrest. The majority of patients who will survive will be converted from ventricular fibrillation or pulseless ventricular tachycardia. Once the patient has deteriorated from VF/VT to asystole, the chance of survival is drastically decreased.

▶ **Remember: With each passing minute, the chance of the VF/VT deteriorating into a nonviable rhythm increases significantly. Also, the success of the defibrillation decreases with each minute that passes**.

▶ The treatment for ventricular fibrillation and pulseless ventricular tachycardia is defibrillation. It is imperative to maintain a patent airway and provide adequate ventilation and chest compressions. However, the method to terminate

VF/VT to a perfusing rhythm is defibrillation and not tracheal intubation, intravenous therapy, or drug administration. Those are considered only adjuncts to defibrillation and should be performed after defibrillation has been attempted.

▶ Initially, three stacked shocks are delivered to the patient at 200 J, 300 J, and 360 J or the equivalent biphasic amount of energy. These should be delivered in as rapid a sequence as possible, with safety to the resuscitation team a key consideration. A pulse check is done following the third defibrillation and *not* between shock 1, shock 2, and shock 3 unless the rhythm is converted after one of the shocks. If paddles are being used to perform the defibrillation, the paddles should be left on the chest and the rhythm reanalyzed quickly as the paddles are being charged for the next defibrillation.

▶ Quick-look paddles can be used to quickly assess the rhythm for VF/VT and deliver defibrillation without the delay associated with connecting monitor lead cables. The paddles are already on the chest and can be immediately charged if VF/VT is identified. Be careful of artifact associated with use of paddles. "Hands-off" defibrillation pads are also widely available and eliminate the paddles.

▶ Remove nitroglycerin patches from the patient's chest prior to defibrillation. The patch may cause the electrical current to arc. The nitroglycerin substrate will not explode or burn.

▶ Do not place the defibrillator paddles over the generator of an implanted automatic defibrillator or pacemaker. The paddles should be placed approximately 5 inches from the generator. Energy discharged from paddles over an implanted device can damage, disable, or misprogram the implanted device. Also, the defibrillation current may be blocked by the implanted device.

▶ If an implanted automatic defibrillator is in place and not delivering a shock to the patient in VF/VT, proceed with normal defibrillation.

▶ Following the first set of stacked shocks and drug administration, an alternative consideration is to deliver the proceeding shocks in a set of three. The sequence would be shock, shock, shock–drug–shock, shock, shock–drug–shock, shock, shock. The shocks that follow the first set of three stacked shocks are to be delivered at 360 joules or the biphasic equivalent.

▶ The person delivering the defibrillation must ensure team safety by clearing all personnel prior to defibrillation. You must look from head to toe and say aloud, "One, I'm clear. Two, you're clear. Three, everybody's clear," assessing for and clearing personnel in contact with the patient.

▶ Following the stacked defibrillations, CPR is initiated, the patient is intubated, and an intravenous line established.

▶ Epinephrine is the first drug of choice administered after the defibrillation at 1 mg every 3 to 5 minutes. If an intravenous line is not established, the epinephrine can be administered down the tracheal tube at 2 to 2.5 times the normal dose. Vasopressin can be administered as an alternative vasopressor drug only in ventricular fibrillation or pulseless ventricular tachycardia. The one-time dose is 40 units intravenous push. If vasopressin is used, epinephrine could be administered 10 to 20 minutes after the vasopressin administration.

▶ You should defibrillate at 360 J or the equivalent biphasic energy within 30 to 60 seconds following the administration of each drug. The sequence is drug–shock, drug–shock.

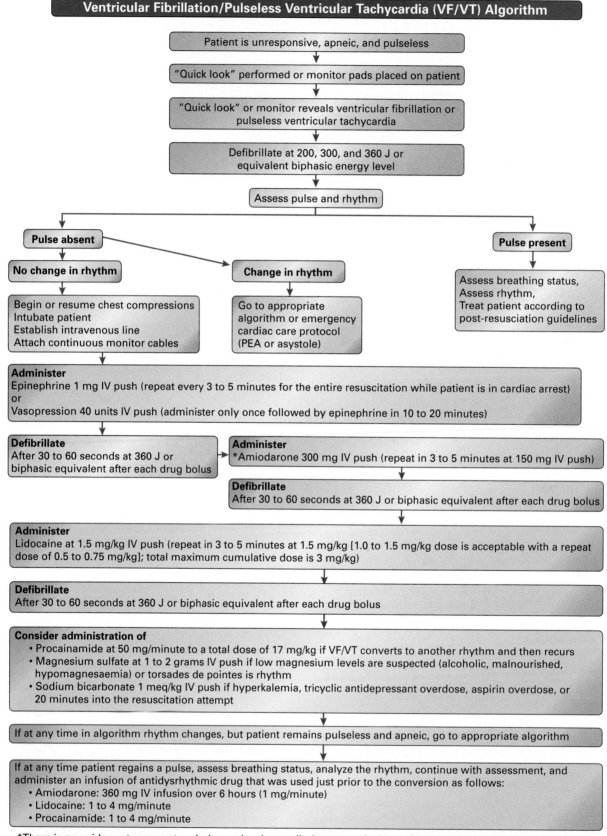

FIGURE 10-2
Algorithm for ventricular fibrillation/pulseless tachycardia (VF/VT).

▶ Antidysrhythmic medications that can be used in VF/VT are:

– *Amiodarone*: 300 mg intravenous push (two 6 ml ampules diluted in 20 to 30 ml of normal saline), repeat at 150 mg in 3 to 5 minutes if ventricular fibrillation or pulseless ventricular tachycardia recurs or persists. The maximum dose is 2.2 grams over 24 hours.

– *Lidocaine*: 1.0 to 1.5 mg/kg intravenous push initial dose repeated in 3 to 5 minutes at 1.0 to 1.5 mg/kg to a maximum dose of 3 mg/kg.

– *Magnesium sulfate:* 1 to 2 grams intravenous push for torsades de pointes, suspected hypomagnesemia states (alcoholic, malnourished)

– *Procainamide:* 50 mg/minute to a total dose of 17 mg/kg for refractory VF in patients who respond to defibrillation, regain a pulse, and then deteriorate back into ventricular fibrillation or pulseless ventricular tachycardia.

▶ Lower maintenance doses of lidocaine should be used in patients of advanced age and those with liver dysfunction. A single loading dose of 1 mg/kg is administered.

▶ Amiodarone, lidocaine, and procainamide are only administered as a bolus during cardiac arrest. Once circulation has been restored, an infusion of the drug used to convert the rhythm is initiated.

▶ Only one antidysrhythmic drug should be used at a time. The maximum drug dose should be reached before switching to the next antidysrhythmic drug.

▶ Once the circulation has been restored, an infusion of the antidysrhythmic agent that was effective in aiding in the conversion of the rhythm should be initiated. The infusion medications are:

– *Amiodarone:* 360 mg IV infusion over 6 hours (1 mg/minute)

– *Lidocaine:* 1 to 4 mg/minute

– *Procainamide:* 1 to 4 mg/minute

▶ Consider the administration of sodium bicarbonate at 1 meq/kg IV push if after 10 to 20 minutes of cardiac arrest or if hyperkalemia, tricyclic antidepressant overdose, or aspirin overdose is suspected.

▶ If intubation, initiation of an intravenous line, or drug administration is delayed, a second set of stacked shocks should be delivered.

Emergency Cardiac Care Protocol: Ventricular Fibrillation and Pulseless Ventricular Tachycardia

1. Ensure the scene is clear of safety hazards. Call for additional resources as necessary.

2. Perform an initial assessment and determine or confirm that the patient is unresponsive, apneic, and pulseless.

3. If a defibrillator is available, immediately perform a "quick look" with the defibrillator paddles or attach the "hands off" defibrillator pads and analyze the patient's rhythm. If the defibrillator is not immediately available, begin chest compressions and positive pressure ventilation. Defibrillation is the primary critical intervention that must be done as soon as possible. Do not delay analysis of the rhythm or defibrillation for any other intervention.

4. Upon confirmation of ventricular fibrillation or pulseless ventricular tachycardia, immediately deliver three defibrillations at 200, 300, and 360 joules or the biphasic equivalent.

(continued)

5. Intubate the patient, establish an intravenous line, and connect the patient to a continuous cardiac monitor.

6. Administer 1 mg of epinephrine IV push every 3 to 5 minutes during the entire resuscitation.

   OR

   Administer 40 units of vasopressin IV push. Vasopressin is only administered once during the resuscitation. Ten to twenty minutes after its administration resume with the administration of epinephrine at 1 mg IV push.

7. After each administration of epinephrine, wait 30 to 60 seconds, then defibrillate at 360 joules or the biphasic equivalent.

8. Administer 300 mg of amiodarone IV push. Amiodarone can be repeated at 150 mg IV push in 3 to 5 minutes. There is no current evidence to suggest amiodarone has a better patient discharge survival benefit in cardiac arrest as compared to lidocaine. Therefore, lidocaine can also be used as the first-line antidysrhythmic drug.

9. After each administration of amiodarone, wait 30 to 60 seconds, then defibrillate at 360 joules or the biphasic equivalent.

10. Administer 1.5 mg/kg of lidocaine IV push. Repeat in 3 to 5 minutes at 1.5 mg/kg. Lidocaine can also be administered at 1.0 to 1.5 mg/kg and repeated at 0.5 to 0.75 mg/kg. The recommended VF/VT dose is 1.5 mg/kg. The total maximum cumulative dose is 3 mg/kg.

11. After each administration of lidocaine, wait 30 to 60 seconds, then defibrillate at 360 joules or the biphasic equivalent.

12. Consider the administration of procainamide rapid IV infusion at 50 mg/minute to a total dose of 17 mg/kg if the ventricular fibrillation or pulseless ventricular tachycardia converts to a different rhythm and then recurs back to VF/VT. After the administration of procainamide, wait 30 to 60 seconds, then defibrillate at 360 joules or the biphasic equivalent.

13. Consider magnesium sulfate at 1 to 2 grams IV push if low magnesium levels are suspected (alcoholic, malnourished, or hypomagnesemia) or torsades de pointes is the rhythm. After the administration of magnesium sulfate, wait 30 to 60 seconds, then defibrillate at 360 joules or the biphasic equivalent.

14. Consider sodium bicarbonate at 1 meq/kg IV push if hyperkalemia, tricyclic antidepressant overdose, aspirin overdose, or 10 to 20 minutes has passed since the beginning of the resuscitation.

15. If at any time the rhythm changes but the patient remains pulseless and apneic, go to that appropriate emergency cardiac care protocol.

16. If at any time the patient regains a pulse, assess the breathing status, continue positive pressure ventilation as necessary, analyze the rhythm, go to the appropriate algorithm if necessary, and administer an infusion of the antidysrhythmic drug that was used just prior to the successful conversion of the rhythm. Administer the infusion as follows:
    – Amiodarone 360 mg IV infusion over 6 hours (1 mg/minute)
    – Lidocaine 1 to 4 mg/minute
    – Procainamide 1 to 4 mg/minute

17. Amiodarone may precipitate hypotension and bradycardia; thus, be sure that an adequate blood pressure and heart rate is established prior to infusion. Procainamide may precipitate hypotension, thus, be sure an adequate blood pressure is present prior to administration. The lidocaine infusion should be reduced by one-half in the elderly and those suffering from liver dysfunction or failure.

Pulseless Electrical Activity (PEA) Algorithm

When electrical activity is identified on the monitor, other than VF or VT, in the absence of a pulse, it is termed pulseless electrical activity (Figure 10-3). There are a myriad of conditions that may cause PEA.

Key Points

▶ PEA is comprised of a group of rhythms previously identified as:
  – electro-mechanical dissociation (EMD)
  – pseudo-EMD
  – idioventricular rhythms
  – ventricular escape rhythms
  – post-defibrillation idioventricular rhythms
  – bradyasystolic rhythms

▶ EMD is characterized by a condition in which electrical depolarization occurs without shortening of the myocardial fibers and no mechanical contraction.

▶ Pseudo-EMD is associated with electrical depolarization with subsequent mechanical contraction that does not produce a measurable or detectable pulse. The most common cause is severe hypovolemia.

▶ The major key to PEA management is to find the possible cause. Etiologies of PEA include:
  – hypovolemia
  – hypoxia and hypoventilation
  – cardiac tamponade
  – tension pneumothorax
  – hypothermia
  – massive pulmonary embolism
  – drug overdose
  – hyperkalemia or hypokalemia
  – acidosis
  – massive myocardial infarction

▶ Fluid challenges are used to manage or rule out hypovolemia. A trial bolus of 500 ml of normal saline is appropriate in PEA even if the hypovolemia is not evident.

▶ Ventilation and aggressive oxygenation are used to combat hypoventilation and hypoxia. Hypoxemia and hypoventilation are common causes of PEA.

▶ Drug overdoses of tricyclic antidepressants, beta blockers, calcium channel blockers, and digitalis are only a few of the drugs that may precipitate PEA.

▶ A Doppler ultrasound should be used to detect possible blood flow not obtainable by regular palpation. If a pulse is detected by Doppler in PEA, it indicates pseudo-PEA. These patients should be treated with fluid boluses, dopamine, or both. If the heart rate is bradycardic, transcutaneous pacing is recommended.

▶ Atropine is used in PEA rhythms that have underlying rates of less than 60 complexes per minute, assuming that the undetectable BP may be rate

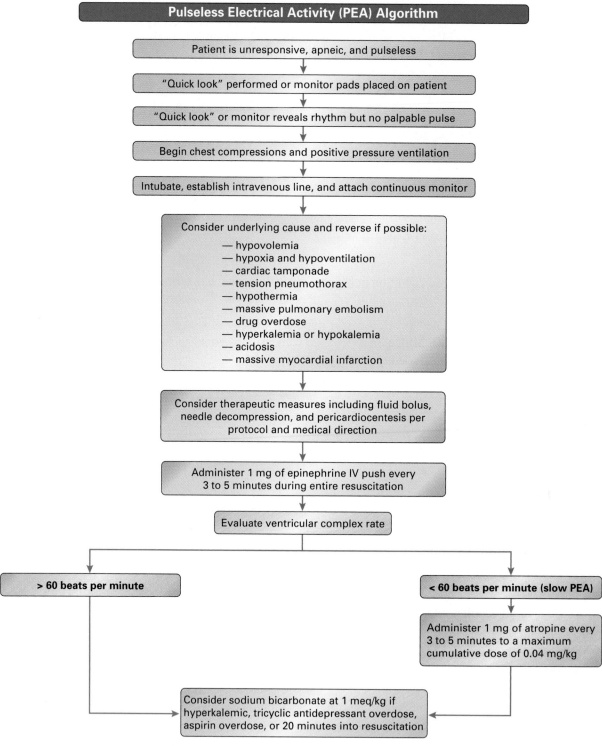

FIGURE 10-3
Algorithm for pulseless electrical activity (PEA).

dependent and reversible. If the rate is greater than 60 complexes per minute, atropine is not typically administered.

▷ Pericardiocentesis is the treatment of choice for suspected pericardial tamponade.

▷ If a tension pneumothorax is suspected, perform a needle decompression by inserting a 14-gauge 2″ angiocath in the second intercostal space at the midclavicular line on the affected side.

▷ The primary drug used in PEA is epinephrine at 1 mg IV push repeated every 3 to 5 minutes.

▷ Atropine should be administered in PEA when the ventricular complex rate is less then 60 beats per minute. Atropine is administered at 1 mg every 3 to 5 minutes to a total maximum cumulative dose of 0.04 mg/kg.

▷ Sodium bicarbonate could be considered at 1 meq/kg in hyperkalemia, tricyclic antidepressant overdose, and 10 to 20 minutes into the resuscitation.

Emergency Cardiac Care Protocol: Pulseless Electrical Activity (PEA)

1. Ensure the scene is clear of safety hazards. Call for additional resources as necessary.

2. Perform an initial assessment and determine or confirm that the patient is unresponsive, apneic, and pulseless.

3. If a defibrillator is available, immediately perform a "quick look" with the defibrillator paddles or attach the "hands off" defibrillator pads and analyze the patient's rhythm. If the defibrillator is not immediately available, begin chest compressions and positive pressure ventilation. Analyze the rhythm as quickly as possible.

4. Pulseless electrical activity is confirmed on the monitor by identifying ventricular complexes with no palpable pulses. Begin or resume chest compressions and positive pressure ventilation. Ensure good ventilation and aggressive oxygenation since PEA is frequently caused by hypoventilation and hypoxemia.

5. Attempt to identify and manage the underlying cause:
   – hypovolemia (administer 500 ml normal saline bolus, repeat if response or hypovolemia evident)
   – hypoxia and hypoventilation (ensure a good airway, provide positive pressure ventilation and oxygen)
   – cardiac tamponade (rapid transport for pericardiocentesis)
   – tension pneumothorax (needle decompression of the affected hemithorax)
   – hypothermia (begin passive rewarming and transport rapidly)
   – massive pulmonary embolism
   – drug overdose (beta blockers—consider glucagon; calcium channel—consider calcium chloride; tricyclic antidepressant—consider sodium bicarbonate)
   – hyperkalemia or hypokalemia (consider sodium bicarbonate in hyperkalemia)
   – acidosis (ensure adequate ventilation and consider sodium bicarbonate 10 to 20 minutes into the resuscitation)
   – massive myocardial infarction

6. Intubate, establish an intravenous line, and attach the patient to a continuous cardiac monitor.

7. Administer 1 mg of epinephrine IV push at every 3 to 5 minutes during the entire resuscitation.

(continued)

8. If the ventricular complex rate is less than 60 beats (slow PEA) per minute, administer 1 mg of atropine every 3 to 5 minutes until the rate increases to greater than 60 beats per minute, the rhythm changes, or 0.04 mg/kg of the drug has been administered.

9. Consider a 500 ml fluid bolus of normal saline as a trial even if no obvious signs of hypovolemia are present.

10. Consider sodium bicarbonate at 1 meq/kg IV push if hyperkalemia, tricyclic antidepressant overdose, aspirin overdose, or 10 to 20 minutes has passed since the beginning of the resuscitation.

Asystole Algorithm

Asystole is associated with no electrical activity. The prognosis of survival is very poor when a patient presents in this rhythm (Figure 10-4). Management of asystole is very similar to PEA.

Key Points

▶ Determining the etiology of the cardiac arrest and possible causes of the rhythm must be aggressively pursued during the differential diagnosis phase of the secondary ABCD survey.

▶ Asystole should be confirmed in more than one lead to ensure that the patient is not truly in a fine or medium ventricular fibrillation.

▶ Be sure the monitor leads are connected, the correct lead or paddle selector is set, and the ECG gain is turned up.

▶ Atropine is administered as a routine medication in asystole. A strong parasympathetic tone may eliminate ventricular and supraventricular pacemaker activity and lead to asystole. Since atropine is a parasympatholytic, also known as a vagolytic, it will block the parasympathetic tone and may restore pacemaker activity.

▶ Defibrillation of asystole produces parasympathetic discharge and may prevent any spontaneous pacemaker activity. Defibrillation of asystole is strongly discouraged and will worsen the chance of a successful resuscitation.

▶ To be effective, pacing must be initiated immediately after the cardiac arrest. If pacing is to be initiated, it should be done early along with CPR and the administration of medications.

▶ When tracheal intubation, intravenous access, CPR, and medication have been successfully performed or administered, but there has been no response, cessation of resuscitation should be considered. Exceptions include hypothermia, electrocution, and drug overdose.

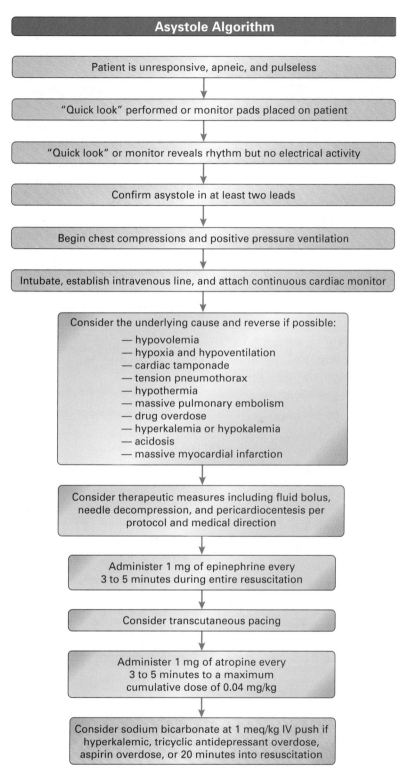

FIGURE 10-4
Algorithm for asystole.

Emergency Cardiac Care Protocol: Asystole

1. Ensure the scene is clear of safety hazards. Call for additional resources as necessary.

2. Perform an initial assessment and determine or confirm that the patient is unresponsive, apneic and pulseless.

3. If a defibrillator is available, immediately perform a "quick look" with the defibrillator paddles or attach the "hands off" defibrillator pads and analyze the patient's rhythm. If the defibrillator is not immediately available, begin chest compressions and positive pressure ventilation. Analyze the rhythm as quickly as possible.

4. Confirm asystole in at least two leads. Be sure the cables are connected, the lead selector switch is set to the appropriate lead or paddles, and be sure the ECG gain is turned up high. Upon confirmation of asystole, begin or resume chest compressions and positive pressure ventilation.

5. Attempt to identify and manage the underlying cause:
   – hypovolemia (administer 500 ml normal saline bolus, repeat if response or hypovolemia evident)
   – hypoxia and hypoventilation (ensure a good airway, provide positive pressure ventilation, and oxygen)
   – cardiac tamponade (rapid transport for pericardiocentesis)
   – tension pneumothorax (needle decompression of the affected hemithorax)
   – hypothermia (begin passive rewarming and transport rapidly)
   – massive pulmonary embolism
   – drug overdose (beta blockers—consider glucagon; calcium channel—consider calcium chloride; tricyclic antidepressant—consider sodium bicarbonate)
   – hyperkalemia or hypokalemia (consider sodium bicarbonate in hyperkalemia)
   – acidosis (ensure adequate ventilation and consider sodium bicarbonate 10 to 20 minutes into the resuscitation)
   – massive myocardial infarction

6. Intubate, establish an intravenous line, and attach the patient to a continuous cardiac monitor.

7. Consider transcutaneous pacing. Set the pacing rate at 80 beats per minute and the milliamps at the highest setting. Administer the epinephrine and atropine while pacing.

8. Administer 1 mg of epinephrine IV push at every 3 to 5 minutes during the entire resuscitation.

9. Administer 1 mg of atropine every 3 to 5 minutes until a cumulative maximum dose of 0.04 mg/kg has been administered.

10. Consider sodium bicarbonate at 1 meq/kg IV push if hyperkalemia, tricyclic antidepressant overdose, aspirin overdose, or 10 to 20 minutes has passed since the beginning of the resuscitation.

POSTRESUSCITATION PATIENT MANAGEMENT IN THE PREHOSPITAL SETTING

The time following post cardiac arrest is critical to patient survival and requires interventions to keep the patient from reverting back to cardiac arrest. The postresuscitation period is considered the time between the resuscitation of the patient and restoration of a spontaneous pulse until the transfer to the emergency department. Patient management during this period is critical and may influence patient survival and neurological outcome.

Following resuscitation, the patient's response may range from being alert, awake, and hemodynamically stable to being deeply comatose and hemodynamically unstable. Aggressive management must ensure that the patient's condition does not deteriorate because of lack of attention to the airway, breathing, or circulation. Perform the primary ABCD survey and secondary ABCD survey (as discussed in Chapter 2) to allow for a systematic and organized evaluation of the patient.

Restoration and maintenance of circulation to the brain and other tissue is the key goal of patient management.

The tachycardia and bradycardia algorithms should not be applied to the postresuscitation period tachycardias and bradycardias. As a general rule, postresuscitation dysrhythmias are not treated during the immediate postresuscitation period unless the patient is significantly symptomatic by showing signs of severe hypotension and poor perfusion.

Postresuscitation Interventions

Following successful resuscitation of the patient, it is imperative to perform certain interventions to ensure the patient does not deteriorate into cardiac arrest. The following critical actions must be taken following successful cardiac arrest.

Airway

Reassess the airway to ensure it is patent. Reverify tracheal tube placement by reassessment of breath sounds, chest rise and fall, and use of an end-tidal CO_2 detector and esophageal tube detection device.

Breathing

Administer supplemental oxygen. Continue to provide positive pressure ventilation as necessary by bag-valve or other ventilation device if the rate or tidal volume is ineffective. Assess bilateral breath sounds and chest wall movement during ventilation. Monitor oxygen saturation by pulse oximetry.

If spontaneous respirations do not return, consider the use of an automatic transport ventilator to provide the necessary ventilatory support and oxygenation. Assess the patient closely for potential complications that may have resulted from the resuscitation. Pneumothorax, fractured ribs, sternal fracture, and a misplaced tracheal tube are all possible complications that must be assessed for following the resuscitation.

Circulation

It is necessary to assess vital signs. Establish an intravenous line if one was not established during the resuscitation. Continuously monitor the ECG rhythm, blood pressure, and pulse oximeter reading.

If an antidysrhythmic agent (amiodarone, lidocaine, or procainamide) was administered during the resuscitation, initiate an infusion of the agent that was successful in converting the VF or VT to a perfusing rhythm.

If possible, obtain a 12-lead ECG tracing. If acute coronary ischemia is present, consider a bolus and infusion of lidocaine. If the systolic blood pressure is greater than 100 mmHg, consider administration of nitroglycerin or a beta blocker to reduce the adrenergic stimulation associated with resuscitation medications.

Differential Diagnosis
Attempt to determine the etiology of the cardiac arrest. Identify any potential complications that may have occurred secondary to the cardiac arrest. Perform a detailed physical examination and gather and review the history.

Special Considerations in Postresuscitation Care

The postresuscitation period presents a very delicate time for patient management. Special considerations must be taken for certain conditions that may arise. The following are special considerations that may be encountered in the postresuscitation care of the patient.

Cerebral Perfusion
The whole goal of resuscitation is to restore the patient to as nearly the normal neurologic prearrest state as possible. Protect cerebral function by ensuring a patent airway, adequate ventilation, and effective perfusion. Normothermia should be maintained since hyperthermia increases oxygen requirements. Seizures also increase cerebral oxygen requirements; therefore, they must be controlled. Elevate the head to 30 degrees to decrease intracranial pressure and increase cerebral venous drainage.

Hypotension
Consider the etiology of low blood pressure to be associated with either a volume, a rate, or a pump problem. A fluid bolus of 250 to 500 ml of normal saline is appropriate to administer, unless fluid overload or pump failure is suspected. Hypotension that persists following fluid administration may need to be treated with inotropic (dopamine) and vasopressor (epinephrine) agents. The goal is to maintain adequate cerebral perfusion.

Recurrent VF/VT
Following successful resuscitation, if ventricular fibrillation or pulseless ventricular tachycardia recurs, consider the administration of procainamide at 50 mg/minute to a total of 17 mg/kg.

Tachycardia in Postresuscitation
Supraventricular tachycardias in the postresuscitation period should be left untreated unless the patient becomes severely hypotensive with evidence of poor perfusion. High amounts of circulating catecholamines are usually the cause of tachycardia.

Bradycardia in Postresuscitation
Atropine, pacing, and catecholamine infusions should be considered only in profound bradycardia with hypotension and evidence of hypoperfusion. Otherwise, reevaluate the airway, breathing, oxygenation, and circulation status and do not immediately administer atropine.

Premature Ventricular Contractions in Postresuscitation
Most often, PVCs are an indication that there is an existing problem in the secondary ABCDs. Increase oxygenation if possible. Monitor the patient closely as the acid-base and catecholamine levels normalize.

PREHOSPITAL ALGORITHMS FOR PATIENTS NOT IN CARDIAC ARREST

It is just as critical to be able to manage the patient who is not in cardiac arrest but has the potential to deteriorate to cardiac arrest. The following conditions must be managed to prevent cardiac arrest from occurring:

▶ Serious nonlethal dysrhythmias that are too fast or too slow

▶ Acute MI

▶ Hypotension, cardiogenic shock, and acute pulmonary edema

The general approach to cardiac care algorithm, introduced earlier in this chapter for patients in cardiac arrest, also applies to the patient who is not in cardiac arrest. Reassessment of the airway and ventilation is a critical consideration in this particular patient. Management of the patient should include the following critical actions:

▶ Administer supplemental oxygen.

▶ Initiate intravenous access.

▶ Maintain continuous ECG monitoring.

▶ Continuously evaluate and reassess the airway and ventilation.

▶ Perform tracheal intubation as necessary.

▶ Assess vital signs.

▶ Obtain and evaluate the patient's medical history.

▶ Perform a primary and secondary survey.

▶ Acquire a 12-lead ECG, especially if the patient is complaining of chest pain.

▶ Monitor the pulse oximetry level.

Like the patient in cardiac arrest, it is necessary to concentrate on the whole patient and not the rhythm, blood pressure, or findings of the 3-lead or 12-lead ECG. The following conditions are most likely to lead to cardiac arrest if not rapidly diagnosed and managed:

▶ Acute MI

▶ Acute pulmonary edema

▶ Dysrhythmias

▶ Hypotension and shock

Rhythms can be simply classified into two broad categories. Cardiac arrest (lethal) rhythms and non-cardiac arrest (nonlethal) rhythms. The cardiac arrest rhythms are segregated into the four basic types discussed earlier in this chapter:

▶ Ventricular fibrillation

▶ Pulseless ventricular tachycardia

▶ Pulseless electrical activity

▶ Asystole

The non-cardiac arrest (nonlethal) rhythms are separated into two broad categories:

▶ Too slow—bradycardias (less than 60 beats per minute)

▶ Too fast—tachycardias (greater than 100 beats per minute)

When evaluating these rhythms it is necessary to concentrate on the patient and not the ECG rhythm. Look for evidence of physiologic instability such as hypotension, decreased mental status, chest pain, and other signs and symptoms. Use the primary and secondary ABCD survey to identify clinical compromise.

The algorithms for AED use and synchronized cardioversion were discussed in Chapter 7. The algorithm for acute ischemic chest pain was discussed in Chapter 9.

Bradycardia Algorithm

This algorithm is used for patients who are not in cardiac arrest (Figure 10-5). The bradycardia is categorized into either absolute or relative bradycardia. *Absolute bradycardia* is referred to as a heart rate less than 60 beats per minute. *Relative bradycardia* is a low rate, 68 for example, in a patient who is symptomatic. It is important to determine if the patient is symptomatic, that is, displaying signs and symptoms of physiologic instability.

Signs and symptoms of physiologic instability associated with bradycardia are:

- ▶ Chest pain
- ▶ Shortness of breath
- ▶ Decreased mental status
- ▶ Hypotension
- ▶ Evidence of poor perfusion and shock
- ▶ Weakness and fatigue
- ▶ Lightheadedness
- ▶ Syncope
- ▶ Diaphoresis
- ▶ Pulmonary congestion (crackles or rales)
- ▶ Congestive heart failure
- ▶ PVCs
- ▶ Acute myocardial infarction

Key Points

- ▶ As with all other rhythms, treat the patient and not the rhythm. Continue to assess the patient for evidence of physiologic instability. Concentrate on treating the symptomatic patient.
- ▶ Assess for signs and symptoms of physiologic instability in bradycardia. This determines the need and extent of the patient management. You must determine if the slow rate is the actual etiology of the signs and symptoms or if the signs and symptoms are due to some other cause.
- ▶ Heart transplant patients have denervated hearts that will not respond to atropine. Thus, proceed directly to pacing or catecholamine infusion in the intervention sequence. Isoproterenol can stimulate the denervated heart and should only be used until a transcutaneous pacemaker is available. Isoproterenol is contraindicated in the hypotensive patient.
- ▶ Atropine is administered at 0.5 mg to 1 mg every 3 to 5 minutes to a total dose of 0.03 mg/kg (0.04 mg/kg is a higher vagolytic dose recommended in asystole and PEA). If the patient is severely symptomatic, use the 3-minute dosing

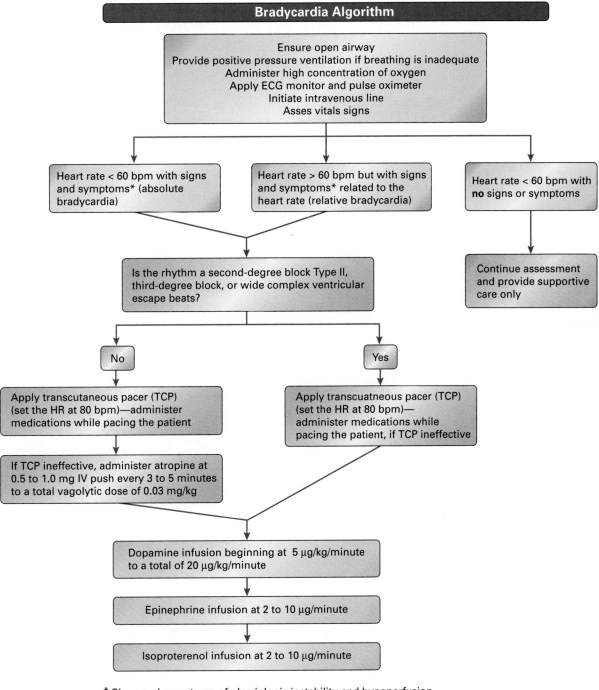

Bradycardia Algorithm

Ensure open airway
Provide positive pressure ventilation if breathing is inadequate
Administer high concentration of oxygen
Apply ECG monitor and pulse oximeter
Initiate intravenous line
Asses vitals signs

Heart rate < 60 bpm with signs and symptoms* (absolute bradycardia)

Heart rate > 60 bpm but with signs and symptoms* related to the heart rate (relative bradycardia)

Heart rate < 60 bpm with **no** signs or symptoms

Continue assessment and provide supportive care only

Is the rhythm a second-degree block Type II, third-degree block, or wide complex ventricular escape beats?

No

Yes

Apply transcutaneous pacer (TCP) (set the HR at 80 bpm)—administer medications while pacing the patient

Apply transcuatneous pacer (TCP) (set the HR at 80 bpm)—administer medications while pacing the patient, if TCP ineffective

If TCP ineffective, administer atropine at 0.5 to 1.0 mg IV push every 3 to 5 minutes to a total vagolytic dose of 0.03 mg/kg

Dopamine infusion beginning at 5 μg/kg/minute to a total of 20 μg/kg/minute

Epinephrine infusion at 2 to 10 μg/minute

Isoproterenol infusion at 2 to 10 μg/minute

* Signs and symptoms of physiologic instability and hypoperfusion
• Chest pain
• Shortness of breath
• Decreased mental status
• Hypotension
• Evidence of poor perfusion and shock
• Weakness and fatigue
• Lightheadedness
• Syncope
• Diaphoresis
• Pulmonary congestion (crackles or rales)
• PVCs
• Acute myocardial infarction

FIGURE 10-5
Algorithm for bradycardia.

interval. Atropine is not indicated in the patient suffering from a second-degree Type II AV block, third-degree block, or wide complex escape beats.

▶ Never use lidocaine to treat a third-degree heart block or any other ventricular rhythm or wide complex rhythm.

▶ Atropine will rarely accelerate the atrial rate in a second-degree Mobitz Type II block and may increase the AV nodal block. This will decrease the ventricular rate and blood pressure and worsen the patient's condition.

▶ If the signs and symptoms associated with bradycardia are only mild, atropine should be considered the first-line drug of choice. The dose is 0.5 mg to 1.0 mg IV every 3 to 5 minutes up to a total dose of 0.03 mg/kg.

▶ Dopamine, at a rate of 5 to 20 µg/kg/minute, should be used if hypotension is associated with the bradycardia. You can proceed directly to an epinephrine infusion if the signs and symptoms are severe. Infuse epinephrine at an initial rate of 2 to 10 µg/minute. Isoproterenol may also be considered and administered at 2 to 10 µg/minute.

▶ Transcutaneous pacing is a primary intervention in the symptomatic bradycardia patient. In a severely unstable patient, you should move immediately to transcutaneous pacing. A trial of atropine may be administered while the transcutaneous pacer is prepared.

▶ Patients with right ventricular infarction may present with bradycardia and hypotension. The hypotension is due to reduction in preload and not the bradycardia. Suspect it in patients with a 12-lead ECG showing inferior wall MI. A judicial fluid challenge may increase the right ventricular filling pressure with a subsequent increase in the force of right ventricular contractions, based on Starling's law.

▶ The Type II second-degree AV block can rapidly convert to a third-degree AV block. The patient needs to be prepared for transvenous pacing while the transcutaneous pacer is used as an immediate intervention.

▶ Atropine is relatively contraindicated in the third-degree AV block patient. Consider transcutaneous pacing, dopamine, and an epinephrine infusion.

Emergency Cardiac Care Protocol: Bradycardia

1. Ensure the scene is clear of safety hazards. Call for additional resources as necessary.
2. Perform an initial assessment. Provide positive pressure ventilation if the breathing is inadequate. Administer a high concentration of oxygen. Apply the ECG monitor and pulse oximeter.
3. Establish an intravenous line.
4. Assess the vital signs.
5. If the heart rate is < 60 bpm and no signs or symptoms of physiologic instability are present, continue with the assessment and provide supportive care. Continue to reassess for signs and symptoms of physiologic instability.[*]
6. If the heart rate is <60 bpm with signs and symptoms of physiologic instability[*] (absolute bradycardia) or if the heart rate is >60 bpm but a relative bradycardia exist with signs and symptoms of physiologic instability,[*] begin transcutaneous pacing at a rate of 80 bpm. Set the milliamps at the lowest setting and increase until capture occurs. Continue pacing as medications are administered concurrently.

(continued)

7. Administer atropine at 0.5 to 1.0 mg IV push every 3 to 5 minutes until a cumulative maximum dose of 0.03 mg/kg is administered. A vagolytic dose of 0.04 mg/kg is used in cardiac arrest patients. A trial of atropine can be administered while the transcutaneous pacer is being set up. Atropine is not indicated if the patient is in a second-degree Type II block, third-degree block, or a wide complex escape beat rhythm. Go directly to transcutaneous pacing. Atropine will not be effective in heart transplant patients due to a denervated heart.

8. Administer a dopamine infusion starting at 5 µg/kg/minute. Titrate to a heart rate > than 60 bpm and an adequate blood pressure. Dopamine can be increased to 20 µg/kg/minute.

9. Administer an epinephrine infusion at 2 to 10 µg/minute.

10. Administer an isoproterenol infusion at 2 to 10 µg/minute.

*Signs and symptoms of physiologic instability and hypoperfusion
- Chest pain
- Shortness of breath
- Decreased mental status
- Hypotension
- Evidence of poor perfusion and shock
- Weakness and fatigue
- Lightheadedness
- Syncope
- Diaphoresis
- Pulmonary congestion (crackles or rales)
- Congestive heart failure
- PVCs
- Acute myocardial infarction

Tachycardia Algorithm

Tachydysrhythmias can be broken into two basic categories based on the morphology (monomorphic or polymorphic wave form) of the ECG tracing: and the width of the QRS complex (narrow complex and wide complex). Each of these types can be further categorized, as shown below.

Tachydysrhythmia Categories Based on Morphology of ECG Tracing and QRS Width

Narrow Complex Tachycardias:	Wide Complex Tachycardias:
• Atrial fibrillation or atrial flutter	• Ventricular tachycardia
• Supraventricular tachycardia	• Wide complex tachycardia of an uncertain type
• Ectopic atrial tachycardia	
• Mutifocal atrial tachycardia	

Tachydysrhythmias are also categorized based on hemodynamic stability, which is primarily determined by signs and symptoms exhibited by the patient. Patients who are exhibiting signs and symptoms of hemodynamic instability are categorized as "unstable," whereas the patient who has no complaints or who is not showing any signs or symptoms that are directly related to the current dysrhythmia is considered to be "stable." Thus, all of the tachydysrhythmias, whether narrow or wide complex, can be clinically categorized as either stable or unstable.

Tachydysrhythmia Categories Based on Patient's Hemodynamic Status

Stable:	Unstable:
• Patient has no complaints, signs, or symptoms or the signs and symptoms are not related to the dysrhythmia	• Patient has signs and symptoms of hemodynamic instability related to the dysrhythmia

You must not only determine the rhythm but also the hemodynamic status of the patient, since the management is significantly different for the stable vs. the unstable patient. This requires you to assess and treat the "whole" patient and not just the rhythm. Whether the rhythm is wide complex, narrow complex, atrial flutter/fibrillation, supraventricular, ventricular, or uncertain, the urgency of management is based on the patient's hemodynamic status and ability to compensate while in the rhythm. Symptomatic, unstable patients require immediate intervention.

The signs and symptoms of hemodynamic instability are the same for tachycardias as for bradycardias. Signs and symptoms of an unstable tachycardia requiring immediate intervention are:

▶ Hypotension

▶ Congestive heart failure

▶ Decreased level of consciousness

▶ Chest pain

▶ Acute MI

▶ Shortness of breath

▶ Evidence of poor perfusion and shock

▶ Pulmonary congestion

The wide complex tachydysrhythmias are further categorized by the morphology of the wave form. Specifically, ventricular tachycardia is categorized as either monomorphic ventricular tachycardia or polymorphic ventricular tachycardia. *Monomorphic* refers to a wave form that remains constant and does not change in its morphology. *Polymorphic* refers to a wave form that changes in morphology. Torsades de pointes is an example of a polymorphic wave form where the waves change deflection from above the isoelectric line to below the isoelectric line.

Treatment of wide complex tachycardias is also dependent on the cardiac function of the patient. If there is evidence of left ventricular dysfunction with clinical signs and symptoms of congestive heart failure, the drug preference changes to ensure a medication with no negative inotropic effects is administered.

When treating a patient with an unstable (symptomatic) tachydysrhythmia, it is important to determine whether the tachycardia is a result of an underlying condition that is also producing the signs and symptoms (for example, both tachycardia and chest pain resulting from an MI) or if the signs and symptoms are a result of the tachycardia (for example, chest pain resulting from tachycardia).

When considering management of the patient based on the algorithm approach it is best to categorize the patient and rhythm into one of the following:

▶ Stable narrow complex tachycardia

▶ Unstable narrow complex tachycardia

▶ Stable wide complex tachycardia (monomorphic)

- Stable wide complex tachycardia (polymorphic)
- Unstable wide complex tachycardia (monomorphic and polymorphic)

Atrial Fibrillation/Atrial Flutter: Key Points

- Avoid immediate cardioversion in the atrial fibrillation/atrial flutter patient unless serious signs and symptoms of hemodynamic instability are present. Cardioversion may precipitate formation of emboli and lead to a stroke.
- Atrial fibrillation and atrial flutter may not require any intervention unless the patient develops serious signs and symptoms of hemodynamic instability. This usually occurs as the result of a rapid ventricular response. The management is geared toward slowing the ventricular response and not converting the rhythm to normal sinus.
- Atrial flutter is a less stable rhythm than atrial fibrillation.
- Amiodarone can be used to control the rate in atrial fibrillation and atrial flutter. Avoid the use of calcium channel blockers since they may block the AV node and cause an increase in the conduction through an accessory pathway leading to an increase in the ventricular rate. Adenosine has a similar effect as verapamil on the accessory pathways; however, the risk of its use is much lower due to the short half life. Diltiazem is also used to control the rate in atrial fibrillation. Refer to your local protocols.
- Cardioversion should be performed if the patient develops severe signs and symptoms of hemodynamic instability. Atrial flutter usually requires a lower energy level to cardiovert, starting at 50 joules.

Narrow Complex Tachycardia: Key Points (Figure 10-6)

- Immediate cardioversion is needed if serious signs and symptoms of hemodynamic instability are evident.
- If the complexes are wide, treat the tachycardia like ventricular tachycardia.
- Vagal maneuvers should be performed prior to medications in the stable patient. Pressure on the eyeball as a vagal maneuver should not be used.
- If a vagal maneuver changes the heart rate in a narrow complex tachycardia, the origin of the dysrhythmia is probably supraventricular.
- Do not perform a carotid sinus massage on middle-aged or elderly patients due to the risk of atherosclerotic disease and embolization of plaque.
- Adenosine is an effective agent in the conversion of narrow complex tachycardias. It produces less hypotension and has a much shorter half-life than verapamil. Adenosine, at a dose of 6 mg, must be administered as a rapid IV push followed by a 20 ml saline bolus as a flush. It can be repeated twice after 1 to 2 minutes at 12 mg.
- Narrow complex tachycardia has typically two difference etiologies: 1) reentry; and 2) automatic focus. PSVT has a reentry etiology and typically responds well to drugs and cardioversion since the rhythm is proliferated by a reentry circuit or pathway. Multifocal atrial tachycardia, ectopic atrial tachycardia, and junctional tachycardia have an automatic foci etiology. Cardioversion does not work in these tachydysrhythmias since a foci and not a reentry pathway is the cause of the tachydysrhythmia. Beta blockers, calcium channel blockers and amiodarone are usually effective agents in tachydysrhythmias with an automatic focus etiology.

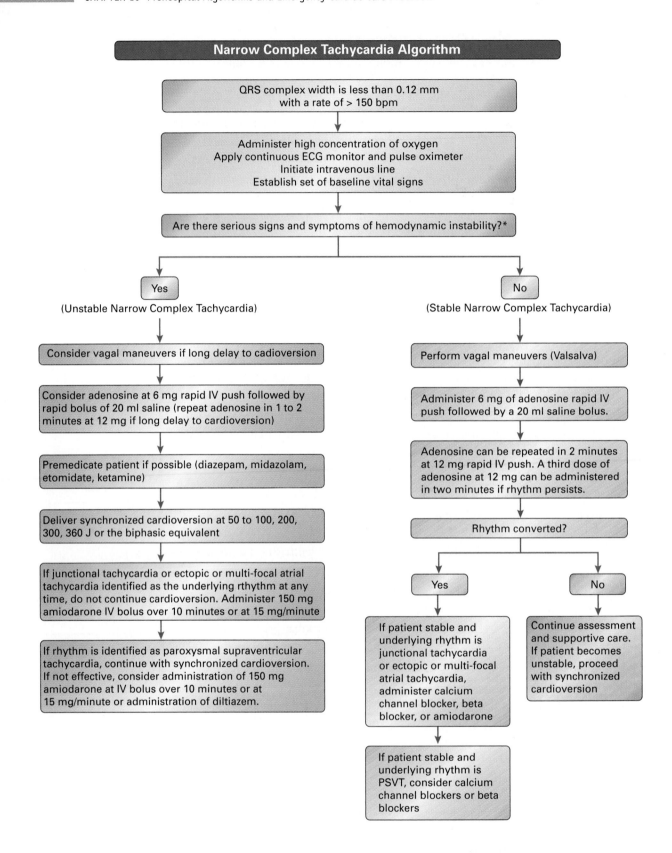

*Serious signs or symptoms of hemodynamic instability include chest pain, dyspnea, decreased mental status, hypotension, hypoperfusion, shock, pulmonary congestion (rales or crackles), and congestive heart failure.

FIGURE 10-6
Algorithm for narrow complex tachycardia.

▶ If the unstable narrow complex tachycardia is junctional tachycardia, multi-focal atrial tachycardia, or ectopic atrial tachycardia after cardioversion, do not continue with cardioversion or do not administer beta blockers or calcium channel blockers since these drugs may cause the hemodynamic status of the patient to deteriorate further. Amiodarone is the drug of choice in these patients.

▶ If the unstable narrow complex tachycardia is identified as paroxysmal supraventricular tachycardia after cardioversion, continue with synchronized cardioversion then consider amiodarone or diltiazem.

▶ Antidysrhythmics may actually worsen the cardiac function and may precipitate hemodynamic instability. The use of two or more antidysrhythmic drugs in the treatment of tachydysrhythmias may actually do more harm than good. Your goal should be to use only one antidysrhythmic drug and avoid the use of two different drugs.

Emergency Cardiac Care Protocol: Stable Narrow Complex Tachycardia

1. Ensure the scene is clear of safety hazards. Call for additional resources as necessary.

2. Perform an initial assessment. Administer a high concentration of oxygen. Apply the ECG monitor and pulse oximeter.

3. Establish an intravenous line.

4. Assess the vital signs.

5. Ensure that the QRS complex is less than 0.12 mm and the rate is >150 bpm and the patient is not displaying serious signs and symptoms of hemodynamic instability.

6. Perform a vagal maneuver. Valsalva maneuver is appropriate for all adult ages. If the patient is middle-aged or elderly, do not do a carotid sinus massage.

7. Administer adenosine at 6 mg rapid IV push followed by a rapid bolus of 20 ml of normal saline. Adenosine can be repeated twice at 12 mg rapid IV push in two minutes after previous bolus.

8. If the rhythm is converted and the patient is hemodynamically stable, attempt to identify the underlying rhythm. Treat the underlying rhythm as follows:
   – **PSVT**—Administer calcium channel blockers or beta blockers
   – **Junctional Tachycardia**—Administer calcium channel blockers, beta blockers, or amiodarone
   – **Ectopic Atrial Tachycardia**—Administer calcium channel blockers, beta blockers, or amiodarone
   – **Multi-focal Atrial Tachycardia**—Administer calcium channel blockers, beta blockers, or amiodarone

9. If the rhythm is *not* converted with vagal maneuvers or adenosine, consider synchronous cardioversion at 50 to 100 J, 200 J, 300 J, 360 J or the equivalent biphasic energy levels. Prior to synchronous cardioversion, consider premedication with an analgesic or sedative drug. Serious consideration must be given to avoiding cardioversion of a stable patient after the medications have been exhausted. Follow your local protocol.

10. If at any time the patient becomes hemodynamically unstable, go to the unstable narrow complex tachycardia algorithm.

Emergency Cardiac Care Protocol: Unstable Narrow Complex Tachycardia

1. Ensure the scene is clear of safety hazards. Call for additional resources as necessary.

2. Perform an initial assessment. Administer a high concentration of oxygen. Apply the ECG monitor and pulse oximeter.

3. Establish an intravenous line.

4. Assess the vital signs.

5. Ensure that the QRS complex is less than 0.12 mm and the rate is >150 bpm and the patient is displaying serious signs and symptoms of hemodynamic instability. Serious signs or symptoms of hemodynamic instability include chest pain, dyspnea, decreased mental status, hypotension, hypoperfusion, shock, pulmonary congestion (rales or crackles), and congestive heart failure.

6. If there is a delay in performing synchronized cardioversion, consider a vagal maneuver. Valsalva maneuver is appropriate for all adult ages. If the patient is middle-aged or elderly, do not do a carotid sinus massage.

7. If there is a delay in synchronized cardioversion or adenosine is immediately available, administer adenosine at 6 mg rapid IV push followed by a rapid bolus of 20 ml of normal saline. If synchronized cardioversion is still not available, adenosine can be repeated twice at 12 mg rapid IV push in one to two minutes after previous bolus.

8. Premedicate patient with analgesic or sedative agent if possible. (Avoid in hypotensive patients.)

9. Perform synchronized cardioversion at 50 to 100 J, 200 J, 300 J, and 360 J or the equivalent biphasic energy level.

10. If the tachydysrhythmia is identified, continue with the rhythm as follows:
    - **Junctional Tachycardia**—Do not continue with cardioversion. Administer 150 mg amiodarone over 10 minutes or at 15 mg/minute.
    - **Ectopic Atrial Tachycardia**—Do not continue with cardioversion. Administer 150 mg amiodarone over 10 minutes or at 15 mg/minute.
    - **Multi-focal Atrial Tachycardia**—Do not continue with cardioversion. Administer 150 mg amiodarone over 10 minutes or at 15 mg/minute.
    - **Paroxysmal Supraventricular Tachycardia**—Continue with synchronized cardioversion. If not effective, consider amiodarone 150 mg over 10 minutes or 15 mg/minute. Diltiazem could also be administered.

Wide-Complex Tachycardias: Key Points (Figure 10-7)

▶ Wide complex tachycardia should be considered ventricular tachycardia and be treated as such until proven otherwise.

▶ Verapamil should *never* be given to a patient with a wide-complex tachycardia of an uncertain type. Administration of verapamil to a patient in ventricular tachycardia can be lethal.

▶ Ventricular tachycardia with a pulse is categorized as either monomorphic or polymorphic wide complex tachycardia. The patient may present as either stable or unstable.

▶ Pulseless ventricular tachycardia is managed exactly the same as ventricular fibrillation.

▶ A patient in a wide complex tachycardia with hypotension, shortness of breath, chest pain, altered level of consciousness, or pulmonary edema is considered to be unstable. Immediate synchronized cardioversion is the treatment of choice. Amiodarone can be administered while preparing for the cardioversion.

▶ The stable wide complex tachycardia that is monomorphic is treated with antidysrhythmic agents. Procainamide is the first line drug of choice if there is no evidence of congestive heart failure or left ventricular dysfunction. Procainamide is administered at 20 mg/minute to a maximum cumulative dose of 17 mg/kg. If signs and symptoms of congestive heart failure or left ventricular dysfunction are present, or if the patient has a history of congestive heart failure, amiodarone is the drug of choice. Procainamide is not used because of its negative inotropic properties. Only one bolus of amiodarone is administered at 150 mg IV bolus over 10 minutes or at 15 mg/minute. DO NOT repeat the amiodarone. If the rhythm fails to convert and the clinical status of the patient remains unchanged, administer lidocaine at 1.0 to 1.5 mg/kg. If the patient fails to convert or becomes clinically unstable, go to the unstable wide complex algorithm or emergency care protocol.

▶ If the wide complex tachycardia is of an unknown type, administer procainamide and then amiodarone. If there is evidence of left ventricular dysfunction or congestive heart failure, do not administer procainamide due to the negative inotropic effects. You should only administer amiodarone.

▶ A stable polymorphic wide complex tachycardia is commonly known as torsades de pointes or multi-axial ventricular tachycardia. This rhythm commonly degrades into ventricular fibrillation.

▶ Stable polymorphic wide complex tachycardia is managed based on the QT interval. If the QT interval is prolonged during an episode of a sinus rhythm, magnesium sulfate is the drug of choice. Magnesium sulfate is administered at 1 to 2 grams mixed in 100 ml of D_5W and administered over 5 to 60 minutes. Follow this bolus with a maintenance infusion of 0.5 to 1.0 gram per hour. Other treatment may include overdrive pacing, isoproterenol, phenytoin, or lidocaine. Realistically, for most EMS systems, the alternative to magnesium sulfate would be phenytoin or lidocaine. Administer phenytoin at 100 mg over 5 minutes via an infusion or slow IV push. Administer until a maximum dose of 1,000 mg is reached or the dysrhythmia is abolished. Administer lidocaine at 0.5 to 0.75 mg/kg every 5 to 10 minutes to a maximum cumulative dose of 3 mg/kg over one hour. If conversion occurs with lidocaine, initiate a maintenance infusion at 3 mg/minute. If at any time the patient becomes unstable, go to the unstable wide complex algorithm or emergency care protocol.

▶ If the QT interval is normal in the stable polymorphic wide complex tachycardia, go to the monomorphic stable wide complex algorithm or emergency cardiac care protocol.

▶ Polymorphic wide complex tachycardia usually requires higher energy levels to cardiovert (200 joules).

▶ Antidysrhythmics may actually worsen the cardiac function and may precipitate hemodynamic instability. The use of two or more antidysrhythmic drugs in the treatment of tachydysrhythmias may actually do more harm than good. Your goal should be to use only one antidysrhythmic drug and avoid the use of two different drugs.

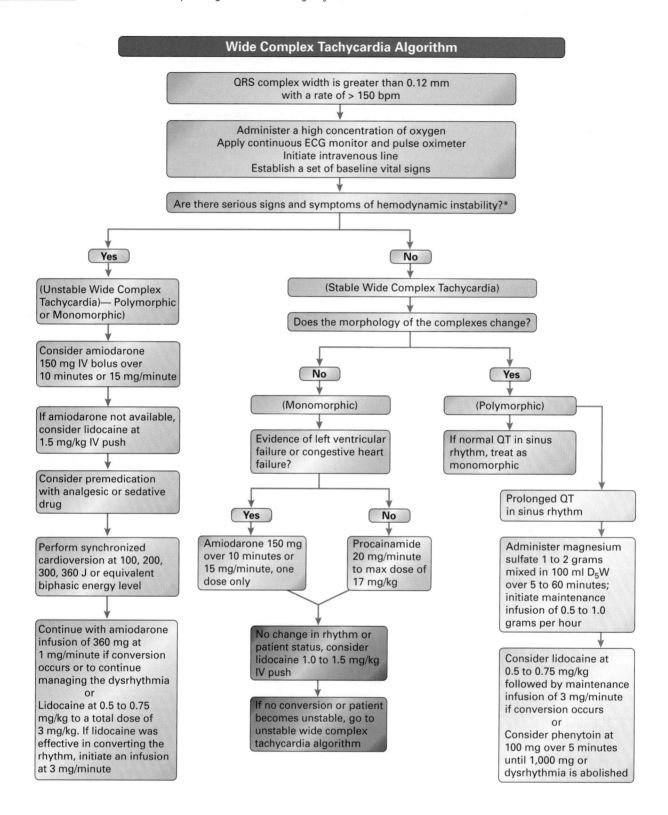

FIGURE 10-7
Algorithm for wide complex tachycardia.

Emergency Cardiac Care Protocol: Stable Wide Complex Tachycardia (Monomorphic)

1. Ensure the scene is clear of safety hazards. Call for additional resources as necessary.

2. Perform an initial assessment. Administer a high concentration of oxygen. Apply the ECG monitor and pulse oximeter.

3. Establish an intravenous line.

4. Assess the vital signs.

5. Ensure that the QRS complex is greater than 0.12 mm and the rate is >150 bpm and the patient is not displaying serious signs and symptoms of hemodynamic instability. Be cautious since monomorphic wide complex tachycardia can easily deteriorate into an unstable wide complex tachycardia or pulseless ventricular tachycardia.

6. If there are **no** signs and symptoms of acute onset congestive heart failure, left ventricular dysfunction, or unstable congestive heart failure, administer procainamide at 20 mg/minute to a maximum dose of 17 mg/kg or until the QRS widens by 50% the original width, hypotension ensues, or the dysrhythmia is abolished. Do not administer procainamide if signs and symptoms of CHF or left ventricular function is present.

7. If procainamide is ineffective in converting the dysrhythmia, or if signs and symptoms of congestive heart failure or left ventricular function are present, administer amiodarone at 150 mg over 10 minutes or 15 mg/minute. Only administer one dose.

8. If the dysrhythmia is not abolished, consider the administration of lidocaine at 1.0 to 1.5 mg/kg IV push.

9. If the dysrhythmia persists or the patient becomes hemodynamically unstable, proceed to the unstable wide complex tachycardia algorithm or emergency cardiac care protocol. (Avoid cardioversion in the stable patient in the prehospital setting, if possible.)

Emergency Cardiac Care Protocol: Stable Wide Complex Tachycardia (Polymorphic)

1. Ensure the scene is clear of safety hazards. Call for additional resources as necessary.

2. Perform an initial assessment. Administer a high concentration of oxygen. Apply the ECG monitor and pulse oximeter.

3. Establish an intravenous line.

4. Assess the vital signs.

5. Ensure that the QRS complex is greater than 0.12 mm and the rate is >150 bpm and the patient is not displaying serious signs and symptoms of hemodynamic instability. Polymorphic wide complex tachycardia is also known as torsades de pointes or multi-axial ventricular tachycardia. Be cautious since polymorphic wide complex tachycardia can easily deteriorate into ventricular fibrillation.

6. If the QT interval is normal during any periods of the normal or sinus rhythm, manage the polymorphic stable wide complex tachycardia as a monomorphic stable wide complex tachycardia.

7. If the QT interval is prolonged during any periods of the normal or sinus rhythm, consider administering magnesium sulfate at 1 to 2 grams mixed in 100 ml D_5W over 5 to 60 minutes followed by a maintenance infusion of 0.5 to 1.0 grams per hour titrated to control the rhythm.

(continued)

8. Other dysrhythmia management control measures include:
    – Phenytoin sodium at 100 mg over 5 minutes via infusion or slow IV push to a maximum dose of 1,000 mg or until the dysrhythmia is abolished.
    – Lidocaine at 0.5 to 0.75 mg/kg every 5 to 10 minutes to a maximum dose of 3 mg/kg over 1 hour. If conversion occurs, start a maintenance infusion at 3 mg/minute.
    – Overdrive pacing
    – Isoproterenol hydrochloride infusion at 2 to 10 µg/minute.

9. If the patient becomes unstable, proceed to unstable wide complex algorithm or emergency cardiac care protocol.

CASE STUDY FOLLOW-UP

You are frantically summoned by an elderly man to attend to his wife who is found lying supine on the bedroom floor. The elderly woman is ashen gray and motionless. You immediately call for a backup unit.

Basic Life Support

You kneel next to the elderly woman and shout, "Hey, ma'am, can you hear me?" You shake her shoulder and get no response. You open her airway and assess for breathing. The patient is breathless. You deliver two quick ventilations with a bag-valve-mask device. You assess for a carotid pulse and find none.

Advanced Life Support

You immediately perform a quick look with the defibrillation paddles and identify ventricular fibrillation on the oscilloscope. You place defibrillation pads on the chest and scan the patient while shouting, "I'm clear, you're clear, everyone's clear," as you begin to charge the defibrillator to 200 J. You deliver the first shock and hold the paddles firmly on the chest as you wait for the rhythm to return to the isoelectric line on the oscilloscope. The monitor shows ventricular fibrillation. You charge to 300 J as you again shout to clear the patient. You deliver the shock and reassess the rhythm. It remains V-fib. You charge to 360 J and deliver the third shock in the stacked shock sequence. You check for the carotid pulse and do not find one.

By this time, your backup crew in on the scene and enters the room. You instruct Mike to continue chest compressions. Heather is at the airway and resumes bag-valve-mask ventilation. You instruct her to hyperoxygenate the patient and perform tracheal intubation. George is establishing intravenous access in an antecubital vein in the right arm. You hook up the continuous monitoring ECG cable.

Heather yells, "Tubes in." You check for chest rise and fall while you listen to the epigastrium. No sounds are heard in the stomach, so you proceed to assess breath sounds over the lungs. You indicate, "Breath sounds are equal and clear bilaterally." You place an end-tidal CO_2 detector on the end of the tracheal tube and ventilate six times. The $EtCO_2$ monitor is showing CO_2 in the exhalation by both a LED readout and waveform. You order Heather to, "Secure the tube."

You ask, "George, where's my IV line?" George states, "This lady has bad veins. The IV just blew." You instruct Heather to administer 2 mg of epinephrine down the tracheal tube and aggressively hyperoxygenate for 30 to 60 seconds. After the 30 to 60 seconds, you clear the patient and defibrillate at 360 J. You check for a carotid pulse and find none.

You order, "Continue compressions and ventilations." George has now established a patent IV line. You estimate the patient's weight at 80 kg. You instruct him to administer 300 mg amiodarone IV push. You wait 60 seconds following the drug administration, clear the patient, and defibrillate at 360 J. No pulse is found. The monitor now shows asystole. You switch to Leads I and III to be sure the patient is not still in V-fib in another lead. The monitor shows asystole in each lead.

continued on next page

You order continuation of the compressions and ventilations while you administer 1 mg of atropine IV push. After 2 minutes you stop and assess the rhythm. You find V-fib on the oscilloscope. You immediately defibrillate at 360 J. No pulse is found, so CPR is continued. You administer another bolus of 1 mg of epinephrine, followed by another 150 mg of amiodarone. After 30 seconds, you defibrillate at 360 J. You find a faint pulse upon assessment, and the monitor shows a sinus rhythm at a rate of 82. The blood pressure is 102/64. You instruct George to mix an amiodarone infusion and run it at 1 mg/minute. The patient remains unresponsive with no spontaneous ventilation. You reassess the tracheal tube and IV line and ensure that the amiodarone infusion is running properly. You prepare the patient for transport. During transport you contact the emergency department and provide an oral report. You continue to assess the patient en route. The patient is transferred to the emergency department without further incident.

SUMMARY

In this chapter we have provided algorithms and emergency cardiac care protocols for managing patients who are in cardiac arrest or suffering from other common dysrhythmias. The algorithms and emergency cardiac care protocols are to be used only as guidelines and not as a legal standard of care. You must use your clinical judgment and expertise when making patient management decisions, since all patients are different and require individual consideration.

When managing the patient in cardiac arrest or one who is suffering from a dysrhythmia, it is imperative that you treat the whole patient and not just the rhythm. Developing tunnel vision and managing rhythms will only lead to unsuccessful resuscitation attempts. Assess your patient and consider conditions that may have led to the cardiac arrest or conditions that are preventing you from successfully converting the rhythm. Get to the etiology of the problem, save the heart, and most importantly save the brain!

REVIEW QUESTIONS

1. The most common initial presenting rhythm in the cardiac arrest patient is
   a. asystole.
   b. pulseless ventricular tachycardia.
   c. ventricular fibrillation.
   d. pulseless electrical activity.

2. Which of the following medications **cannot** be administered tracheally?
   a. amiodarone
   b. naloxone
   c. lidocaine
   d. epinephrine

3. Which of the following would be considered an acceptable alternative vasopressor agent to be used in ventricular fibrillation or pulseless ventricular tachycardia?
   a. vasopressin
   b. amiodarone
   c. isoproterenol
   d. phenytoin sodium

4. In which of the following conditions is sodium bicarbonate **not** recommended as an intervention?
   a. prolonged cardiac arrest in an intubated patient
   b. a patient with suspected hypoxic lactic acidosis
   c. a tricyclic antidepressant overdose
   d. a patient found to be hyperkalemic

5. Immediately upon identifying ventricular fibrillation on the monitor, you should
   a. defibrillate at 200 joules or the biphasic equivalent.
   b. begin chest compression and ventilation.
   c. establish an intravenous line and intubate the patient.
   d. attach the continuous ECG monitor and check a second lead.

6. During the resuscitation, the rhythm converts to asystole. You should immediately
   a. defibrillate at 200 joules, since it may be a fine ventricular fibrillation.
   b. check a second lead to ensure that it is not ventricular fibrillation.
   c. stop chest compression and decompress the chest.
   d. administer a bolus of sodium bicarbonate.

7. You have provided the initial three stacked defibrillations to a patient in ventricular fibrillation. The patient regains a pulse for a few minutes, then suddenly reverts back into ventricular fibrillation. You should immediately
   a. administer a bolus of lidocaine at 1 mg/kg.
   b. defibrillate at 200 joules or the biphasic equivalent.
   c. defibrillate at 360 joules or the biphasic equivalent.
   d. hyperventilate and perform tracheal intubation.

8. The appropriate dose of amiodarone when used for a patient in ventricular fibrillation, is
   a. 300 mg IV push repeated in 3 to 5 minutes at 150 mg IV push.
   b. 150 mg IV push repeated in 3 to 5 minutes at 300 mg IV push.
   c. 30 mg/kg repeated in 10 minutes at 30 mg/kg.
   d. 5 mg/kg mixed in 50 ml of normal saline repeated every 8 minutes.

9. Following the administration of a medication in the patient in ventricular fibrillation, you should
   a. immediately defibrillate at 360 joules or the biphasic equivalent.
   b. perform CPR for 30 to 60 seconds, then defibrillate at 360 joules or the biphasic equivalent.
   c. perform CPR for 1 to 2 minutes, then defibrillate at 360 joules or the biphasic equivalent.
   d. perform CPR for 30 seconds and repeat the defibrillation at 200 J or the biphasic equivalent.

10. Hypovolemia, hypoxemia, tension pneumothorax, and pericardial tamponade are all possible etiologies of
    a. ventricular fibrillation.
    b. symptomatic bradycardia.
    c. unstable ventricular tachycardia.
    d. pulseless electrical activity.

11. The treatment of choice for a patient in PEA from a tension pneumothorax is
    a. 250 ml fluid bolus of normal saline.
    b. needle thoracentesis.
    c. administration of 1 mg of epinephrine.
    d. transcutaneous pacing.

12. The total cumulative dose of atropine in a 70 kg patient in asystole is
    a. 1.0 mg.
    b. 2.1 mg.
    c. 2.8 mg.
    d. 4.0 mg.

13. Following successful resuscitation, the patient's blood pressure remains hypotensive. Your first consideration in management of the blood pressure would be to
    a. administer a fluid bolus of 250 to 500 ml if fluid overload is not suspected.
    b. initiate a norepinephrine infusion at 20 µg/minute.
    c. initiate a dopamine infusion starting at 1 to 2 µg/kg/minute.
    d. begin transcutaneous pacing at a rate of 80 and 100 milliamp.

14. The patient you have just successfully resuscitated is in a narrow complex tachycardia. He is normotensive and perfusing well. The treatment of choice for the narrow complex tachycardia in this case is
    a. administration of adenosine at 6 mg rapid IV bolus.
    b. to leave the rhythm untreated unless the patient becomes hypotensive.
    c. synchronized cardioversion starting at 50 joules.
    d. administration of verapamil at 5 mg, then repeated in 15 minutes at 10 mg.

15. You encounter a patient who is in a third-degree heart block at a ventricular rate of 30 beats/minute. The monitor shows couplets of premature ventricular contractions. Your treatment of choice is
    a. administration of a lidocaine bolus of 1 to 1.5 mg/kg.
    b. administration of atropine at 1.0 mg.
    c. initiation of transcutaneous pacing.
    d. initiation of an epinephrine infusion at 2 to 10 µg/minute.

16. You are treating a symptomatic patient in a second-degree Mobitz Type I heart block. You have attached the external pacer, adjusted the milliamps, and there is still no capture occurring. Your next intervention should be
    a. continue with external pacing.
    b. administer a bolus of epinephrine at 1 mg.
    c. initiate an infusion of dopamine starting at 5 µg/kg/minute.
    d. initiate an epinephrine infusion at 2 µg/minute.

17. A patient comes into the emergency department complaining of palpitations. The patient denies any chest pain, weakness, dyspnea, or any other complaints. He is alert and oriented to person, place, and time. His skin is warm and dry. His vital signs are: blood pressure 142/66, respirations 16, and pulse 196/minute. You attach the monitor and it reveals a narrow complex tachycardia at a rate of 196. The treatment of choice is
    a. administer 6 mg of adenosine IV push.
    b. perform a vagal maneuver.
    c. administer 5 mg of verapamil IV push.
    d. perform synchronized cardioversion at 50 joules.

18. While treating a stable narrow complex tachycardia patient, she suddenly becomes weak, lightheaded, and severely pale and complains of chest discomfort. Your next immediate action should be
    a. perform synchronized cardioversion at 50 to 100 joules.
    b. defibrillate at 200 joules.
    c. try another vagal maneuver.
    d. administer Verapamil at 5 mg slow IV push.

19. The treatment of choice for the patient in torsades de pointes is
    a. administration of lidocaine at 1.0 to 1.5 mg/kg IV push.
    b. initiation of electrical pacing.
    c. administration of magnesium sulfate at 1 to 2 grams IV.
    d. perform vagal maneuvers.

20. You find a patient in a monomorphic wide complex tachycardia. The patient is complaining of some respiratory distress. Upon assessment you find crackles in the dependent lung fields. The blood pressure is 108/88 mmHg and the respiratory rate is 32 per minute. You would manage the dysrhythmia by
    a. administering procainamide at 20 mg/minute to a total of 17 mg/kg.
    b. administer lidocaine at 1.0 mg/kg to a total dose of 3 mg/kg.
    c. administer amiodarone at 150 mg IV bolus over 10 minutes or at 15 mg/minute.
    d. perform synchronized cardioversion at 50 to 100 joules or the biphasic equivalent.

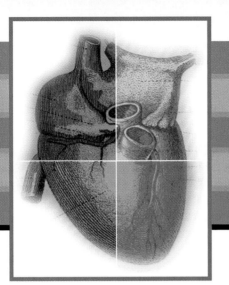

Prehospital Cardiac Emergency Scenarios: Application Exercises

It has no doubt occurred to you that you can learn all about a variety of advanced-cardiac-life-support topics—how to perform an intubation, how to gain IV access, how to read an ECG, and so on—and yet have no idea how, or if, you will be able to apply it all when a real patient is becoming severely cyanotic in front of you, lights are flashing, the noise level is rising, people are running around, and panic threatens to destroy your thinking processes.

During your ACLS course, you will work through a set of scenarios that provide a framework to practice functioning as part of an ACLS team in simulated cardiac emergencies. This chapter presents core scenarios to help you apply the advanced-cardiac-life-support concepts and skills you have studied in the preceding chapters.

Core scenarios in this chapter are:

- Respiratory Arrest
- Ventricular Fibrillation with AED Intervention
- Adult Ventricular Fibrillation/Pulseless Ventricular Tachycardia
- Pulseless Electrical Activity
- Asystole
- Acute Coronary Syndrome
- Bradycardia
- Unstable Wide Complex Tachycardia
- Stable Narrow Complex Tachycardia
- Stable Wide Complex Tachycardia

⊞ INTRODUCTION

The typical cardiac arrest team requires emergency response personnel to perform the responsibilities listed below. Ideally, your initial response will include enough emergency response personnel to perform these functions immediately after initiating the resuscitation. However, in many EMS systems only two EMS providers arrive on the scene and must initiate the resuscitation and wait for a response from a backup crew. If this is the case, utilize personnel at the scene to maximize your effectiveness in the resuscitation. Be sure not to forget the vital basic skills, such as chest compressions and ventilation. You may encounter some paramedics who want to forgo chest compressions or ventilations in order to perform more advanced skills. Without these basic procedures, however, advanced interventions will be futile. Without chest compressions, drugs will remain in the peripheral vein. Without ventilation and oxygenation, the heart becomes more hypoxic and acidotic and less likely to react to conversion, while brain cells continue to die.

Responsibilities at the Cardiac Arrest Scene

The following responsibilities should be assumed at the scene of a cardiac arrest.

- ▶ **Team leader**—the individual who leads the arrest, performs the patient assessment, interprets ECGs, uses the monitor/defibrillator, and directs and oversees the actions of the team members. The team leader makes all of the clinical decisions *with input and suggestions from the team.* It is *not* necessary for the team leader to be the most highly certified, senior, or experienced member of the team. In fact, it is beneficial for less-experienced individuals to serve as the team leader to gain experience and become better team members.

- ▶ **Airway and ventilation**—one individual to manage the airway and ventilate the patient, as directed by the team leader. This usually includes intubating the patient.

- ▶ **IV and medications**—one individual to gain IV access and administer medications, as directed by the team leader

- ▶ **External chest compressions**—one individual to perform external chest compressions, as directed by the team leader

- ▶ **Record keeper (if possible)**—one individual to record the times and all pertinent assessment findings, patient status, interventions performed, medications given, and events of the resuscitation

There will be circumstances where there are not enough individuals to form a complete team. In fact, it is generally true that you have *either* too few *or* too many people on the arrest team. In the case of too few people, some members of the team will assume multiple roles. If too many people become distracting, the team leader should take control and ask those not directly involved in the treatment of the patient to leave the immediate scene and maybe prepare the cot and ambulance for transport. These additional personnel may be used to assist the family members at the scene by providing an explanation of what is occurring and giving comfort to the family.

⊞ CORE EMERGENCY CARDIAC SCENARIOS

Each scenario follows a standard format:

Overview: An overview of the scenario and a list of the algorithms that are used

Psychomotor Skills: A list of the skills that are covered

Background Patient Information: Background information on the hypothetical patient who is at the center of the scenario

Assessment and Management Priorities: The pertinent assessment findings and appropriate management of the patient. In real life, assessment and management are often done concurrently. It is difficult to represent this fact by words printed on paper. The following icons will be used to organize the flow of the scenario.

 assessment icon

 management icon

Key Points: The major considerations for this kind of scenario

In this scenario, you MUST: The critical actions and skills necessary to maximize the patient's chance for survival

Unacceptable Actions: Actions that represent common mistakes made in managing these situations. Any of these reduce the patient's probability of survival and are considered to be unacceptable.

An important note: Patient care is *not* linear. Assessment and management, especially in emergency situations, occur simultaneously. Multiple individuals perform skills and interventions concurrently. The scenarios, by design, attempt to describe a non-linear process in a linear fashion.

This textbook is intended to be used interactively. Use a note card or ruler to cover the management steps as you read each case. At each step, think of what you would do based on the assessment information.

⊞ RESPIRATORY ARREST

Overview

This case is used to emphasize progressive and sequential airway management, ventilatory support, and IV access for the patient in respiratory arrest who still has a pulse. The order of airway management techniques in the patient in respiratory arrest is identical to that for the patient in cardiac arrest. Using the patient in respiratory arrest as an example offers you an opportunity to focus on airway management and IV priorities and skills. This case uses the following algorithm to establish these priorities:

▶ General Approach to the Suspected Cardiac Arrest Patient (see Chapter 10, Figure 10-1)

Psychomotor Skills

▶ Noninvasive airway techniques

– pocket face mask

– bag-valve mask

> – oropharyngeal airway
> – barrier methods
> – oxygen delivery systems
> ▶ Invasive airway techniques
> – tracheal intubation
> ▶ Intravenous access

Background Patient Information

You arrive on the scene of a residence and find a 70-year-old-female who presents with a long history of heavy smoking and a past medical history of COPD. Her daughter at the scene explains that her mother has experienced severe dyspnea that began approximately three hours ago and gradually worsened. As you approach the patient and begin your general impression, you do not see any chest wall movement.

Assessment and Management Priorities

Time	Assessment and Management	See Pages
01:12	**A** Perform an initial assessment (ABCD survey): The patient is unresponsive, cyanotic, and appears to be not breathing.	17–18, 303–306
	M Open the patient's airway using the head-tilt, chin-lift maneuver. If there is any suspicion of a spine injury, perform a jaw-thrust maneuver. Quickly assess the oral cavity for any obvious obstruction such as vomitus, food, and blood.	18–22
01:12	**A** Breathing: With the airway maneuver maintained, look for chest rise and fall, and listen and feel for air movement. Estimate the respiratory rate and tidal volume. There are no respirations and no movement of air noted.	22–24
01:13	**M** You must immediately begin positive pressure ventilation. If possible, insert an oropharyngeal airway and begin bag-valve-mask ventilation. A pocket mask or other ventilation device may be used if readily available and if it does not delay the initiation of ventilation. If no oxygen is attached to the ventilation device or less than 40% oxygen concentration is being delivered, deliver a tidal volume of 10 ml/kg with each ventilation delivered over a 2-second period. Once oxygen has been connected to the ventilation device and a concentration of greater than 40% is being delivered, reduce the tidal volume of each ventilation to 6 to 7 ml/kg delivered over a 1- to 2-second period.	23–24, 81–91
01:13	**A** Circulation: The patient has a carotid pulse. Therefore, you realize, defibrillation and chest compressions are not appropriate.	24
01:15	**M** Continue to ventilate the patient and ensure a high concentration of oxygen is being delivered. Prepare for advanced airway management. If you are trained and skilled in tracheal intubation, prepare the patient for intubation. If you are not skilled in tracheal intubation, consider an	46–64

Time	Assessment and Management	See Pages
	alternative airway device such as the ETC or LMA. You elect to perform tracheal intubation.	
01:16	A Immediately upon placement of the tracheal tube, you inspect the chest for rise and fall with each ventilation. Upon identifying chest rise and fall, you immediately assess for gurgling sounds over the epigastrium and then for breath sounds over the midaxillary region at the 4th intercostal space and over the anterior chest at the 2nd intercostal space on both the right and left chest. Upon primary confirmation of tracheal tube placement, you apply a colorimetric end-tidal CO_2 detector. You ventilate six times and get a positive color change indicating exhalation of CO_2. You also apply a pulse oximeter to the patient. You note the tracheal tube marking at the level of the teeth to be 21 cm.	59–62
01:19	M You secure the tracheal tube with a commercial tracheal tube holder. You then establish an IV lifeline of normal saline running at a TKO rate. This is a routine part of advanced life support and should be performed as soon as possible. Often, other people can start an IV while you are managing the airway or intubating.	62, 106–107
01:21	A You continue with a rapid medical assessment, obtain a complete set of baseline vital signs, ascertain a history from the daughter, attach the continuous ECG monitor, and obtain a 12-lead ECG.	26, 29
01:34	M Based on the information found in the history and physical assessment, continue with your prehospital management as appropriate. Begin transport and continue your reassessment and management en route to the medical facility.	

Key Points

▶ The assessment of and attention to the airway are a priority in any unresponsive patient.

▶ Use the General Approach to the Suspected Cardiac Arrest algorithm. This is the standard patient approach utilizing the scene size up and initial assessment.

▶ Use the initial assessment (ABCD survey) to establish the basic priorities of management in the arrested and nonarrested patient.

▶ Use noninvasive airway techniques for the initial management of the airway. These include manual positioning, oropharyngeal airway, and suctioning.

▶ Basic techniques are used to initially ventilate the nonbreathing patient. These include bag-valve mask and pocket face mask.

▶ Simple face masks, nonrebreathing masks, and nasal cannulas are used to provide supplemental oxygen to the patient who is breathing and has both an adequate tidal volume and respiratory rate.

▶ Invasive airway management is used for the definitive management of the airway.

▶ A peripheral IV of normal saline is established.

▶ Continued assessment is required in every scenario.

▶ IV, cardiac monitor, pulse oximeter, vital signs, history, physical, and 12-lead ECG are part of the routine assessment and management of cardiac emergencies.

In this Scenario, You MUST

1. Perform the steps of the initial assessment (ABCD survey).
2. Use the General Approach to the Suspected Cardiac Arrest algorithm.
3. Open the airway.
4. Assess the adequacy of the respiratory rate and tidal volume. Ventilate as necessary.
5. Perform tracheal intubation or consider insertion of an ETC or LMA if necessary to effectively manage the airway and provide effective ventilation.
6. Assess the placement of the tracheal tube using both primary and secondary confirmation techniques. Also assess the adequacy of ventilation.
7. Establish IV access.
8. Continue assessment and management of the patient focusing on the etiology of the respiratory compromise.
9. Consider the need for an automatic transport ventilator.
10. Transport your patient with continued assessment and management en route.

Unacceptable Actions

▶ Failure to adequately assess the patient

▶ Initiating an intervention before appropriate assessment

▶ Performing external chest compressions in a patient with a pulse

▶ Interruption in ventilation with the exception for intubation or reassessment (no longer than 30 seconds)

▶ Failure to deliver high concentration oxygen

▶ Using an inappropriate oxygen delivery device (e.g., a nasal cannula, simple face mask)

▶ Failure to identify a malpositioned tracheal tube (mainstem intubation, esophageal intubation)

▶ Taking more than 30 seconds to intubate the trachea or insert an alternative airway device

 # VENTRICULAR FIBRILLATION WITH AED INTERVENTION

Overview

One of the major goals in the management of an out-of-hospital cardiac arrest patient is to quickly identify and manage ventricular fibrillation. It is important that you think of ventricular fibrillation or pulseless ventricular tachycardia as a survivable rhythm and treat it aggressively. The most important intervention for the patient in ventricular fibrillation or pulseless ventricular tachycardia is defibrillation. The possibility of survival drops with every second that passes. This case emphasizes the use of the automated external defibrillator. This case uses the following algorithms:

▶ General Approach to the Suspected Cardiac Arrest (see Chapter 10, Figure 10-1)

▶ AED (see Chapter 7, Figure 7-6)

Psychomotor Skills

▶ Cardiopulmonary resuscitation

▶ Automated defibrillation

▶ Noninvasive airway techniques

Background Patient Information

You are volunteering at the local rural fire department in a first responder capacity when you are called for a 58-year-old male patient who is at the local shopping mall. Witnesses claim that he suddenly clutched his chest and fell to the floor. You and another volunteer EMT-Basic arrive at the mall at the same time.

Assessment and Management Priorities

Time		Assessment and Management	See Pages
10:48	A	Perform an initial assessment (ABCD survey): The EMT-Basic responder performs the survey and finds that the patient is unresponsive, apneic, and pulseless.	17–18, 303–306
10:48	M	The EMT-Basic responder begins positive pressure ventilation and chest compression as you access and prepare the automated external defibrillator (AED). Turn on the AED and follow the prompts. Immediately place the electrode/defibrillator pads on the patient's chest. Stop CPR and clear the patient for rhythm analysis.	24–26
10:49	A	The AED announces that a shock is indicated.	190–192
10:50	M	Clear the patient by saying "I'm clear, you are clear, everyone is clear" as you look from head to toe to be sure no one is in contact with the patient. Press the shock button to deliver the defibrillation. Stay clear of the patient and allow the AED to reanalyze the rhythm. Deliver up to three shocks if the patient remains in a shockable rhythm.	190–192
10:51	A	Following the initial three shocks, the AED indicated to check a pulse and breathing. You assess the carotid artery and find that the patient has a pulse. You assess the ventilatory status and find no chest rise or fall and no air movement. The EMT-Basic responder assesses the blood pressure and gets a reading of 98/60 mmHg.	190–192
10:52	M	DO NOT continue chest compression, but ventilate the patient once every 5 seconds. Leave the AED in place and call for an ALS unit. Continue to reassess the patient.	

Key Points

▶ Use the General Approach to a Suspected Cardiac Arrest and AED algorithms.

▶ Use the initial assessment (ABCD survey) for every cardiac arrest scenario.

▶ The use of the AED is a psychomotor skill that requires regular practice with the equipment that you will be using. You must be familiar with the operation, method of attachment of the pads, safety, shock delivery, and troubleshooting of the defibrillator.

▶ You must know how to turn on the power, attach the AED, analyze the ECG, and safely deliver the shock.

▶ If the patient regains a pulse, immediately assess the ventilatory status and measure the blood pressure.

In this Scenario, You MUST

1. Perform the steps of the initial assessment (ABCD survey).
2. Use the General Approach to a Suspected Cardiac Arrest and AED algorithms.
3. Initiate CPR if a defibrillator is not immediately available. **DO NOT** delay defibrillation to perform CPR, airway management, ventilation, or to gain IV access.
4. Deliver the first defibrillation immediately upon arrival of the AED.
5. Maintain the airway and ventilate the patient.
6. Check the pulse. If the patient has a pulse, check blood pressure.
7. Support ventilations after the return of a pulse.

Unacceptable Actions

▶ Unsafe operation of the AED

▶ Failure to clear during AED attempts

▶ Delay defibrillation to perform other interventions.

ADULT VENTRICULAR FIBRILLATION/ PULSELESS VENTRICULAR TACHYCARDIA

Overview

The management of ventricular fibrillation and pulseless ventricular tachycardia are major focuses of ACLS. Many patients who have VF or pulseless VT have little or no myocardial damage and can survive and live long, productive lives after their cardiac event. This case uses the following algorithms:

▶ General Approach to the Suspected Cardiac Arrest (see Chapter 10, Figure 10-1)

▶ Ventricular Fibrillation/Pulseless Ventricular Tachycardia (VF/VT) (see Chapter 10, Figure 10-2)

Psychomotor Skills

▶ CPR during cardiac arrest

▶ Assessment and reassessment of the cardiac arrest patient

▶ Recognition of VF or pulseless VT

▶ Repeated defibrillation with a standard manual defibrillator

▶ Attachment and use of monitoring ECG leads

▶ Leading a cardiac arrest team

▶ Use of the tracheal tube to deliver medications

▶ Use of alternative airway skills if tracheal intubation is unsuccessful

▶ Gaining IV access and delivering medications to the patient in cardiac arrest

▶ Use of epinephrine, vasopressin, amiodarone, lidocaine, magnesium sulfate, procainamide, and sodium bicarbonate in cardiac arrest

Background Patient Information

You respond to the scene for a 45-year-old male at the local unemployment office. Upon your arrival, the security guard informs you that the patient is in cardiac arrest. He said two employees are performing CPR. He leads you back into the lobby area where the patient is lying supine on the floor.

Assessment and Management Priorities

Time		Assessment and Management	See Pages
15:39	A	Stop the CPR being performed by the workers and conduct an initial assessment (ABCD survey): The patient is unresponsive, apneic, and pulseless.	17–18, 21–24, 303–306
15:39	M	Immediately do a "quick look" with the monitor/defibrillator paddles.	306–310
15:40	A	You identify the following rhythm:	
15:40	M	Immediately charge the defibrillator to 200 joules and deliver the first defibrillation. The rhythm remains the same, so deliver a second defibrillation at 300 joules and then again at 360 joules.	24–26, 190–193
15:41	A	Following the third defibrillation, you assess the carotid pulse and the breathing. There is no pulse and no breathing. The rhythm remains the same on the monitor.	
15:41	M	You immediately direct the office worker at the scene to resume chest compressions. Your partner begins to ventilate the patient as he also prepares for intubation. You attach the ECG continuous monitoring electrodes and prepare to initiate an intravenous line. The backup EMS crew arrives on the scene. You instruct one crew member to take over the chest compressions and the other to go ahead and start the IV line.	106

Time	Assessment and Management	See Pages
	Your partner states "I have the tube." You inspect the chest for rise and fall and assess for epigastric sounds. Seeing rise and fall of the chest and hearing no epigastric sounds, you assess breath sounds. Breath sounds are equal bilaterally. You quickly attach an electronic end-tidal CO_2 detector to the end of the tube. CO_2 is present in the expired air. The tracheal tube is secured. The intravenous line is established. You instruct the team to administer 1 mg of epinephrine rapid IV push.	59–62, 213–215
15:42	**A** After 60 seconds, you stop CPR and assess the rhythm and pulse. The patient remains pulseless and apneic. The ECG rhythm is as follows:	
15:42	**M** You immediately charge the defibrillator to 360 joules and deliver the defibrillation ensuring everyone is clear of the patient.	
15:43	**A** You assess the carotid pulse, breathing, and ECG rhythm. There is no pulse or breathing and the ECG rhythm is as follows:	
15:43	**M** You instruct the crew to continue chest compressions and ventilation. You direct the team to administer 300 mg of amiodarone IV push.	
15:44	**A** After 60 seconds, you stop CPR and assess the rhythm and pulse. The patient remains pulseless and apneic. The ECG rhythm is as follows:	

Time	Assessment and Management	See Pages
15:44	M You defibrillate the patient at 360 joules.	
15:45	A You assess the carotid pulse, breathing, and ECG rhythm. There is no pulse or breathing and the ECG rhythm is as follows:	

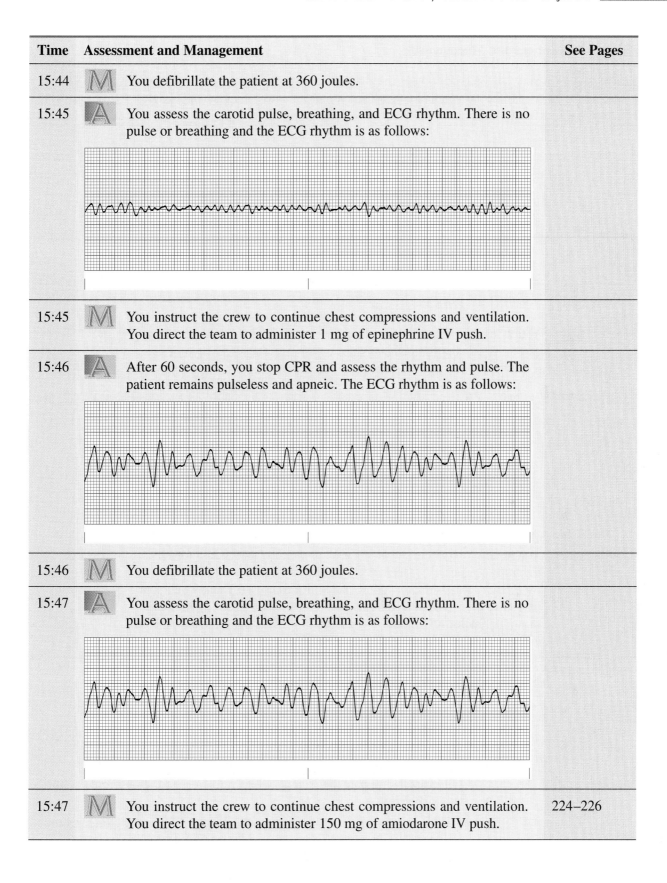

Time	Assessment and Management	See Pages
15:45	M You instruct the crew to continue chest compressions and ventilation. You direct the team to administer 1 mg of epinephrine IV push.	
15:46	A After 60 seconds, you stop CPR and assess the rhythm and pulse. The patient remains pulseless and apneic. The ECG rhythm is as follows:	
15:46	M You defibrillate the patient at 360 joules.	
15:47	A You assess the carotid pulse, breathing, and ECG rhythm. There is no pulse or breathing and the ECG rhythm is as follows:	
15:47	M You instruct the crew to continue chest compressions and ventilation. You direct the team to administer 150 mg of amiodarone IV push.	224–226

Time	Assessment and Management	See Pages
15:48	**A** Sixty seconds following the drug administration, you stop CPR and assess the rhythm and pulse. The patient remains pulseless and apneic. The ECG rhythm is as follows:	

Time	Assessment and Management	See Pages
15:48	**M** You defibrillate the patient at 360 joules.	
15:49	**A** You assess the carotid pulse, breathing, and ECG rhythm. There is a carotid pulse, but the patient is not breathing. The ECG rhythm is as follows:	

Time	Assessment and Management	See Pages
15:49	**M** You resume ventilation and obtain a set of baseline vital signs. You check tracheal tube and IV placement to ensure both are patent. You instruct two crew members to prepare the patient for transport. You instruct your partner to prepare an amiodarone infusion by mixing 360 mg in 500 ml of normal saline and running it at 1 mg/min. You transport the patient with no change in the patient condition en route.	224–226

Key Points

▶ Use the General Approach to the Suspected Cardiac Arrest Patient and VF/VT algorithms.

▶ Perform the steps of the initial assessment (ABCD survey).

▶ Immediately intubate the patient who is refractory to the first three defibrillatory shocks.

▶ Start an IV of normal saline for the patient in cardiac arrest. Drugs given in cardiac arrest should be followed by a 20 ml fluid flush.

▶ Defibrillate 30–60 seconds after each drug administration.

▶ Repeat epinephrine every 3 to 5 minutes at 1 mg throughout the entire resuscitation.

▶ Lidocaine can be used as a first line antidysrhythmic drug.

▶ 40 units of Vasopressin can be administered once only in ventricular fibrillation or pulseless ventricular tachycardia.

▶ A biphasic defibrillator that delivers the equivalent energy level can be used.

In this Scenario, You MUST

1. Perform the steps of the initial assessment (ABCD survey) and frequently reassess the patient's condition.
2. Follow the General Approach to the Suspected Cardiac Arrest Patient and VF/VT algorithms.
3. Assure uninterrupted chest compressions and ventilations.
4. Attach the ECG monitor.
5. Recognize ventricular fibrillation.
6. Direct the resuscitation team.
7. Deliver defibrillation at the proper energy setting and in the proper sequence.
8. Deliver shocks 30–60 seconds after drug administration.
9. Demonstrate the proper transfer of care from BLS to ALS.
10. Intubate and obtain IV access at the proper time in the arrest management.
11. Administer the proper sequence and dose of pharmacological agents.

Unacceptable Actions

▶ Failure to perform CPR when indicated

▶ Failure to effectively ventilate the apneic patient

▶ Failure to intubate the patient at the appropriate time

▶ Any unsafe or ineffective operation of the defibrillator

▶ Failure to "clear" during defibrillation attempts

▶ Failure to shock 30–60 seconds after each drug

▶ Medication errors

▶ Failure to assess pulse after rhythm cardioversion

▶ Withholding defibrillation until other interventions (e.g., intubation, IV access) are performed

▦ PULSELESS ELECTRICAL ACTIVITY

Overview

Pulseless electrical activity (PEA) is not a specific dysrhythmia. PEA is used to describe the situation when a cardiac rhythm does not produce mechanical evidence of contraction. There are a number of causes of this condition, including electromechanical dissociation (EMD), pseudo-EMD (pulse is detected by Doppler device only and not by palpation), idioventricular rhythms, ventricular escape rhythms, bradyasystolic rhythms, and post defibrillation idioventricular rhythms. The prognosis for survival from PEA is very poor. The best chance for resuscitation is to find and treat the cause of the PEA. The patient history and your physical exam provide clues to the underlying problems. This case uses the following algorithms:

▶ General Approach to the Suspected Cardiac Arrest (see Chapter 10, Figure 10-1)

▶ Pulseless Electrical Activity (PEA) (see Chapter 10, Figure 10-3)

Psychomotor Skills

▶ Physical examination for hypovolemia, pericardial tamponade, and tension pneumothorax, hypoventilation, pericardial tamponade, hypothermia, drug overdose, acidosis, massive myocardial infarction, hyperkalemia, hypokalemia, and pulmonary embolism

▶ Fluid resuscitation

▶ Needle chest decompression

Background Patient Information

You are treating a 28-year-old female who was shot in the right anterior chest with a small-caliber handgun. There is an entrance wound at the level of the 4th intercostal space just lateral to the mid-clavicular line. You cannot find an exit wound.

Assessment and Management Priorities

Time		Assessment and Management	See Pages
00:14	A	Perform the initial assessment (ABCD survey): The patient is pulseless and apneic. There is obvious external blood loss.	17–18, 21–24, 303–306
00:14	M	Manually control the airway and immediately begin positive pressure ventilation and external chest compressions.	39–40, 41, 81–91
00:15	A	You perform a "quick look" and reveal the following ECG rhythm:	119–120
00:15	M	Resume chest compressions and ventilation. Attach monitoring electrodes for continuous ECG monitoring. Intubate immediately, obtain IV access, and administer 1.0 mg of epinephrine followed by a fluid bolus of 250 ml of normal saline.	303–306
00:16	A	Following your intubation, the breath sounds remain absent on the right hemithorax. Your partner who is ventilating with a bag-valve-mask device indicates that there is some resistance to bagging that appears to be worsening.	
00:16	M	You immediately insert a 14-gauge 2-inch IV catheter in the 2nd intercostal space at the midclavicular line on the right side of the chest. You note air escape from the catheter.	311–313

Time		Assessment and Management	See Pages
00:17	A	The rhythm remains the same; however, a faint carotid pulse is palpated. The blood pressure is 72/58 mmHg.	
00:18	M	You continue to ventilate and administer normal saline for fluid resuscitation to improve the blood pressure. You immediately prepare the patient for transport and notify the receiving hospital to alert the trauma team.	

Key Points

▷ Use the General Approach to the Suspected Cardiac Arrest Patient and PEA algorithms.

▷ Perform the steps of the initial assessment (ABCD survey).

▷ Search for one of the reversible causes of PEA (hypovolemia, hypoxia, cardiac tamponade, tension pneumothorax, hypothermia, massive pulmonary embolism, drug overdose, hyperkalemia, hypokalemia, acidosis, massive myocardial infarction).

▷ Epinephrine is used to increase myocardial and cerebral blood flow during the resuscitation of patients in PEA.

▷ Atropine is used to treat absolute or relative bradycardia in patients who are in PEA.

In this Scenario, You MUST

1. Perform the steps of the initial assessment (ABCD survey).
2. Use the General Approach to the Suspected Cardiac Arrest Patient and PEA algorithms.
3. Initiate CPR.
4. Properly operate and attach the monitor.
5. Recognize pulseless electrical activity.
6. Direct the team members to intubate and start an IV.
7. Be able to list the common conditions which cause PEA, the signs/symptoms, and emergency treatment for each.
8. Be able to perform a needle thoracentesis (chest decompression).

Unacceptable Actions

▷ Failure to assess the patient

▷ Failure to consider the various causes of PEA

▷ Treating PEA only with epinephrine

▷ Failure to properly ventilate the patient or failure to intubate quickly

▷ Failure to administer volume to resuscitate the patient

▷ Defibrillating the patient

▷ Failure to perform proper CPR

▷ Failure to perform a needle thoracentesis (chest decompression) upon recognition of the absent breath sounds

▞ ASYSTOLE

Overview

Asystole is an ominous cardiac rhythm. Although it may represent the end point of resuscitative efforts, it may also result from a variety of reversible causes. One of the main considerations in the treatment of asystole is to search for reversible causes. When asystole results or persists after a prolonged resuscitation effort, you should consider terminating the code. This case uses the following algorithms:

▶ General Approach to the Suspected Cardiac Arrest (see Chapter 10, Figure 10-1)

▶ Asystole (see Chapter 10, Figure 10-4)

Psychomotor Skills

▶ Recognition of the role of ventilation on acid-base balance in cardiac arrest

▶ Assessment of causes of asystole (hypovolemia, pericardial tamponade, tension pneumothorax, hypoventilation, hypothermia, drug overdose, acidosis, massive myocardial infarction, hyperkalemia, hypokalemia, and pulmonary embolism)

▶ Identifying the appropriate point to terminate the resuscitation

Background Patient Information

You are called to the scene for a 20-year-old male at the local university dormitory. His roommate indicated that he thinks has taken an overdose of his medication. The roommate left for an exam about an hour ago and that was the last time he saw the patient, until now.

Assessment and Management Priorities

Time	Assessment and Management		See Pages
20:54	A	Perform an initial assessment (ABCD Survey): The patient is unresponsive, pulseless, and apneic. You perform a "quick look" and it reveals the following:	17–18, 21–24, 134, 303–306
20:54	M	Confirm the asystole in two leads. Immediately begin chest compressions and ventilation. Intubate and obtain IV access. Attach a continuous ECG monitor.	314–315

Time		Assessment and Management	See Pages
20:56	A	You consider the differential diagnosis of asystole (hypovolemia, pericardial tamponade, tension pneumothorax, hypoventilation, hypothermia, drug overdose, acidosis, massive myocardial infarction, hyperkalemia, hypokalemia, and pulmonary embolism) and look for evidence of any of the etiologies in your assessment. Try to determine what drug was used to overdose.	316
20:56	M	Immediately attach the transcutaneous pacer (TCP) and administer 1.0 mg epinephrine. Continue chest compressions and ventilation.	198–202, 213–215
20:58	A	Stop CPR and reassess pulse, breathing, and rhythm. There is no response. The patient remains pulseless and apneic.	
20:58	M	Administer atropine at 1.0 mg.	232–236
20:59	A	Stop CPR and reassess pulse, breathing, and rhythm. There is no response. The patient remains pulseless and apneic.	
20:59	M	Repeat epinephrine at 1.0 mg. Continue chest compressions and ventilation.	213–215
21:00	A	Stop CPR and reassess pulse, breathing, and rhythm. There is no response. The patient remains pulseless and apneic	
21:01	M	Administer atropine at 1.0 mg. You estimate the patient's weight to be 165 lbs (75 kg). You can administer a total of 3 mg of atropine to reach the 0.04 mg/kg total vagolytic dose.	232–236
21:02	A	Stop CPR and reassess pulse, breathing, and rhythm. There is no response. The patient remains pulseless and apneic.	
21:04	M	Continue to administer epinephrine at 1.0 mg every 3 to 5 minutes throughout the entire resuscitation. One more dose of atropine can be administered at 1.0 mg. Consider the administration of sodium bicarbonate at 1 meq/kg early if tricyclic antidepressant overdose is suspected. Consider contacting medical direction to terminate the resuscitation effort following another set of drug administrations.	213–215, 253–255

Key Points

▶ Use the General Approach to the Suspected Cardiac Arrest Patient and Asystole algorithms.

▶ Perform the steps of the initial assessment (ABCD survey).

▶ Proper ventilation is the best way to maintain acid-base balance in cardiac arrest.

▶ Search for treatable causes of asystole.

▶ Asystole is usually considered an endpoint of resuscitation. If no treatable cause is identified, consider termination of the resuscitation.

▶ The reversible causes of asystole are hypovolemia, pericardial tamponade, tension pneumothorax, hypoventilation, hypothermia, drug overdose, acidosis, massive myocardial infarction, hyperkalemia, hypokalemia, and pulmonary embolism.

▶ Transcutaneous pacing should be instituted as soon as possible in the resuscitation.

▶ Epinephrine, atropine, and sodium bicarbonate are used in the management of asystole.

▶ Defibrillation of asystole may increase the parasympathetic tone and decrease the likelihood of conversion of the rhythm.

In this Scenario, You MUST

1. Perform the steps of the initial assessment (ABCD survey).
2. Use the General Approach to the Suspected Cardiac Arrest Patient and Asystole algorithms.
3. Initiate CPR.
4. Recognize and confirm asystole in two different leads.
5. Recognize the role of ventilation in acid-base balance.
6. Properly monitor the IV access site.
7. List and describe the treatment for the causes of asystole.
8. List the proper dose of epinephrine, atropine, and sodium bicarbonate.
9. Perform TCP early and concurrently with medications.
10. Perform a pulse check one minute following drug administration and with every rhythm change.
11. Describe the considerations in terminating the resuscitation.

Unacceptable Actions

▶ Diagnosing asystole in only one lead
▶ Use of TCP too late or without the concurrent use of medications.
▶ Defibrillating asystole.

ACUTE CORONARY SYNDROME

Overview

Most of the previous algorithms focus on reversing cardiac arrest. The remaining algorithms are designed to *prevent* cardiac arrest. Recent therapeutic options have lead to a significant reduction in the morbidity and mortality from acute coronary syndromes. This case uses the following algorithm:

▶ Suspected Ischemic Chest Pain (see Chapter 9, Figure 9-7)

Psychomotor Skills

▶ Rhythm analysis
▶ 12-lead ECG

Background Patient Information

You are called to a local car dealership for a 56-year-old car salesman complaining of chest discomfort. He began to have chest discomfort while closing a deal that would make him Bob Smith's Salesman of the Year. He was thinking of the all-expense-paid trip to Hawaii when he started to look dusky and sweaty, and the caring customers insisted that he sit down and rest. When he felt no relief after 2 minutes, some concerned coworkers insisted that they immediately dial 911. Upon your arrival at the scene, you find the patient sitting upright in a chair. He has his hand clutched over the center of his chest. He is severely diaphoretic and pale. He immediately describes his chest discomfort as a real heavy pressure in the center of his chest, a steady ache between his shoulder blades, and pain down his left arm.

Assessment and Management Priorities

Time		Assessment and Management	See Pages
10:22	A	Perform an initial assessment (ABCD survey): The patient is alert and oriented. He is complaining of severe, "pressure-type" chest pain, radiating to his back and down his left arm. He says it started about 10 minutes ago. He is pale and diaphoretic and is having some shortness of breath. He has no pertinent medical history.	17–18, 21–24, 273
10:23	M	Begin the MONA (morphine, oxygen, nitroglycerin, and aspirin) management sequence. Place the patient on the ECG monitor, administer oxygen, and initiate an intravenous line of normal saline at a TKO rate. Obtain baseline vital signs.	209–211, 242–245, 248, 280–286
10:26	A	The baseline vitals are: pulse: 80 bpm, strong and regular; respirations: 16/min with no evidence of respiratory distress; BP: 154/88 mmHg; SpO_2, 98% while on room air. You see the following on the monitor:	119–120

Time		Assessment and Management	See Pages
10:28	M	Have the patient chew two 80 mg baby aspirin. Administer 1 sublingual tablet or spray of 0.3–0.4 mg nitroglycerin and contact medical direction for consultation. Medical direction requests that you repeat the nitroglycerin and obtain a 12-lead ECG. You begin to prepare the patient for transport.	155–157, 244–245, 248, 284–286
10:30	A	The pain is not relieved. A second set of vital signs are: pulse: 92 bpm, strong and regular; respirations: 19/min with no evidence of respiratory distress; BP: 160/90 mmHg; SpO_2, 99% while on a nasal cannula at 4 lpm. The 12-lead ECG indicates a probable acute inferior wall myocardial infarction. (See Figure 11-1.) The patient continues to complain of severe discomfort.	276–279, 357

Time	Assessment and Management	See Pages
10:32	**M** You begin immediate transport and transmit the ECG to the hospital by cellular phone. Medical direction requests that you screen the patient for fibrinolytic therapy and administer 2.0 mg of morphine sulfate for pain control.	242–243, 252–253
10:34	**A** You question the patient from a predefined checklist about his medical history. He has no contraindications to fibrinolytic therapy.	253, 287–288
10:36	**M** You administer 2.0 mg of morphine sulfate slow IV push for pain control, contact the receiving hospital, and report the fibrinolytic checklist results.	242–243
10:38	**A** During your ongoing assessment en route to the emergency department, the patient states the pain has subsided significantly. You reassess the vital signs and check all of your interventions.	
10:38	**M** You arrive at the emergency department and transfer the care of the patient to the emergency department staff.	

Key Points

▶ Use the Suspected Ischemic Chest Pain algorithm.

▶ Perform the steps of the initial assessment (ABCD survey).

▶ The most effective strategy for decreasing the morbidity and mortality from AMI is early recognition and early care.

▶ Learn your local protocols for managing an acute coronary syndrome patient.

▶ The prehospital interventions for the acute coronary syndrome patient are:

– Attach a continuous ECG monitor and analyze the rhythm.

– Initiate an intravenous line.

– Administer oxygen at 4 l/min, aspirin at 160 to 325 mg, nitroglycerin tablet or spray, and morphine sulfate IV (MONA).

– Obtain a 12-lead ECG.

– Inform the receiving facility of the patient and his status.

– Rapidly transport patient to an appropriate facility.

– Screen the patient for possible fibrinolytic therapy.

▶ You should be able to treat the following dysrhythmias in the setting of the acute coronary syndrome patient:

– normal sinus rhythm, sinus bradycardia, sinus tachycardia

– AV nodal blocks: first-degree, second-degree (Mobitz I and II), and third-degree blocks

– multiple PACs, atrial tachycardia, atrial tachycardia with block, atrial flutter with various degrees of block, PVCs, and ventricular ectopy

– ventricular fibrillation and ventricular tachycardia

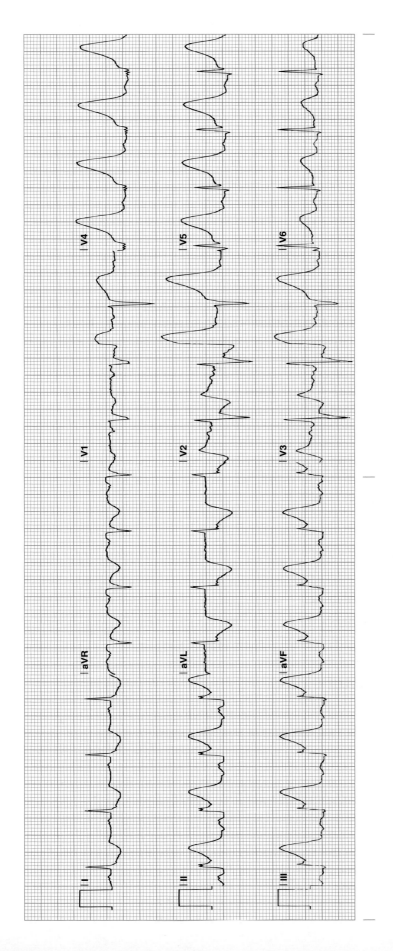

FIGURE 11–1
12-lead ECG indicating acute inferior wall myocardial infarction.

In this Scenario, You MUST

1. Perform a rapid, focused history and physical exam including vitals, continuous ECG monitoring, and a 12-lead ECG.
2. Use the Suspected Ischemic Chest Pain algorithm.
3. Initiate general treatment to include oxygen, aspirin, intravenous line, nitroglycerin, and morphine sulfate.
4. Obtain the necessary information on the checklist for fibrinolytic therapy.
5. List the major actions, indications, and contraindications for the medications used to treat the acute coronary syndrome patient.
6. Identify and treat dysrhythmias in the setting of an acute coronary syndrome.

Unacceptable Actions

▶ Failure to consider and properly evaluate a patient with acute chest pain consistent with an acute coronary syndrome.

▶ Failure to obtain a 12-lead ECG in a timely fashion

▶ Failure to administer oxygen, aspirin, nitroglycerin, or morphine when indicated

▶ Failure to control pain

▶ Failure to recognize exclusion criteria for fibrinolytics

▶ Administering medications that are contraindicated in the scenario

■ BRADYCARDIA

Overview

Bradycardia rhythms are common pre-arrest and postarrest presentations. Properly managing a bradycardia may prevent cardiac arrest and reduce the possibility that a patient will re-arrest. It is extremely important to determine if the patient is symptomatic as a result of the bradycardia. Be sure to treat the patient and not the rhythm since some patients may present with a bradycardia but will not present as being physiologically unstable. This case uses the following algorithm:

▶ Bradycardia (see Chapter 10, Figure 10-5)

Psychomotor Skills

▶ Operation of the transcutaneous pacer

▶ Administering a dopamine and epinephrine infusion

▶ Interpretation of bradycardia

Background Patient Information

You are called to the scene of a residence for a 62-year-old female who is complaining of severe weakness and dizziness. Upon your arrival, you find the patient lying supine on the living room couch. She state that she gets "really lightheaded" if she tries to sit up. She also complains of some minor chest discomfort and moderate shortness of breath.

Assessment and Management Priorities

Time	Assessment and Management	See Pages
11:33	**A** Perform an initial assessment (ABCD survey): The patient is responsive to verbal stimuli, but disoriented to time and day. Her baseline vital signs are: pulse 39 bpm; blood pressure 72/48 mmHg; respirations 26/min and slightly labored; skin is pale, cool, and clammy; SpO_2 is 84% on room air. The lungs reveal crackles (rales) in the dependent zones.	17–18, 21–24
11:35	**M** Administer oxygen at 15 l/min via a nonrebreather mask, start an intravenous line of normal saline at a TKO rate, attach a continuous cardiac monitor.	303–306
11:37	**A** Upon placement of the ECG monitor, the rhythm is as follows: 	122–123
11:40	**M** You administer 1.0 mg of atropine IV push as your partner prepares the transcutaneous pacer.	320–323
11:42	**A** The patient's heart rate and rhythm do not change after administration of the atropine. The blood pressure drops to 68/42 mmHg.	
11:45	**M** Your partner applies the pacer pads and sets the heart rate on the TCP to 80 bpm and gradually increases the output until you have electrical capture.	200
11:48	**A** At 60 mA, you note that the patient's heart rate is 80, her blood pressure increases to 86/64 mmHg, and her level of consciousness is improving. She is complaining about the pain from the pacer.	
11:53	**M** You contact medical direction to consider the administration of either a narcotic or benzodiazepine to control the pain associated with the pacer.	

Key Points

▶ Use the Bradycardia algorithm, which is used to treat relative and absolute bradycardias.

▶ Perform the steps of the initial assessment (ABCD survey).

▶ Bradycardia should be treated only if it is symptomatic. Symptomatic bradycardia causes any of the following: chest pain, dyspnea, weakness/dizziness, syncope, decreased level of consciousness, hypotension, ventricular ectopy, pulmonary congestion, congestive heart failure, and acute MI.

▶ Atropine is used in the initial management of symptomatic bradycardia.

▶ The transcutaneous pacer is set up while you are awaiting the actions of atropine.

▶ Dopamine or epinephrine infusions are used if the patient is unresponsive to atropine and the transcutaneous pacer is unavailable or fails to produce mechanical capture.

▶ Isoproterenol is rarely used.

▶ Do not use lidocaine, amiodarone, or procainamide to treat a ventricular escape rhythm in a bradycardia rhythm.

In this Scenario, You MUST

1. Recognize symptomatic bradycardia from your assessment and physical exam findings.
2. Use the Bradycardia algorithm.
3. Obtain IV access and place the patient on oxygen and a cardiac monitor.
4. Administer the appropriate dose of atropine.
5. Apply the transcutaneous pacer while awaiting the actions of the atropine.
6. Know the dose for a dopamine infusion.
7. Identify second-degree type II and third-degree AV blocks.
8. Recognize the need for transcutaneous pacing.
9. Order a 12-lead ECG.
10. Perform checklist for the use of fibrinolytics if the patient has signs and symptoms suggestive of AMI.

Unacceptable Actions

▶ Failure to prepare for transcutaneous pacing while waiting for atropine to work

▶ Failure to recognize the need for transcutaneous pacing for second-degree type II block, third-degree block, or wide complex ventricular escape beats

▶ Inappropriately using dopamine, epinephrine, or isoproterenol

▶ Using lidocaine, amiodarone, or procainamide to treat ventricular escape rhythms

▶ Treating an asymptomatic bradycardia

▦ UNSTABLE WIDE COMPLEX TACHYCARDIA

Overview

The management of any unstable tachycardia, regardless of its type, is primarily by synchronized cardioversion. The wide complex may be polymorphic or monomorphic. If the synchronized cardioversion is delayed, it is appropriate to administer a trial of antidysrhythmic medications prior to the synchronized cardioversion. This case uses the following algorithms:

▶ Wide Complex Tachycardia (see Chapter 10, Figure 10-7)
▶ Synchronized Cardioversion (see Chapter 7, Figure 7-7)

Psychomotor Skills

▶ Identification of unstable wide complex tachycardia

- ▶ Synchronized cardioversion
- ▶ Switching from synchronized to unsynchronized cardioversion

Background Patient Information

You respond to a pillow factory for a 38-year-old female who suddenly became "faint" and had a syncopal episode while at work. Upon your arrival, she is dizzy and lightheaded and is complaining of a "funny feeling" in her chest.

Assessment and Management Priorities

Time	Assessment and Management	See Pages
14:02	**A** Perform an initial assessment (ABCD survey): The patient responds sluggishly to your commands; her skin is pale, cool, and clammy; her radial pulse is very weak at 180 bpm; she complains of shortness of breath; her blood pressure is 72/40 mmHg.	
14:05	**M** You immediately administer oxygen at 15 lpm via a nonrebreather mask, start an intravenous line of normal saline at a TKO rate, attach a continuous ECG monitor, pulse oximeter, and automatic blood pressure monitor.	303–306
14:05	**A** The SpO$_2$ is 92%; BP is 74/44 mmHg; and the monitor shows:	128, 131–134
14:06	**M** You immediately prepare the defibrillator for synchronized cardioversion.	195
14:07	**A** Your partner reassesses patient's level of responsiveness as you finalize your preparation for synchronized cardioversion.	195
14:07	**M** You perform the first synchronized cardioversion at 100 joules.	194–196
14:08	**A** You reassess the heart rate and blood pressure. The heart rate is 118 bpm, and the blood pressure is 86/64 mmHg. The patient becomes more responsive. The ECG rhythm is as follows:	

Time	Assessment and Management	See Pages
14:18	M Your partner prepares an amiodarone infusion of 360 mg and prepares to run it at 1 mg/min. You continue to reassess the patient and prepare her for transport.	224–226

Key Points

▶ Use the Wide Complex Tachycardia and Synchronized Cardioversion algorithms.

▶ Perform the steps of the initial assessment (ABCD survey).

▶ Patients in a wide complex tachycardia who present with chest pain, dyspnea, decreased level of consciousness, hypotension, shock, pulmonary congestion, or CHF are unstable and need to be cardioverted immediately.

▶ Be sure to become familiar with the operation of the defibrillator that you will be using; specifically, learn where the synchronize button is located.

In this Scenario, You MUST

1. Perform the initial assessment including ABCs, attach the cardiac monitor, and take baseline vital signs.

2. Use the Wide Complex Tachycardia and Electrical (Synchronized) Cardioversion algorithms.

3. Identify patients who present with wide complex tachycardia and who are unstable.

4. Reassess the patient (pulse, respiration, blood pressure) and administer antidysrhythmic agents after cardioversion.

5. Administer oxygen, start an IV, and place the patient on continuous cardiac monitoring.

6. Change from synchronized cardioversion to unsynchronized cardioversion if the patient goes into ventricular fibrillation or if delays in cardioversion occur because of difficulty with synchronization.

Unacceptable Actions

▶ Failure to resynchronize the defibrillator after cardioversion

▶ Failure to differentiate between stable and unstable tachycardia

▶ Failure to attempt to determine the cause of the tachycardia after treatment

▶ Failure to provide antidysrhythmic therapy after cardioversion

■ STABLE NARROW COMPLEX TACHYCARDIA

Overview

In the narrow complex tachycardia it is important to determine whether the patient is stable or unstable. If unstable, synchronized cardioversion is an intervention of choice to reverse the rhythm. If the rhythm is a junctional tachycardia, multi-focal atrial tachycardia, or an ectopic atrial tachycardia, cardioversion is not indicated since the rhythm is due to an abnormal foci and not a reentry pathway. Paroxysmal supraventricular tachycardia is due to a reentry pathway and should be cardioverted. Often, it is impossible to determine the rhythm until the ventricular rate is slowed down. Thus, follow the standard treatment algorithm for a narrow complex tachycardia until the underlying rhythm can be determined. This case uses the following algorithm:

▶ Narrow Complex Tachycardia (see Chapter 10, Figure 10-6)

Psychomotor Skills

▶ Rhythm diagnosis

▶ Vagal maneuvers

▶ Synchronized cardioversion

Background Patient Information

You are called to a residence for an unknown problem. Upon arrival, you find a 52-year-old female who is complaining of a sudden onset of heart palpitations. She is alert and oriented and in no obvious distress. She denies chest discomfort or dyspnea.

Assessment and Management Priorities

Time	Assessment and Management	See Pages
14:14	**A** Perform an initial assessment (ABCD survey): The patient has had similar episodes in the past and is taking Verapamil. Her blood pressure is 128/82 mmHg; heart rate is 180 bpm; and her respirations are 14/min with no evidence of respiratory distress.	
14:16	**M** You place the patient on oxygen at 4 lpm via a nasal cannula. You start an intravenous line of normal saline in a large antecubital vein and place the patient on a continuous cardiac monitor, pulse oximeter, and automatic blood pressure monitor.	303–306
14:18	**A** The blood pressure is 130/80mmHg; SpO$_2$ is 98%. The monitor shows:	128, 129, 131–134
14:19	**M** You instruct the patient how to perform a Valsalva maneuver. The patient does the vagal maneuver.	325–327

Time	Assessment and Management	See Pages

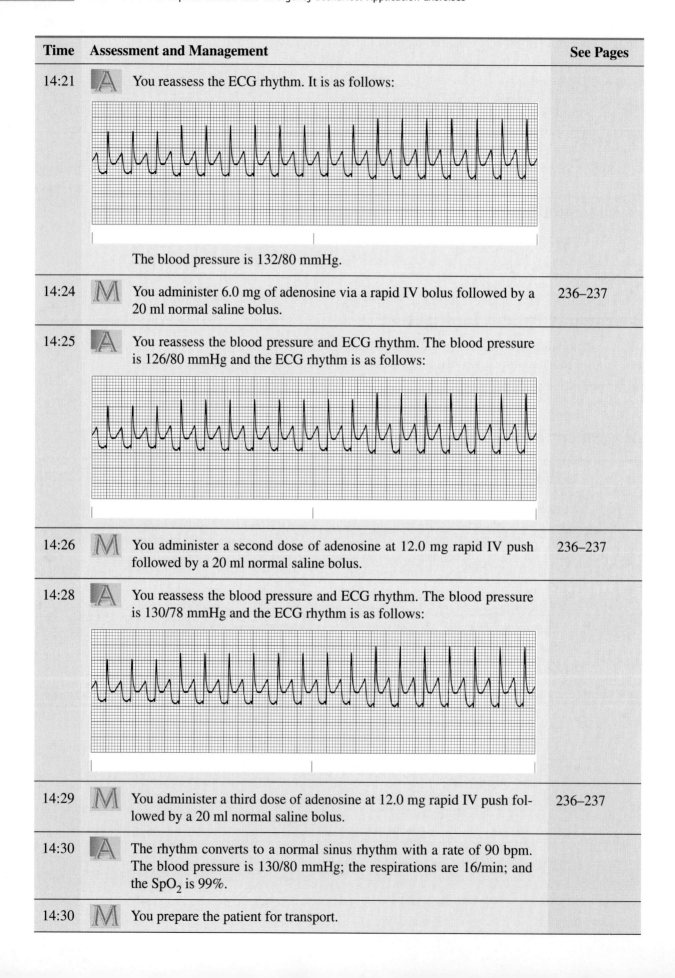

14:21 **A** You reassess the ECG rhythm. It is as follows:

The blood pressure is 132/80 mmHg.

14:24 **M** You administer 6.0 mg of adenosine via a rapid IV bolus followed by a 20 ml normal saline bolus.   236–237

14:25 **A** You reassess the blood pressure and ECG rhythm. The blood pressure is 126/80 mmHg and the ECG rhythm is as follows:

14:26 **M** You administer a second dose of adenosine at 12.0 mg rapid IV push followed by a 20 ml normal saline bolus.   236–237

14:28 **A** You reassess the blood pressure and ECG rhythm. The blood pressure is 130/78 mmHg and the ECG rhythm is as follows:

14:29 **M** You administer a third dose of adenosine at 12.0 mg rapid IV push followed by a 20 ml normal saline bolus.   236–237

14:30 **A** The rhythm converts to a normal sinus rhythm with a rate of 90 bpm. The blood pressure is 130/80 mmHg; the respirations are 16/min; and the SpO$_2$ is 99%.

14:30 **M** You prepare the patient for transport.

▦ STABLE WIDE COMPLEX TACHYCARDIA

Overview

The wide complex tachycardia can present as unstable monomorphic or polymorphic or as stable monomorphic or stable polymorphic. The unstable wide complex tachycardia is treated the same regardless if it is monomorphic or polymorphic. It is necessary to determine if there is any evidence of left ventricular failure or congestive heart failure when treating the stable monomorphic wide complex tachycardia. If there is evidence of left ventricular failure or congestive heart failure, amiodarone is the first line drug of choice. If no evidence of left ventricular failure or CHF is present, procainamide is administered first. If the rhythm is a polymorphic stable wide complex tachycardia with a normal QT interval during a period of normal sinus rhythm, the patient is treated the same as the monomorphic stable wide complex tachycardia. If the polymorphic wide complex tachycardia has a prolonged QT interval, the patient is treated with magnesium sulfate, lidocaine, phenytoin, isoproterenol, or overdrive pacing. If at any time the stable wide complex tachycardia becomes unstable, synchronized cardioversion becomes the treatment of choice. This case uses the following algorithm:

▶ Wide Complex Tachycardia (see Chapter 10, Figure 10-7)

Psychomotor Skills

▶ Rhythm diagnosis

▶ Synchronized cardioversion

Background Patient Information

You arrive on the scene and find a 62-year-old male patient sitting next to his car on the side of the road. As you approach the patient, you note he is alert and responding appropriately to your questions. He states he was driving his car when suddenly he began to feel this funny feeling in his chest and his heart appears to be beating to fast. He was afraid to continue driving so he pulled over to the side of the road and called for EMS on his cell phone.

Assessment and Management Priorities

Time	Assessment and Management		See Pages
22:59	A	Perform an initial assessment (ABCD survey): The patient reports he has had similar episodes in the past. His blood pressure is 128/82 mmHg; heart rate is 170 bpm; and respirations are 14/min with no evidence of respiratory distress.	
23:00	M	You place the patient on a nasal cannula at 4 lpm, start an intravenous line of normal saline running TKO, place the patient on a continuous cardiac monitor, pulse oximeter, and automatic blood pressure monitor.	303–306

Time	Assessment and Management	See Pages
23:01	**A** The blood pressure is 130/80 mmHg, and the SpO$_2$ is 98%. The lungs are clear, there is no JVD, and the perfusion status appears to be stable. The monitor shows:	132–133

| 23:02 | **M** You administer procainamide at 20 mg/min as an infusion to a total of 17 mg/kg. | 230–231, 328–332 |
| 23:07 | **A** The blood pressure is 132/80 mmHg. The ECG rhythm is as follows: | |

23:07	**M** You continue with the infusion of procainamide at 20 mg/min and carefully monitor the blood pressure and the QRS width. You begin transport.	230–231
23:16	**A** En route, the rhythm converts. The ECG monitor shows a normal sinus rhythm with a rate of 98 bpm. The blood pressure is 134/82 mmHg, and the SpO$_2$ is 98%. The patient states that he feels much better.	
23:16	**M** You stop the infusion of procainamide at 20 mg/min and prepare a maintenance infusion by mixing 2 grams of procainamide in 500 ml of normal saline. You initiate the procainamide maintenance infusion at 2 mg/min. You continue to monitor the patient en route.	230–231

Key Points

▶ Use the Narrow Complex and Wide Complex Tachycardia algorithms.

▶ Perform the steps of the initial assessment (ABCD survey).

▶ The first step in the tachycardia algorithm is to rule out instability. Stable tachycardia may be a narrow complex tachycardia or a wide complex tachycardia.

▶ Determine if the stable wide complex tachycardia is monomorphic or polymorphic.

▶ Look for signs and symptoms of left ventricular failure or congestive heart failure in the monomorphic stable wide complex tachycardia.

▶ If there is evidence of left ventricular failure or congestive heart failure in monomorphic wide complex tachycardia, do not administer procainamide due to the negative inotropic properties. Amiodarone would be the first line drug of choice.

▶ A polymorphic wide complex tachycardia with a prolonged QT is treated with magnesium sulfate, lidocaine, phenytoin, isoproterenol, and overdrive pacing. If the QT interval is normal, treat it the same as a monomorphic wide complex tachycardia.

In this Scenario, You MUST

1. Perform initial assessment, apply the ECG monitor, and assess vital signs.
2. Use the Narrow Complex and Wide Complex Tachycardia algorithms.
3. Determine the type of tachycardia and whether it is stable or unstable.
4. Assess for signs of left ventricular failure or congestive heart failure.
5. Perform synchronized cardioversion or administer medications to manage the tachycardia.
6. Correctly perform synchronized cardioversion.
7. Reassess the patient after synchronized cardioversion and medication administration.

Unacceptable Actions

▶ Failure to perform an ABCD survey and determine the stability of the patient

▶ Incorrect rhythm interpretation

▦ SUMMARY

This chapter has introduced the concept of case-based instruction. Each scenario provides you with a sequence of integrated assessments and interventions based on the assessments. Key points and unacceptable actions for each scenario are listed. This kind of practical applicable instruction will increase your confidence in managing cardiac emergencies.

REVIEW QUESTIONS

1. What is the first step that should be taken upon your arrival at the scene of a potential cardiac emergency?
   a. Ensure the scene is safe.
   b. Open the airway.
   c. Assess the breathing.
   d. Assess the pulse.

2. What is the initial method of opening the airway for any non-trauma patient?
   a. oropharyngeal airway
   b. tracheal intubation
   c. chin lift without head tilt
   d. head tilt, chin lift

3. You must be able to deliver the first defibrillation within _____ seconds of the arrival of an AED.
   a. 30
   b. 60
   c. 90
   d. 120

4. If you have a monitor/defibrillator immediately available, what should you do once you determine that a patient is unresponsive?
   a. Defibrillate at 200 joules.
   b. Begin 1 minute of CPR and then defibrillate.
   c. Insert a tracheal tube and an intravenous line.
   d. Open the airway, and assess the breathing and pulse.

5. What is the next immediate step you should do after inflating the cuff of the tracheal tube?
   a. Confirm tube placement by evaluating the pulse oximeter reading.
   b. Confirm tube placement by inspection and auscultation.
   c. Secure the tube.
   d. Insert a bite block.

6. How long should you wait to defibrillate after administering a medication to a patient in ventricular fibrillation.
   a. 5 seconds
   b. 15–30 seconds
   c. 30–60 seconds
   d. 60–90 seconds

7. Which of the following is **not** an appropriate antidysrhythmic in the treatment of recurrent ventricular fibrillation?
   a. procainamide
   b. bretylium
   c. lidocaine
   d. magnesium sulfate

8. Which of the following is used in cardiac arrest of any origin or presenting rhythm?
   a. epinephrine
   b. amiodarone
   c. atropine
   d. sodium bicarbonate

9. What is the likely cause of PEA in a patient with chest trauma, distended neck veins, and muffled heart tones?
   a. tension pneumothorax
   b. hypovolemia
   c. hypoxia
   d. cardiac tamponade

10. What should you do if a patient in asystole fails to respond to transcutaneous pacing, repeated administration of epinephrine, and the total vagolytic dose of atropine?
    a. Administer sodium bicarbonate.
    b. Consider the termination of resuscitation.
    c. Use high dose epinephrine.
    d. Administer a 300 cc fluid bolus.

11. What should guide the amount of oxygen delivered to a patient with signs and symptoms of an acute coronary syndrome?
    a. blood gasses
    b. pulse oximetry and physical assessment findings
    c. the level of respiratory distress and the severity of the complaint of dyspnea
    d. ECG changes and the baseline vital signs

12. A patient with a polymorphic wide complex tachycardia with a prolonged QT interval should be treated with?
    a. magnesium sulfate
    b. adenosine
    c. amiodarone
    d. nitroglycerin

13. At what heart rate should you set the transcutaneous pacer to treat symptomatic bradycardia?
    a. 60
    b. 70
    c. 80
    d. 90

14. What is the treatment for unstable wide complex tachycardia?
    a. lidocaine
    b. adenosine
    c. procainamide
    d. synchronized cardioversion

15. Which of the following unstable narrow complex tachycardia rhythms should be preferentially treated with synchronized cardioversion?
    a. junctional tachycardia
    b. paroxysmal supraventricular tachycardia
    c. multi-focal atrial tachycardia
    d. ectopic atrial tachycardia

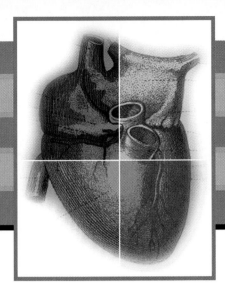

Acute Stroke

The emergency assessment and management of stroke has evolved drastically over the last several years. Previously, the stroke patient was basically provided supportive care and assessed for maximal neurologic deficit. However, management of the acute ischemic stroke, known today as a "brain attack," has taken on a new aggressive assessment approach and treatment plan in an attempt to reduce the neurologic deficit and disability associated with its incidence. Early and prompt recognition of the signs and symptoms of stroke, expeditious transport by EMS, early notification of designated stroke centers, and aggressive assessment and intervention by the emergency department physician and staff is paramount to reducing the morbidity and mortality of an acute ischemic stroke.

Topics in this chapter are:

- Acute Stroke and Transient Ischemic Attack (TIA)
- Initial Assessment of the Patient with an Acute Stroke or TIA
- Treatment Strategies for the Acute Stroke Patient

CASE STUDY

You are called to a residence for a 56-year-old male patient whose wife called EMS because her husband suffered a sudden onset of weakness to one side of his body. As you arrive, you find the patient in the living room sitting in a recliner. His wife states that her husband, John, was relaxing and watching television when he began to complain that his right arm was getting numb. She noticed that his speech was slurred and his facial expression appeared to be asymmetrical. Having just recently read a pamphlet on the signs and symptoms of stroke, she recognized the urgency of his condition and immediately called 911. You approach John as he explains, with slurred speech, that his arm is numb. You note a droop to the right side of his face. He is holding his right arm with his left hand while attempting to make gross motor movements. He is upset and frightened.

How would you proceed to assess and care for this patient? This chapter will describe the assessment and management of a patient suffering from an acute ischemic stroke. Later we will return to the case and apply the information learned.

INTRODUCTION

An acute stroke (or brain attack) is yet another cardiovascular emergency that, like a myocardial infarction (heart attack), can cause airway, breathing, and circulation compromises and, on occasion, cardiac arrest. It is the third leading cause of death behind cardiac disease and cancer, accounting for more than 150,000 deaths annually in the United States. Sadly, for those that survive, they are often times left with severe neurological impairments that may drastically alter their daily lives. However, with fibrinolytic therapy for some ischemic stroke patients we can intervene and limit or reverse many of their neurological deficits.

ACUTE STROKE AND TRANSIENT ISCHEMIC ATTACK (TIA)

The term acute ischemic stroke (sometimes called a cerebral vascular accident, or CVA) refers to an acute onset of signs and symptoms of stroke with evolving brain ischemia and injury. This is also termed a "brain attack" because, like a heart attack, it results in ischemia and injury that require immediate assessment and treatment in order to limit the amount of damage associated with the ischemic event—in this case damage to the brain. A *transient ischemic attack (TIA)*, has a similar etiology and presentation to a stroke; however, the signs and symptoms are temporary and the patient suffers no permanent neurologic dysfunction. It is, however, often the precursor to a full acute ischemic stroke.

Etiology of an Acute Stroke

Stroke is an emergency that arises when a blood vessel that perfuses the brain becomes occluded or ruptures. This leads to a disruption of blood flow that results in ischemia and necrosis in the area of the brain perfused by that vessel. Ischemia of the brain tissue results in local edema as well as abnormal nerve function and transmission, which in turn causes characteristic signs and symptoms of a stroke. Ischemic strokes (occlusive strokes) occur because of an occlusion, whereas, hemorrhagic strokes are due to a ruptured vessel. Thrombotic and embolic strokes are considered to be ischemic.

Causes of occlusive stroke include thrombus formation at the site of the infarct that occur at locations of pre-existing atherosclerotic plaque, or thrombus formation in the heart, carotids or other peripheral vessels, which then embolizes into the cerebral vessels. Emboli can also be formed from atherosclerotic plaques, cardiac valvular vegetations, air or other gases (e.g., nitrogen from diving accidents), amniotic fluid, tumors, bone marrow (from fractures), parasites, or fat.

Hemorrhagic strokes result from subarachnoid hemorrhage (SAH) or intracerebral hemorrhage (ICH). SAH often occurs from a ruptured cerebral aneurysm, with the blood then filling the subarachnoid space and compressing adjacent brain tissue. ICH generally occurs from hypertensive bleeds (rupture of small vessels within the brain that have been damaged by long-standing hypertension), or from ruptured arterio-venous malformations (AVM).

Etiology of a Transient Ischemic Attack (TIA)

A transient ischemic attack (TIA) is thought to occur when there is a temporary disruption in cerebral blood flow. Once circulation is restored spontaneously, symptoms resolve. The most common etiology is a small thrombotic embolus traveling through the cardiovascular system that becomes lodged in a cerebral blood vessel too small for it to pass through. A TIA is only temporary because the body is able to lyse, or dissolve, the clot causing the obstruction, or the thromboembolus will fragment into clinically insignificant micro emboli and pass through to a more distal site, thereby returning normal perfusion and abating the signs and symptoms.

Although a TIA is a "temporary" emergency, it is extremely important for TIAs to be recognized. About one-third of all TIA patients experience a full acute ischemic stroke shortly after the "transient" event. Therefore, a TIA in the adult patient should be viewed as a warning sign of an impending acute ischemic stroke until proven otherwise.

Upon identification of a TIA, a physician should carefully evaluate the patient so that additional diagnostic tests can be completed to determine the likelihood of an acute ischemic stroke and preventive management initiated. If carotid atherosclerotic plaques are found to be the etiology of the TIA symptoms, there is also a strong possibility of coronary artery disease in the same patient, which also places that person at risk for future myocardial ischemic events.

Clinical Presentation of an Acute Stroke or TIA

Clinically, strokes of hemorrhagic etiology have some distinguishing characteristics from those of occlusive (ischemic) origins. A hemorrhagic stroke will typically be of abrupt onset (seconds), occur during stress or exertion, and rapidly progress to maximal deficit. Patients with severe hemorrhage may progress rapidly through a stuporous state to coma and death. If able to give a history, these patients will often describe a "pistol-shot headache," which is an abrupt-onset headache of maximal intensity. Some patients may present with atypical findings; therefore, any patient with a new onset of headache or change in a typical headache must be taken seriously. Other common symptoms include nausea and vomiting.

If subarachnoid hemorrhage (SAH) occurs, there may be no lateralizing features. The blood may distribute in the subarachnoid space of both cerebral hemispheres, leading to bilateral symptoms of compression and/or herniation. These patients may have findings of nuchal rigidity (neck stiffness) or complain of neck pain. Conversely, intracerebral hemorrhage (ICH), which occurs in one of the cerebral hemispheres, does tend to show initial lateralizing findings. These findings persist until enough blood or swelling causes a shift of the midline producing contralateral compression, coma, and herniation syndromes.

Acute ischemic strokes and TIAs may present with very insidious, nonspecific symptoms such as memory loss, auditory disturbances, vertigo, gait disturbances, very focal weakness or paresthesias that go unreported or unrecognized by patients and their families. They may also present with more specific symptoms or characteristic patterns that may suggest the vessel of origin.

Strokes or TIAs involving occlusion of the anterior circulation (carotid artery) typically present with weakness and numbness of the face and extremities on the opposite side of the body from the damaged cerebral cortex. If the dominant hemisphere is involved there may also be aphasia (speech impairment). If the posterior circulation (vertebro-basilar artery) is the occluded vessel, there may be bilateral findings such as facial numbness on one side of the body with contralateral weakness. Vertigo, bilateral blindness, ataxia (impaired muscular coordination), and general weakness are also possibilities as these vessels supply the cerebellum, occipital lobe, and brainstem (including cranial nerves). The Circle of Willis connects the two major blood supplies of the brain and, if intact, often limits the degree of damage done by the acute ischemic stroke.

Understanding what a stroke is, and knowing the common indicators, will help you identify the acute ischemic stroke or TIA early in its progression when treatment will be most beneficial. Early recognition is critical to successful management with minimal residual effects. There is a correlation between the length of time between onset of the acute ischemic stroke and successful treatment. The longer the stroke exists without proper management, the worse the prognosis and the overall severity of the emergency.

The signs and symptoms of an acute ischemic stroke and of a TIA are essentially the same, since both result from inadequate perfusion to an area of the brain. The difference is that the signs and symptoms seen during a TIA resolve spontaneously, usually within minutes, however, almost always within 24 hours of onset. During the initial stages of a stroke or TIA, it is usually not feasible (nor absolutely necessary with regard to initial supportive management) to delineate between the two. Table 12-1 identifies some common signs and symptoms seen with an acute ischemic stroke or TIA.

TABLE 12-1 Signs and Symptoms of Acute Stroke or TIA

- Headache (possibly severe, may be associated with neck pain/rigidity)
- Paralysis (usually hemiplegic)
- Paresis (weakness to one or more extremities)
- Ataxia (lack of coordinated muscle movement)
- Dysphagia (difficulty in swallowing)
- Aphasia (difficulty with speech due to brain impairment)
- Dysarthria (difficulty with speech due to impairment of the muscles of speech)
- Diplopia (double vision)
- Disturbances in sensory perception (in one or more parts of the body)
- Amaurosis fugax (temporary blindness due to thromboembolus in ophthalmic artery)
- Vertigo (dizziness)
- Changes in cognition (anything from mild confusion to unresponsiveness)
- Loss of muscle tone to one side of the face, with paralysis to opposite extremities
- Possible seizures, incontinence, vomiting

An acute ischemic stroke or TIA should be suspected in any patient who has experienced a rapid onset of neurologic deficits or an alteration in mental status. The additional physical findings listed in Table 12-1 may exist alone or in combination with each other. As well, they may progressively worsen, wax and wane, or be maximally severe at onset.

INITIAL ASSESSMENT OF THE PATIENT WITH AN ACUTE STROKE OR TIA

As with any cardiovascular emergency, only a good patient assessment can lead to sound medical treatment. Even though acute cardiovascular decompensation is rare with strokes, oftentimes the health care provider will be faced with airway maintenance challenges, which do occur frequently in the acute stroke patient who is unresponsive.

Airway

In conjunction with initial airway management, remember to stabilize the spine if trauma is suspected. Remember, also, that the decreasing mental status or unresponsiveness of the acute stroke patient may result in a loss of the patient's ability to protect his airway. The mandible will become relaxed and fall posteriorly while the person lies supine. As the mandible is displaced posteriorly, so are the muscles that support the tongue and epiglottis. This can lead to a partial or total obstruction as the tongue falls against the posterior wall of the hypopharynx and the epiglottis partially occludes the glottic opening. Another threat is the accumulation of saliva, blood, or vomitus in the hypopharynx. Thoroughly assess the airway and apply suction, if necessary, to remove any secretions, blood, vomitus, or foreign materials.

You may need to insert a simple mechanical device, such as an oropharyngeal airway (OPA) or a nasopharyngeal airway (NPA) in the absence of a gag reflex, to help keep the airway open while positive pressure ventilation is initiated. Eventually, any acute stroke patient in need of ventilatory support should be intubated, if necessary using a rapid sequence induction intubation technique (described later), and manually or mechanically ventilated until further diagnostic or interventional procedures are employed. Care must be taken to provide appropriate ventilation guidelines that ensure adequate oxygenation and ventilation rates. Hyperventilation, as suggested in the past, may actually worsen the neurologic status of the patient. It should be reserved for severe cases of increased intracranial pressure (ICP) states and even then it should be a carefully controlled hyperventilation (also described later).

Vital Signs

Vital sign changes are not usually very clear indicators of the presence of an acute stroke and depend on the severity and location of the stroke. Commonly, an acute stroke will not cause hypotension or shock. If the patient shows signs of shock you should seek an alternative cause (for example, internal hemorrhage). An acute stroke more commonly causes hypertension, occasionally severe enough to require pharmacological therapy. This is one reason why the monitoring of vital signs is an integral part of emergency stroke management. Also be alert for dysrhythmias, as they are more likely to occur as the stroke progresses and involves more and more of the brain stem. Treat any life-threatening dysrhythmias with the appropriate pharmacological therapy.

Respiratory Effort

Abnormal breathing patterns are another possible finding in an acute stroke. They are one of the most useful indicators of brainstem function. *Cheyne-Stokes respiratory pattern* will occur when there is bilateral cerebral hemisphere damage resulting from a large hemorrhagic stroke. It indicates bilateral cerebral cortical injury, functionally disconnecting cerebral influence on the brainstem respiratory centers. This breathing pattern is characterized by a waxing and waning hyperpneic (full and deep breaths) respiratory pattern, followed by a short period of apnea before repeating itself. The apneic period occurs after CO_2 levels decrease from the hyperpneic phase.

Central neurogenic hyperventilation is characterized by increased rate and depth of respiration resulting from early herniation or primary damage to the pons or lower midbrain. The respiratory control centers in the lower brainstem no longer inhibit respiration due to hypocapnea (low CO_2 levels), and this allows for continued hyperventilation and respiratory alkalosis.

Apneustic breathing is a pattern in which there is a 2- to 3-second pause after full inspiration that results from lower pontine lesions seen in basilar artery occlusion. Lastly, if the medulla is compressed or injured, *Biot's breathing* may be noted, characterized by chaotic irregular breathing regularly interrupted by apneic episodes. This progresses to irregular inspiratory gasps and then apnea.

Most patients who die of neurologic insult will die a respiratory death. So, just as you must maintain the airway when the patient cannot, you must also supplement any inadequate respiratory effort with positive pressure ventilation and oxygenation.

Circulatory Status

As mentioned previously, cardiac arrest is an uncommon complication of an acute stroke. When it does occur, it is usually secondary to respiratory arrest associated with the stroke. While the need for chest compressions is rare, cardiac monitoring is imperative, since acute ischemic strokes often cause abnormalities in blood pressure and cardiac rhythms. Hypertension is more commonly caused by an acute stroke than hypotension. Hypertension is thought possibly to be a result of the body's response to the stroke, increasing blood flow to the ischemic areas by increasing its driving pressure. Hypertension may also be a stress response by the body to the cerebral insult, or more likely is one of the contributing factors to the acute stroke itself. (Hypertension is a major risk factor.) For this reason many experts believe that hypertension should not be treated in the prehospital setting. However, it is also well understood that severe hypertension in the presence of acute intracranial hemorrhage (ICH) may worsen outcome. Your medical director should address this or any other special circumstances (e.g., long transport times) in your protocols or standing orders.

If hypotension is seen in conjunction with an acute stroke, you should rapidly seek out other causes for the hypotension. Only with severe brain insults at the terminal stages will the pressure start to drop. Thus, hypotension is not usually an initial finding with an acute stroke.

Neurological Assessment

Constant monitoring of the acute stroke/TIA patient will help you to decide if the patient is improving or deteriorating. While the assessment techniques you use need not be exhaustive, they do need to be reliable, and the most reliable finding in the acute stroke patient is the level of consciousness. A depressed mental status, or a deteriorating mental status, indicates a major insult to the brain. Stroke patients who present or become unresponsive are at the greatest risk of death from the acute stroke.

The Glasgow Coma Scale (Figure 12-1) provides a standardized way to assess the severity of the neurological injury. A benefit of this scale is that it can be used by any health care provider with a high degree of objectivity and accuracy. Any numeric change upon reassessment indicates a general improvement, or worsening, in the patient's condition. The scale uses assessments of three parameters: eye opening, motor response, and verbal response. The total score can range from 3 to 15. In general, a score of 8 or less indicates a severe neurological insult with a poor prognosis.

Since responsiveness requires an intact brain stem, you can infer some type of dysfunction of the brain stem from altered mental status or unresponsiveness. Assess the following to gain an idea about the status of the brain stem:

- Reactivity of the pupils to light
- Size and equality of the pupils (inequality may indicate herniation of the temporal lobe)
- Corneal reflexes
- Gag reflex
- Doll's eyes maneuver (oculocephalic reflex) is used to asses the integrity of the brainstem in a comatose patient. The maneuver should only be performed if the patient has no evidence of a spinal injury and is comatose (not responding to any noxious stimuli). To perform the maneuver, hold the patient's eyelids open so that you can see the eyes, turn the patient's head quickly to one side and then to the other side. In the comatose patient, if the brainstem is intact, the eyes move in the opposite direction of the turned head. For example, if the head is turned to the right, the eyes will move to

Glasgow Coma Scale

Eye opening	Spontaneous	4	
	To Voice	3	
	To Pain	2	
	None	1	
Verbal response	Oriented	5	
	Confused	4	
	Inappropriate Words	3	
	Incomprehensible Sounds	2	
	None	1	
Motor response	Obeys Command	6	
	Localizes Pain	5	
	Withdraw (pain)	4	
	Flexion (pain)	3	
	Extension (pain)	2	
	None	1	
Glasgow coma score total			

FIGURE 12–1
Glasgow Coma Scale.

the left. This is considered to be an intact Doll's eye movement. If the head is turned to the right and the eyes move with the turned head (to the right side), the Doll's eyes movement is absent. This is an indication of a lesion of the pons or midbrain. Thus, eye movement opposite of the turned head is a good sign of an intact brainstem; whereas, eye movement to the same side of the turned head is a sign of a possible brainstem lesion.

The mnemonic *FAST* may be used as a quick assessment tool to help confirm the suspicion of an acute stroke in the conscious patient:

- **F**acial symmetry
- **A**ctive strength/coordination testing
- **S**ensation
- **T**alk/language

Prehospital Specific Neurological Assessments

Recently, two organized screening methods have been shown to be effective in identifying a large number of patients suffering from acute stroke. These methods are simple to employ and may be rapidly performed by EMS personnel. They are the Cincinnati Prehospital Stroke Scale (CPSS) and the Los Angeles Prehospital Stroke Screen (LAPSS).

The Cincinnati Prehospital Stroke Scale (Table 12-2) is an assessment technique that looks at three parameters:

- **Facial droop** (Figure 12-2)
- **Arm drift** (Figure 12-3)
- **Abnormal speech**

The CPSS is interpreted in the following way: If any one of the parameters is determined to be abnormal then the probability of a stroke is 72%.

The Los Angeles Prehospital Stroke Screen (Table 12-3) is a more thorough evaluation tool for the "acute, non-traumatized and non-comatose" patient.

In Table 12.3 if items 1–5 are ALL checked YES (or UNKNOWN) and the patient has obvious asymmetry you should give pre-arrival notification to the hospital of apparent stroke patient contact. If any item is checked NO then you should continue with assessment and look for other etiology of symptoms. *Interpretation:*

TABLE 12–2 Cincinnati Stroke Scale

Sign of Stroke	Patient Activity	Interpretation
Facial Droop	Have patient look up at you, smile, and show teeth.	*Normal:* Symmetry to both sides. *Abnormal:* One side of the face droops or does not move symmetrically.
Arm Drift	Have patient lift arms up and hold them out with eyes closed for ten seconds.	*Normal:* Symmetrical movement in both arms. *Abnormal:* One arm drifts down or asymmetrical movement of the arms.
Abnormal Speech	Have the patient say "you can't teach an old dog new tricks."	*Normal:* The correct words are used and no slurring of words is noted. *Abnormal:* The words are slurred, the wrong words are used, or the patient is aphasic.

Kothari RU, Pancioli A, Liu T, Broderick J. "Cincinnati Prehospital Stroke Scale: Reproductibility and Validity." *Annals of Emergency Medicine.* 1999: 33:373–378.

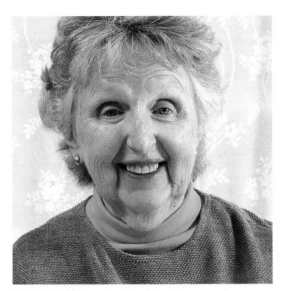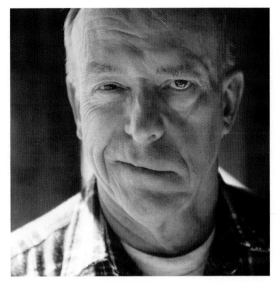

FIGURE 12-2
(A) The face of a non-stroke patient has normal symmetry. (B) The face of a stroke patient often has abnormal, drooped appearance on one side. (*Michal Heron*)

93% of patients with an acute stroke will have a positive LAPSS score (sensitivity = 93%), and 97% of those with a positive LAPSS score will be suffering a stroke (specificity = 97%). NOTE: Based on the study, 7% of patients may still be suffering from an acute stroke despite having the inability to be identified by the Los Angeles Prehospital Stroke Screen.

Hospital Specific Neurological Assessment

The NIH Stroke Scale, or NIHSS (Table 12-4), was developed by the National Institutes of Health and is used as a measure of stroke severity. This scale was utilized by the National Institute of Neurologic Disorders and Stroke (NINDS) for its rt-PA (recombinant tissue plasminogen activator or t-PA) Study. This study demonstrated that the study-group patients receiving fibrinolytics (rt-PA) were 30 percent more likely to have minimal or no deficit at 3 months than patients treated with a placebo. This represented a significant statistical difference in outcome for

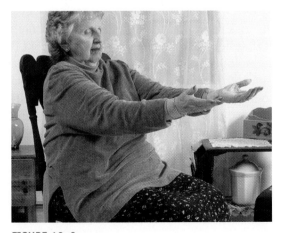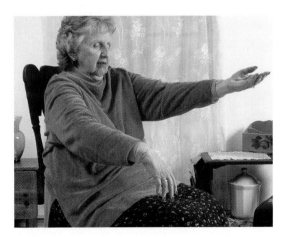

FIGURE 12-3
(A) A patient who has not suffered a stroke can generally hold arms in an extended position with eyes closed. (B) A stroke patient will often display "arm drift" or "pronater drift"; that is, one arm will remain extended when held outward with eyes closed, but the other arm will drift or drop downward and pronate (turn palm downward).

TABLE 12–3 Los Angeles Prehospital Stroke Screen (LAPSS)

Considerations	Yes	Unknown	No
1. Age **greater than** 45 years			
2. **No** history of seizures or epilepsy			
3. Duration of symptoms is **less** than 24 hours			
4. Patient is **not** wheelchair bound or bedridden			
5. Blood glucose level **between 60 and 400 mg/dl**			
Physical exam to determine unilateral asymmetry	**Equal**	**R Weakness**	**L Weakness**
A. Have patient look up, smile, and show teeth		Droop	Droop
B. Compare grip strength of upper extremities		Weak grip No grip	Weak grip No grip
C. Assess arm strength for drift or weakness		Drifts down Falls rapidly	Drifts down Falls rapidly

Kidwell CS, Saver JL, Schubert GB, Eckstein M, Starkman S. "Design and retrospective analysis of the Los Angeles Prehospital Stroke Screen (LAPSS)." *Prehospital Emergency Care.* 1998; 2:267–273.
Kidwell CS, Starkman S, Eckstein M; Weems K, Saver JL. "Identifying stroke in the field: prospective validation of the Los Angeles Prehospital Screen (LAPSS)." *Stroke.* 2000; 31:71–76.

patients suffering from acute stroke symptoms. It is also important to mention that this improvement was not without risk. The study also demonstrated a 10-fold increase in symptomatic hemorrhage (6.4% vs. 0.6%) within 36 hours following study medication administration. There was also a 10-fold increase in the risk of fatal intracranial hemorrhage in the treated group (3% vs. 0.3%).

Differential Diagnosis for Acute Stroke/TIA

Prior to administering any treatment, consider the variety of emergencies that may have precipitated the presenting signs and symptoms in order to avoid administering treatment that may be inappropriate or harmful. For example, a hypoglycemic patient and an acute ischemic stroke patient may both display an altered mental status, focal neurologic deficits such as aphasia (inability to speak), and hemiparesis (partial paralysis), or unresponsiveness. But if dextrose (which is appropriate for a hypoglycemic patient) is administered to an unresponsive patient who is actually suffering an acute ischemic stroke, the neurological damage may be worsened by the dextrose. Also, imagine the risk of administration of rt-PA to a patient who is actually hypoglycemic and NOT suffering from an acute ischemic stroke.

Rapid bedside testing may be employed to help identify certain possible causes of the patient's neurological emergency. For example, a bedside glucose measurement will help identify hypoglycemia, and there are other bedside tests that can determine the presence or absence of drugs. There may also be specific physical findings that point toward certain other etiologies. For example, needle tracks may point to drug abuse and bites on the tongue or inner cheek are common to seizures. Table 12-5 presents the most common differential diagnoses for suspected acute ischemic strokes.

After you have properly assessed and treated threats to the airway, breathing, and circulation, attention must be turned to the underlying cause of the neurologic deficit. It is important for the physician to determine not only the presence or absence of a stroke but also the type of stroke. Since an acute ischemic stroke from a brain infarction (embolus or thrombus) is managed radically differently from a stroke from a cerebral hemorrhage, this determination is imperative.

TABLE 12–4 | NIH Stroke Scale

Level of Consciousness (LOC)	0 = alert 1 = not alert, arousable 2 = not alert, obtunded 3 = nonresponsive
Questions	0 = answers two correctly 1 = answers one correctly 2 = answers neither correctly
Commands	0 = performs 2 tasks 1 = performs 1 task 2 = performs neither task
Gaze	0 = no visual loss 1 = partial gaze palsy 2 = forced deviation
Visual fields	0 = no visual loss 1 = partial hemianopia 2 = complete hemianopia 3 = bilateral hemianopia
Facial palsy	0 = normal 1 = minor paralysis 2 = partial paralysis 3 = complete paralysis
Motor Arm **a - left** **b - right**	0 = no drift 1 = drift before 10 sec. 2 = falls before 10 sec. 3 = no effort against gravity 4 = no movement
Motor Leg **a - left** **b - right**	0 = no drift 1 = drift before 5 sec. 2 = falls before 10 sec. 3 = no effort against gravity 4 = no movement
Ataxia	0 = absent 1 = one limb 2 = two limbs
Sensory	0 = absent 1 = mid to moderate loss 2 = severe to total loss
Language	0 = normal 1 = mild to moderate aphasia 2 = severe aphasia 3 = mute
Dysarthria	0 = normal 1 = mild to moderate 2 = severe
Extinction/Inattention	0 = normal 1 = mild—one modality 2 = severe—more than one modality

Developed by the National Institute of Neurological Disorders and Stroke/National Institutes of Health, Bethesda, Maryland.

TABLE 12–5	Differential Diagnosis for Acute Stroke

- Hemorrhagic versus ischemic stroke
- Meningitis/encephalitis
- Drugs/narcotic overdose
- Intracranial mass (tumor, subdural hematoma)
- Craniocerebral trauma/cervical trauma
- Seizures (although seizures could be caused by a stroke)
- Hypertensive crisis
- Metabolic causes
- Glucose levels (hypoglycemia or hyperglycemia)
- Post-arrest cerebral ischemia
- Drug use/abuse

To assist with this determination, the emergency department physician has advanced diagnostic capabilities at his disposal. While a complete discussion of these alternative diagnostic exams is well beyond the scope of this text, we mention them to help you understand the additional studies the ED physician may be requesting. Table 12-6 identifies these additional diagnostic studies that will help isolate the presence or absence and type of acute stroke.

TREATMENT STRATEGIES FOR THE ACUTE STROKE PATIENT

Acute stroke, or "brain attack" as it is alternatively referred to, is a true medical emergency. Care and treatment depends on rapid evaluation and determination of the cause of the event. If the cause is determined to be a nonhemorrhagic occlusive acute ischemic stroke, then fibrinolytic therapy may be appropriate in certain patient populations. (Refer to Table 12-7 for contraindications for fibrinolytic therapy.) These patients must:

▶ Be thoroughly evaluated
▶ Have a CT scan
▶ Be ready for treatment within 3 hours of symptom onset
▶ Be at least 18 years of age or older

TABLE 12–6	Diagnostic Evaluations for Patients with Acute Stroke

- Computed tomography (CT)
- Magnetic resonance imaging (MRI)
- Cerebral angiography
- Doppler flow studies
- Electrocardiogram
- Serum electrolytes
- Other labs (serum osmolarity, renal, liver, calcium, toxicology screen)
- Glucose levels
- Arterial blood gas levels
- Hematological studies
- Lateral cervical spine x-rays

TABLE 12-7 Contraindications to Fibrinolytic Therapy

- Intracranial hemorrhage diagnosed with CT scan
- Clinical suspicion of subarachnoid hemorrhage (SAH)
- Minor or rapidly improving stroke symptoms
- Recent acute ischemic stroke or head trauma, within preceding 3 months
- Undergone major surgery or major trauma within 14 days
- Uncontrolled systolic BP >185, or diastolic BP >110 with initial treatment
- Lumbar puncture within previous 7 days
- GI or urinary tract hemorrhage within 21 days
- Arterial puncture of a noncompressible vessel within 7 days
- Seizure at onset of stroke
- Anticoagulant therapy within 48 hours with elevated PT or PTT
- Platelet count below 100,000
- Glucose <50 mg/dl or >400 mg/dl
- History of ICH, AVM, or aneurysm

▶ Have an NIH Stroke Scale (NIHSS) score of > 4 and < 22
▶ Not have any "exclusion criteria"

Patients may also be considered with a NIHSS score of < 4 if their neurologic dysfunction is either severe aphasia or hemianopsia (lateralized vision loss or severe vision abnormality). Patients with NIHSS scores > 22 have suffered a severe neurologic insult because a large area of the brain has been infarcted. If given fibrinolytics they are at increased risk of developing an intracranial hemorrhage. Therefore, the risk of hemorrhage must be weighed heavily against the probability of benefit from treatment before fibrinolytic therapy is considered.

TIAs need further diagnostics to determine the need for surgical treatment if carotid stenosis is found to be the etiology. If the patient is not a surgical candidate, then anticoagulant therapy is considered in the high risk patient population (see Table 12-8), or antiplatelet therapy may be utilized if the patient is not a candidate for anticoagulants.

Patients determined to have sustained hemorrhagic strokes will require immediate neurosurgical consultation to determine the appropriateness of surgical intervention and intracranial monitoring.

General Considerations in Initial Care of Acute Stroke

As emphasized earlier, initial management is geared toward supporting the ABCs. In the acute stroke patient this is of paramount concern, since vomiting with subsequent aspiration is common. The airway should initially be assessed for patency, while suctioning as appropriate. If the patient cannot maintain his airway, insert a

TABLE 12-8 High-Risk Patients with TIA Syndrome

- Patients with high-grade carotid stenosis (70–99%) anatomically related to symptoms
- Patients already on antiplatelet therapy
- Patients with chronic atrial fibrillation or other cardiac etiology to emboli
- TIAs occurring with increasing frequency

nasopharyngeal or oropharyngeal airway initially, and consider tracheal intubation. Positive pressure ventilation is appropriate for those patients who have a disturbance in their minute ventilation (a decrease in the respiratory rate, inadequate tidal volume, or ataxic ventilations). Oxygenation should always accompany ventilations. Overzealous hyperventilation must be avoided. Hyperventilation at 20–24/minute should only be used when evidence of brain herniation is present (posturing or fixed and dilated pupil). Monitor oxygenation by applying a pulse oximeter. If the patient has been intubated, an end-tidal CO_2 monitor should be utilized.

Initiate intravenous access with an isotonic solution in a patent vein, and run it at 30 ml/h. Preferably, this should be done with 0.9% NaCl (normal saline), but lactated Ringer's may also be used. Dextrose-containing solutions should be avoided. Dextrose solutions are metabolized by the body causing free water, which is hypo-osmolar (hypotonic), to be left in the intravascular space. This may cause the hypotonic fluid to leave the vascular space and enter the brain tissue, which would potentially cause cerebral edema. As well, large volumes of crystalloid solution (normal saline, lactated Ringer's) should also be avoided unless the patient is hypotensive (generally a systolic BP of less then 90 mmHg). Do not withhold crystalloid solutions from a stroke patient who is hypotensive. Hypotension decreases cerebral perfusion pressure and may worsen the stroke state. In conjunction with initiating the IV, draw blood samples so that a stat lab report may be obtained for the blood values.

The administration of the "rule-out" drugs (dextrose, Narcan®, and thiamine) early in the management regime should be guided by conscious assessments, glucose meter reading, and interpretations, and not a "knee-jerk" reaction. Although relatively safe to use in the normal patient, dextrose administration may worsen neurologic outcome. The administration of 25 grams of D_{50} should be done only after a bedside glucose assessment demonstrates hypoglycemia. Thiamine (vitamin B_1) may be administered at 100 mg IM or IV push for any patient who demonstrates neurologic deficits in conjunction with suspected malnourishment, chronic alcoholism, or thiamine deficiency. Narcan® (naloxone, a narcotic antagonist) may also be considered at a 0.4 to 2.0 mg initial dose for those patients suspected to be under the influence of narcotics.

Prehospital Assessment and Management

The prehospital management of the acute stroke patient emphasizes quick recognition (i.e., CPSS or LAPSS assessment scores), supportive measures, expeditious transport, and notification of the stroke center (preferably) or emergency department. It is essential to provide airway control and ventilatory support when the gag and cough reflexes are diminished or absent. Prehospital management must include the following:

- Determine time of onset of symptoms (Imperative! Guides all future treatment.)
- Oxygen therapy (guided by pulse oximetry to maintain $SpO_2 > 95\%$)
- Immediate transport to a facility with ability to intervene in an acute stroke
- IV normal saline or lactated Ringers KVO (don't delay transport)
- Determine the blood glucose level
- Notify stroke center or emergency department to initiate acute ischemic stroke response team and to report stroke assessment (CPSS or LAPSS) findings

Initial Emergency Department Treatment

A patient suffering from an acute stroke or TIA could potentially be a challenge, since acute strokes may present with neurological abnormalities anywhere on the continuum from alert and oriented to unresponsive with cardiovascular instability. The management of an acute stroke/TIA patient in the initial phases (until advanced diagnostic exams isolate the type of stroke) is geared toward maintaining the airway, breathing, and circulatory status. After that, there are additional interventions, discussed below, that can help limit the acute stroke progression and reduce the intracranial pressure.

After initial stabilization, the advanced diagnostic procedures are conducted to determine the nature of the acute stroke/TIA. If the health care facility is unable to perform these advanced procedures, the patient should be transferred to another facility capable of doing them after the initial stabilization is completed.

Emergency Department Acute Stroke Response Team

Patients determined by exam and CT to have an occlusive acute ischemic stroke, who present within 3 hours of onset of symptoms, might be candidates for fibrinolytic therapy. This therapy has been approved by the FDA but is being implemented with caution due to the risk of intracranial hemorrhage. Some centers are administering intra-arterial fibrinolytics up to 6 hours after the infarct.

The following is a suggested protocol for fibrinolytics in occlusive ischemic stroke:

- ▶ Team approach initiated, with immediate response of emergency nursing personnel and the emergency physician to the bedside for a rapid initial assessment (includes NIH stroke scale score > 4/< 22 and ruling out of contraindications to fibrinolytics); CT Department notified of priority case

- ▶ ABCs appropriately stabilized; 2 peripheral IV lines placed with blood draw for CBC, PT, PTT, electrolytes, liver profile, type and screen, HCG (female of reproductive age), and urinalysis

- ▶ Blood pressure treated if systolic >185, diastolic >110 mmHg (consider nitropaste, labetalol, or nitroprusside)

- ▶ If screening exam confirms suspected acute ischemic stroke, patient immediately sent to CT; neurologist/neurosurgeon and radiologist notified for consultation

- ▶ If all criteria are met and consultants are in agreement, initiation of rt-PA 0.9 mg/kg body weight, with 10% given as a bolus, and the remaining 90% given over 1 hour IV piggyback

- ▶ All anticoagulant therapy and antiplatelet therapy held for 24 hours

- ▶ Admission to ICU for intensive monitoring and serial examinations

If the patient is not a candidate for fibrinolytics, antiplatelet aggregation therapy with aspirin, warfarin (Coumadin), low-molecular-weight anticoagulants (Lovenox) or ticlodipine may provide some benefit to those patients with occlusive/ischemic stroke who have no contraindications to therapy with these agents in preventing recurrent acute ischemic stroke.

Special Considerations in the Management of the Acute Stroke Patient

Each stroke patient presents with a myriad of signs and symptoms and potential complications. Some of the conditions require special treatment considerations.

Common complications and special considerations that may require specific management techniques are discussed in the following segments.

Management of Hypertension

The cranial vault is basically occupied by three items: the brain (80% of space), the vasculature and its contents (10%), and the cerebrospinal fluid (10%). Adequate cerebral blood flow (CBF) is necessary to maintain adequate cerebral functioning. Neurologic abnormalities seen in an acute stroke can be described according to changes in CBF. CBF is dependent upon a normal cerebral perfusion pressure (CPP). CPP is simply a relationship between arterial blood flow and the amount of resistance it meets as it passes through the brain. The relationship is as follows:

$$CPP = \text{mean arterial pressure (MAP)} - \text{intracranial pressure (ICP)}$$

As long as the MAP stays high enough to overcome the ICP, the cerebral blood flow remains adequate. Relating this to an acute stroke, a hemorrhagic stroke would cause an increase in ICP (due to extra blood volume in a closed cranial vault), thereby causing a resistance the MAP might be unable to overcome. Conversely, a MAP that is reduced (from poor cardiac output) will be insufficient to overcome even the normal ICP, which will also lead to inadequate cerebral blood flow.

Here is a quick-reference summary of these abbreviations:

CBF	cerebral blood flow
CPP	cerebral perfusion pressure
ICP	intracranial pressure
MAP	mean arterial pressure

It is important to understand this concept when treating hypertension in an acute stroke patient. If your patient is suffering a hemorrhagic stroke and is also hypertensive, that hypertension may be caused by a reflex response of the body to increase MAP in an attempt to overcome elevated ICP caused by the accumulation of blood in the cranium. In essence, this hypertension is present so the body can maintain a normal CBF. The problem is, the increases in mean arterial pressure can also add to, and worsen, the hemorrhage. So you will want to take actions to reduce the arterial pressure to limit the hemorrhage, but not so much that the MAP cannot overcome the ICP.

Experts still disagree about the specifics of hypertension management. However, there is agreement that hemorrhagic strokes (as identified by advanced diagnostic studies) should be treated with antihypertensives to premorbid (before the hemorrhage) levels if known, to limit the size of the bleed and opportunities for rebleeding. Ischemic thrombotic or embolic strokes do not require the aggressive management of hypertension, because the blood pressure typically decreases within a couple of hours. The only exception to this is if the hypertension is persistent at levels above 220/120 mmHg during serial evaluations every 15 minutes of at least 60–90 minutes duration, or is in association with AMI or left ventricular failure.

A physician who is knowledgeable and experienced in neurologic emergencies should guide the administration of antihypertensives. For your background information, however, Table 12-9 offers the general guidelines for the treatment of hypertension in conjunction with an acute stroke.

TABLE 12–9 Antihypertensive Administration for the Acute Ischemic and Hemorrhagic Stroke

Patients who are NOT Candidates for Fibrinolytic Therapy

1. DBP > 140 mmHg	Reduce diastolic blood pressure by lowering afterload. Consider treatment with sodium nitroprusside at 0.1–5 µg/kg/min (start at 0.1 to 0.5 µg/kg/min). Aim for 10–20% reduction in DBP.
2. SBP > 220, DBP > 120, MAP > 130 mmHg	Examine patient for contraindications to beta-blocker administration. Consider labetalol 10–20 mg only if HR is > 60 bpm. May repeat labetalol or double the dose every 20 minutes to a maximum dose of 150mg. You may also consider treatment with sodium nitroprusside at 0.1–5 µg/kg/min (start at 0.1 to 0.5 µg/kg/min). Aim for 10–20% reduction in DBP.
3. SBP < 220, DBP < 120, or MAP < 130 mmHg	Examine the patient for presence of or suspicion of AMI, aortic dissection, CHF, or encephalopathy. If these conditions are not present then emergent lowering of blood pressure may not be warranted.

Fibrinolytic Therapy Candidates

Pretreatment

1. SBP > 185, or DBP > 110 mmHg	Nitropaste (1–2") or labetalol (10–20 mg) SIVP. May repeat labetalol. If these interventions do not lower BP or maintain it at a level less than 185/110 mmHg then fibrinolytics should not be considered.

During Fibrinolytic Therapy and Immediately Following Administration

1. Monitor vital signs	It is necessary to monitor the vital signs frequently. They should be assessed every 10–15 minutes during and immediately following fibrinolytic administration. Vital signs should then be assessed every 30–60 minutes.
2. DBP > 140 mmHg	Lower diastolic blood pressure by reducing afterload. Consider administration of sodium nitroprusside at 0.1–5 µg/kg/min (start at 0.1 to 0.5 µg/kg/min).
3. SBP > 230, DBP > 120 mmHg	Examine the patient for contraindications to beta blocker DBP administration. If no contraindication, then consider labetalol (10–20 mg) over 2 minutes. May repeat labetalol or double the dose every 10 minutes to a maximum dose of 150 mg. You may consider giving an initial bolus and then initiate a labetalol infusion at 2–8 mg/min. If labetalol is not successful in controlling the BP then you may consider sodium nitroprusside (0.1–5 µg/kg/min).
4. SBP 180–230 DBP 105–120 mmHg	Examine the patient for contraindications to beta blocker administration. Consider labetalol (10–20 mg) SIVP. May repeat labetalol or double the dose every 10–20 minutes to a maximum dose of 150 mg. You may also consider giving an initial bolus and then initiate a labetalol infusion at 2–8 mg/min.

Hemorrhagic Stroke Patients (NOT Fibrinolytic Therapy Candidates) with Hypertension

1. SBP > 230 or DBP > 120 mmHg	Consider administration of sodium nitroprusside (0.5 to 10 µg/kg/min) or nitroglycerin infusion (10–20 µg/min).
2. SBP 180–230 DBP 106–120 mmHg	Examine the patient for contraindications to beta blocker administration. Consider labetalol (10–20 mg) SIVP. May repeat labetalol or double the dose every 10–20 minutes to a maximum dose of 150 mg. You may also consider giving an initial bolus and then initiate a labetalol infusion at 2–8 mg/min.
3. For new onset hypertension related to the hemorrhagic stroke	If the patient's "pre-hemorrhagic stroke" BP is estimated or known to be without hypertension (i.e., 120/80) then treatment of the hypertension may be considered to try to restore near pre-stroke pressures. This is especially important during the first few hours following the onset of a subarachnoid hemorrhage (SAH).

Constant monitoring of the blood pressure is important in titrating the drugs listed in Table 12-9 to achieve the effective response. Labetalol essentially works by dropping cardiac output through its beta-blocking effects (hence causing a drop in MAP), while sodium nitroprusside is a rapid-acting vasodilator, which will also decrease the MAP, but may actually increase ICP by cerebral vasodilation. Intravenous administration of nitrates, other beta-blockers, or calcium channel blockers may be considered as alternatives or adjuncts to therapy.

Management of Increased Intracranial Pressure

As a result of an acute stroke, there may be dramatic increases in the ICP by either a space-occupying hematoma, with a hemorrhagic stroke, or edema that may be seen with ischemic strokes. Referring back to the concept of normal CBF, any increase in ICP without a change in MAP will result in inadequate CPP and a drop in CBF. Or, simply put, an increase in the pressure within the skull, without a reflexive increase in the blood pressure to force the blood through, will cause an inadequate amount of blood flow through the brain.

Common sense would dictate that in an acute stroke, it would **not** be a desirable intervention to purposely make the systolic pressure rise with sympathomimetic drugs. This could actually complicate matters as well as increase myocardial workload. As an alternative, however, certain interventions can be used that will help reduce the excessively high ICP, thereby allowing whatever the systolic pressure is to be more effective in maintaining normal blood flow. These measures can include simple maneuvers like semi-Fowler's positioning, limitation of IV fluids, and effective ventilation and oxygenation following tracheal intubation, to more aggressive interventions including specific drug administration and, on occasion, controlled hyperventilation.

Rapid Sequence Intubation *Rapid sequence intubation (RSI) allows for the patient to be sedated and paralyzed for tracheal intubation with specific pharmacologic agents chosen to lower ICP and blunt the increased ICP response to laryngoscopy. Follow your local protocol.* This procedure must be approved by medical direction. A suggested regimen includes:

▶ Preoxygenation with 100% oxygen, cardiac monitoring, and continuous pulse oximetry
▶ Lidocaine IVP 1.0–1.5 mg/kg
▶ Norcuron® (vecuronium) 0.01 mg/kg IVP as a defasciculating agent
▶ Let above medications circulate 3 minutes with careful monitoring to ensure the quality of rate and depth of respirations
▶ Sodium pentothal 3.0–5.0 mg/kg IVP (not to be used in patients at risk for hypotension). Fentanyl or etomidate may be used.
▶ Sellick's maneuver (cricoid pressure to prevent aspiration of gastric contents)
▶ Succinylcholine 1.5 mg/kg IVP (rapid) or rocuronium 0.6 to 1.2 mg/kg (rapid)
▶ Intubate trachea and inflate cuff
▶ Assess breath sounds bilaterally, confirm presence of $ETCO_2$ and, if correct placement confirmed, may release cricoid pressure and begin ventilation therapy
▶ Consider administration of a longer-acting nondepolarizing muscle relaxant such as Norcuron® 0.10–0.15 mg/kg to keep the patient paralyzed for 30–45 minutes while diagnostics are obtained with consideration for further sedation using a barbiturate or benzodiazepine. (Consult medical direction.)

▶ Ventilation rate should be based on pre-RSI assessment and, if available, continuous monitoring with a quantitative $ETCO_2$ detector.

Hyperventilation   Hyperventilation has been a strong recommendation in the past for treatment of increased intracranial pressure (ICP) caused by conditions such as stroke and traumatic brain injury (TBI). Recent literature has demonstrated the danger of unregulated hyperventilation. It is true that increased ventilation rates do cause a decrease in $PaCO_2$ (hypocarbia), which leads to a reduction in cerebral vessel size (vasoconstriction). It was assumed beneficial that any decrease in vessel size would indirectly lower ICP because of the decreased blood volume within the cranial vault. Although this statement is true, it is only true within very limited parameters. Research has demonstrated that at mild states of hyperventilation we do indeed see a decrease in ICP. However, at lower states of hypocarbia (increased hyperventilation) we actually see detrimental effects with a significant decrease in cerebral blood flow (CBF) resulting in a decreased cerebral perfusion pressure (CPP). It is also suggested that prolonged "mild" hyperventilation may lead to the same situation.

Hyperventilation can be utilized in the treatment of severe cases of increased ICP. In the absence of ICP monitoring (i.e., patients who do not have an intracranial pressure measuring device), controlled hyperventilation should only be employed on those patients who demonstrate witnessed focal neurological changes such as the following:

▶ Unilateral dilated pupil
▶ Sudden decrease in GCS by > 2 points
▶ Decorticate posturing
▶ Decerebrate posturing
▶ Signs of herniation syndrome (increased BP, decreasing HR)

Even when hyperventilation is performed, it must be regulated and utilized for brief periods of time. With the availability of quantitative $ETCO_2$ measuring devices it is now feasible to correlate $ETCO_2$ with the circulating $PaCO_2$ of a patient. Routine ventilation of an acute ischemic or hemorrhagic stroke patient should be performed to maintain a normal carbon dioxide level or "eucapnea" state (35–45 mmHg). Whenever you witness a focal neurological change (as indicated above) the patient should be "mildly hyperventilated" to a hypocapnea state with an $ETCO_2$ of 30–32 mmHg for a brief period of approximately 5 minutes and then re-evaluated for further need. By performing these actions you can ensure adequate oxygenation and ventilation and decrease the likelihood of causing further neurologic injury to the patient. If an $ETCO_2$ monitor is not available, hyperventilation should be performed at 20 to 24 ventilations/minute.

Mannitol   Mannitol is a hyperosmolar agent that will draw interstitial fluid into the vasculature, to eventually be eliminated by the kidneys. This elimination of excessive interstitial fluid in the brain will reduce the ICP and allow the MAP to be more effective in maintaining CBF. Mannitol can be administered at 0.5 g/kg of a 20% solution over a 20-minute period. Its onset is about 20 minutes with a 4–6 hour duration. Repeat dosage can be administered at 0.25 g/kg every 4–6 hours. Exercise caution in those patients who may not tolerate an increase in intravascular volume well (e.g., those with CHF or renal disease) and in hypotension.

Management of Seizures   Seizures are a relatively infrequent, but potentially life-threatening, complication of a stroke. About 1% of thrombotic, 5%–10%

of embolic, and 15% of hemorrhagic stroke patients will suffer from seizures. The reason they are detrimental is that they increase metabolic activity in the brain, increase core temperature, increase waste production, and consume large amounts of energy and oxygen due to the constant muscular contractions. These effects only worsen the ICP, which in turn will reduce the CPP and hence reduce the CBF. The following is an outline of management principles for the acute stroke patient with concurrent seizures:

▶ Protect the airway and provide positive pressure ventilation with supplemental oxygen

▶ Maintain a normal temperature

▶ Administer diazepam 5–10 mg IV push

   [or]

   Administer lorazepam 1–4 mg IV push over 10 minutes

It may be necessary to administer a long-acting anticonvulsant to control seizures in acute stroke patients. Since almost all anticonvulsants depress respirations, attention must be paid to the respiratory status. Intubation with positive pressure ventilation may be necessary. The following therapies have a longer duration of action in controlling seizures:

▶ Administer phenytoin at 50 mg/min until a maximum dose of 16 mg/kg is achieved

   [or]

   Administer IV phenobarbital to a maximum of 20 mg/kg, followed by 30–60 mg every 6–8 hours

▶ If the patient is experiencing intractable seizures that are not terminated by phenytoin or phenobarbital, consider the administration of pentobarbital. Pentobarbital is a very potent drug and should only be administered within intensive care environments.

Anticoagulant and Fibrinolytic Therapy

Heparin administration has been considered under the premise that its anticoagulation properties may help prevent the recurrence or propagation of a thrombus. Likewise, fibrinolytic therapy has proved to be an effective strategy in the management of an acute stroke due to its fibrinolytic actions in selected patients. However, neither heparin nor fibrinolytic therapy has been proven (or disproved) as a universally safe and effective treatment for an acute stroke patient. Therefore, it is still not recommended as a routine treatment for the stroke patient, and its administration, if any, should be under the strict guidance of the patient's neurologist.

Overall Goals of Acute Stroke/TIA Management

During the acute management phase of a patient experiencing either an acute ischemic stroke or TIA, the goals are to support any lost or diminished functions of the airway, breathing, and circulation. Additionally, the care provider should treat any cardiac emergencies according to the appropriate algorithms presented elsewhere in this text, and initiate ICP reduction measures. There should be expedited transfer of the patient to initiate advanced diagnostic studies so that additional treatment, potentially including fibrinolytics, may be appropriately rendered. Figure 12-4 identifies the treatment algorithm for the patient with an acute ischemic stroke.

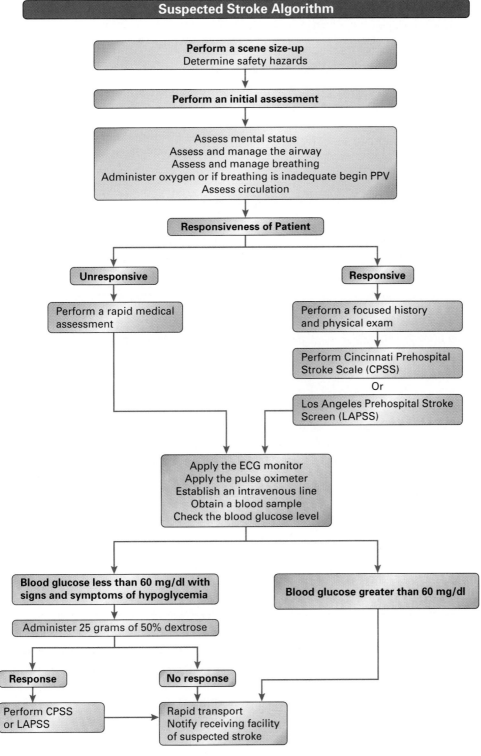

Suspected Stroke Algorithm

Perform a scene size-up
Determine safety hazards

Perform an initial assessment

Assess mental status
Assess and manage the airway
Assess and manage breathing
Administer oxygen or if breathing is inadequate begin PPV
Assess circulation

Responsiveness of Patient

Unresponsive

Perform a rapid medical assessment

Responsive

Perform a focused history and physical exam

Perform Cincinnati Prehospital Stroke Scale (CPSS)
Or
Los Angeles Prehospital Stroke Screen (LAPSS)

Apply the ECG monitor
Apply the pulse oximeter
Establish an intravenous line
Obtain a blood sample
Check the blood glucose level

Blood glucose less than 60 mg/dl with signs and symptoms of hypoglycemia

Blood glucose greater than 60 mg/dl

Administer 25 grams of 50% dextrose

Response

Perform CPSS or LAPSS

No response

Rapid transport
Notify receiving facility of suspected stroke

FIGURE 12–4
Algorithm for initial management of suspected stroke.

CASE STUDY FOLLOW-UP

You are called to the scene for a 56-year-old male patient who is complaining of a sudden onset of weakness to the right side of his body. Noting his slurred speech and facial droop, John's wife recognized the signs of a stroke and called 911.

Assessment

Your initial assessment of John reveals an open airway, adequate ventilation, and good peripheral pulses. His skin is warm and dry. However, the right side of his face droops excessively when he speaks. The monitor shows a normal sinus rhythm at 85 beats per minute. His blood pressure is 178/96, his respiratory rate is 19/minute, and his pulse oximeter reading is 97%.

Recognizing the signs and symptoms of a possible acute stroke, you perform an assessment that will help to confirm your suspicion. You may either perform the Cincinnati Prehospital Stroke Scale (CPSS) or the Los Angeles Prehospital Stroke Screen (LAPSS). You find facial droop, arm drift, and an abnormal speech pattern. His pupils are equal and reactive to light. Initially, John is alert and oriented to person, place, and time; however, as time progresses, his speech becomes more garbled and less comprehensible as his mental status continues to deteriorate.

Treatment

You immediately place John on a nonrebreather mask at 15 lpm and constantly monitor his ventilation status for inadequacy and his airway for the accumulation of secretions. You initiate an intravenous line of normal saline, draw blood, and perform a blood glucose analysis. His glucose reading is 103 mg/dL. You continue to monitor the patient and prepare him for transport. En route, you notify the emergency department of the patient's condition and request that they activate the stroke response team.

Upon arrival at the emergency department, the team rapidly assesses John's condition. The physician conducts an initial assessment and obtains an NIH stroke score. He notifies the CT team that they may need to scan a stroke patient. He orders laboratory studies and establishes a second IV line. The blood pressure remains unchanged. Based on his assessment, the emergency department physician suspects an acute occlusive stroke and sends John for a CT scan. The physician immediately calls for a neurologist and radiologist for a consultation to consider fibrinolytic therapy. The physicians wait for the CT scan results to determine how to proceed with John's treatment.

SUMMARY

The acute stroke, similar to the acute myocardial infarction, is a devastating cardiovascular event that claims more than one hundred thousand lives each year in the United States. It results from ischemic damage to the brain caused by the occlusion or rupture of a blood vessel that perfuses the brain. A transient ischemic attack (TIA) has a similar etiology with similar signs and symptoms, but resolves itself within 24 hours. However, a TIA is often the precursor of a full acute ischemic stroke.

The initial management goals are to support any lost or diminished functions in the airway, breathing, and circulation. Early recognition of the signs and symptoms of stroke, expeditious transport by EMS, and aggressive assessment and intervention by the emergency department physician and staff or stroke center staff are paramount to reducing the morbidity and mortality of an acute ischemic stroke.

REVIEW QUESTIONS

1. While an acute stroke and a TIA may both produce focal neurologic deficits, only an acute ischemic stroke
   a. will have an abatement of signs and symptoms within 24 hours.
   b. is caused by a hemorrhage only, while a TIA is from a thrombus.
   c. will not cause cardiac arrest.
   d. will result in death of brain cells.
   e. none of the above

2. Why is the identification of a TIA so important?
   a. because it may foretell an impending acute ischemic stroke
   b. so anticonvulsant medications can be administered early
   c. to limit the extent of residual damage
   d. so that the patient can be put on a healthy diet and exercise plan

3. Essentially any neurologic abnormality can occur with an acute stroke or a TIA.
   a. true
   b. false

4. Upon noxious stimuli application to a patient suffering an acute stroke, he opens his eyes and tries to push your hand away while making incomprehensible sounds. Based on this limited information, his Glasgow Coma Scale score would be
   a. 3.
   b. 5.
   c. 7.
   d. 9.
   e. 11.

5. Which of the following treatments may be beneficial in reducing ICP early in the management of an acute stroke or TIA patient?
   a. controlled mild hyperventilation for those with focal neurological changes
   b. IV therapy
   c. Trendelenburg positioning
   d. administration of anticonvulsants to prevent seizures

6. Which of the following is a common distinguishing sign or symptom of a hemorrhagic stroke?
   a. hemiparesis and hemiplegia
   b. abrupt onset of a severe headache
   c. pupillary fixation and dilation
   d. nausea and vomiting

7. When bilateral cerebral hemisphere damage has occurred due to a large acute stroke, which respiratory pattern will most likely occur?
   a. central neurogenic hyperventilation
   b. Biot's
   c. Cheyne-Stokes
   d. apneustic

8. The doll's eyes maneuver in the comatose patient provides an indication of
   a. the integrity of the brainstem.
   b. encroachment on the third cranial nerve.
   c. herniation through the tentorial incisura.
   d. cerebellar function.

9. For fibrinolytic therapy to be considered in the acute ischemic stroke patient, the drug must be administered within how many hours from onset of symptoms?
   a. 1
   b. 3
   c. 6
   d. 36

10. Aggressive management of hypertension should be considered in which of the following types of stroke etiology?
    a. embolic
    b. thrombotic
    c. hemorrhagic
    d. none of the above

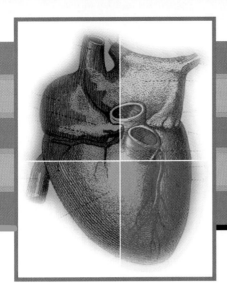

Special Resuscitation Situations

Not every cardiac arrest is precipitated by a problem with the heart. When a person suffers cardiac arrest from a non-cardiac cause, such as trauma or hypothermia, resuscitation must be attempted, just as for any patient in arrest from a cardiac cause. In addition, however, special consideration must be given to the condition that caused the arrest. This is a patient who probably has a healthy heart and has an excellent chance of successful resuscitation if the underlying cause is identified and treated.

Topics in this chapter are:

Traumatic Cardiac Arrests

Cardiac Arrest and Pregnancy

Lightning Strikes

Hypothermia Induced Arrest

Water Submersion Emergencies

Toxicologic Cardiac Emergencies and Arrest

CASE STUDY

It is a cold day in late January, and you are outside your house taking down your Christmas decorations and lights. As you are coiling up a string of lights, you hear the faint pitch of a siren approaching your neighborhood. The siren gets louder and louder until you realize that the ambulance is turning onto your street. As a volunteer for your town's Fire Department/EMS Service, you quickly glance around to the neighbors' houses—trying to see if anything looks awry—when you see your neighbors two houses down waving frantically at the approaching ambulance. They are new to the neighborhood, and you briskly walk across the front yards to ask Mrs. Tieche if you can help.

Through her tears she tells you her nephew David has fallen through the ice in the pond behind the neighbors' house. The paramedics grab their gear and walk past you as Mrs. Tieche leads them behind the house. As a volunteer, you elect to offer your help. As soon as you get to the backyard, you see the limp, blue, cold body of a young man lying supine on the frozen ground. Mr. Tieche is performing CPR.

How would you proceed to assess and care for this patient? In this chapter, you will learn about special patient considerations that may necessitate a change in your routine management for cardiovascular emergencies. Later, we will return to the case study and apply the procedure learned.

INTRODUCTION

This book emphasizes the cardiac arrest that is precipitated by a failure or disturbance in the myocardium itself. This emphasis is deliberate, because the majority of cardiac arrests do occur in an older population who have some form of cardiac disease.

However, it is important to realize that *not all cardiac arrests are caused primarily by heart disease.* The subset of patients who suffer cardiac arrest from other etiologies is small. However, it is extremely important to recognize these patients and understand the physiology behind their arrests—and then understand why they require special assessment and management considerations—in order to appropriately and effectively manage the emergency in the prehospital setting. It is important to remember that many of the patients in this category may still have a healthy heart. And successful resuscitation is likely if they are provided the appropriate treatment aimed at the cause of their arrest.

This chapter is designed to introduce you to these special resuscitation considerations, and provide you with a functional knowledge of how to handle these special emergencies requiring resuscitation.

TRAUMATIC CARDIAC ARRESTS

Assessing and treating a patient in cardiac arrest from a traumatic incident can be most frustrating to the prehospital advanced cardiac life support provider. Unlike the majority of patients with cardiac arrest from a cardiac problem, traumatic arrests can occur from a host of diverse etiologies. Too often prehospital providers look at the patient in terms of *how* he came to be in arrest (e.g., car crash, fall, gunshot), rather than by what *organ systems* have been involved in that traumatic incident. This narrow approach may cause one to overlook certain injuries, or to provide a "knee-jerk" itinerary of interventions that may (or may not) be 100% appropriate for the patient.

TABLE 13–1 Potential Causes of Traumatic Cardiac Arrest

- Acute internal hemorrhage from an abdominal or thoracic injury
- Profound hypoxia from a disturbance of airway patency, or pulmonary efficacy (airway obstruction, laryngeal fracture, pneumothorax, open chest wall injury)
- Severe CNS damage from cervical spinal cord injury or head injury
- Direct trauma to vital organs (lungs, heart, great blood vessels)
- Inadequate cardiac output from excessive mechanical pressure on the heart (tension pneumothorax, pericardial tamponade)
- Acute external hemorrhage (arterial and large venous) from soft tissue injury

The best approach is to first find out how the person was traumatized (the mechanism of injury), and then relate that to the organ system(s) that may be involved in the trauma. This approach will allow you to focus your attention appropriately on the real causative agent(s) of the arrest. Remember these two points regarding traumatic arrests: (1) *The traumatic incident is what caused the organ system failure,* and (2) *the organ system failure is what caused the cardiac arrest.*

Understand, also, that a variety of mechanisms of injury that *seem* to be different are essentially the same and produce similar injuries. Take, for example, an unrestrained driver who crashes his car and sustains severe chest wall injuries. He may go into arrest from a pulmonary injury that causes profound hypoxia, or from pericardial tamponade, or even from acute hemorrhaging into the thorax from a torn aorta. But yet the same chest injuries could be anticipated in a different patient who sustains his injuries when a car falls off a jack-stand and lands on his chest. The point is simply this: Use the mechanism of injury *only* as a clue to give you insight to the organs that are probably involved in the trauma, then focus your assessment and management energy on correcting those deficits.

Table 13-1 lists potential causes of arrest following trauma.

Approach to the Traumatic Cardiac Arrest Patient

The causes of traumatic cardiac arrest are numerous. The cardiac arrest patient from a traumatic cause can have such profound damage that even the best medicine today is incapable of correcting the problems and preventing death. Both blunt and penetrating etiologies of traumatic cardiac arrest carry an extremely poor prognosis. These patients rarely survive, and are usually not resuscitated in the emergency department should they be found in an asystolic or agonal PEA rhythm. But since it is virtually impossible to fully assess the extent of damage in the prehospital phase, most traumatic patients should be extended full cardiopulmonary resuscitation focused on replacing or supporting lost vital functions and correcting underlying abnormalities in oxygenation and circulation.

The limitation to providing full resuscitation to the traumatized cardiac arrest patient is when the cardiac arrest exists in conjunction with a severed head or trunk (decapitation or hemicorporectomy), full body burns, severe blunt trauma with no pupillary response, no vital signs and no shockable cardiac rhythm, deeply penetrating wound to the cranium, or penetrating cranial or trunk wounds with an anticipated transport time of 15 minutes or more (Table 13-2). In these patients, the extent of damage is so grave that attempts at resuscitation are often futile. Since the exact criteria for withholding or initiating resuscitation vary across the nation, it is up to you to become familiar with and adhere to the policy and protocols established by your EMS system.

TABLE 13–2 Traumatic Arrests in which Resuscitation is Unlikely

- Hemicorporectomy or decapitation
- Full body burns
- Severe blunt trauma with absence of all of the following:
  - pupillary response (and)
  - vital signs (and)
  - shockable cardiac rhythms
- Deeply penetrating cranial injury (ies)
- Penetrating cranial and/or truncal wound(s) with prolonged (>15 min) transport time to a health care facility

Treatment of the Traumatic Cardiac Arrest Patient

Specifically, initial prehospital management of the trauma cardiac arrest should include the following:

- Manual cervical spine immobilization until full spinal immobilization is achieved
- Airway management with close attention to supporting inadequate breathing with positive pressure ventilation, oxygen, and tracheal intubation
- Rapid control of external hemorrhage
- Application and interpretation of the ECG monitor
  - If PEA is present, actively look for cause (e.g., fluid loss, tension pneumothorax, tamponade) and treat it.
  - If ventricular fibrillation is present, treat according to the V-fib algorithm.
  - If bradyasystolic rhythms are present, consider severe terminal hypovolemia or significant hypoxemia.
- Intravenous access with an isotonic crystalloid (lactated Ringer's or normal saline) and fluid boluses of 20 ml/kg if hypovolemia is known or suspected
  - If successful resuscitation does occur, attempt to keep systolic pressure about 90 mmHg (not much higher) in order to reduce the possibility of rebleeding.
- Assessment for, and treatment of, injuries leading to the arrest
  - Life threatening injuries to airway, bellows action of the thorax, uncontrolled hemorrhage
- Administration of medications and nonpharmacologic interventions as appropriate for the presenting cardiac ECG tracing
- Rapid transport to emergency department (preferably Level I trauma center)

In conclusion, decisions about appropriate management of the traumatic cardiac arrest must be made in light of the underlying organ failure. In some instances, simple correction of an occluded airway, relief of a tension pneumothorax, or control of external hemorrhage may be all that is necessary to achieve a successful resuscitation. It is of utmost importance for the care provider to assess the mechanism of injury to determine probable body organs involved, and then perform the assessment and treatment necessary to support and/or replace lost functions. However, the care provider must also recognize those situations in which resuscitation of the traumatic arrest patient is futile and would result in a needless expenditure of resources.

⊞ CARDIAC ARREST AND PREGNANCY

Assessment and treatment of a pregnant woman in the prehospital environment is different than for the non-pregnant patient because of the changes that take place in the cardiovascular and respiratory systems during pregnancy. These changes (as discussed below) result in an altered presentation of the common signs and symptoms of certain medical emergencies. When you understand the basic changes in physiology, you can provide more appropriate and efficient assessment and care.

Briefly, the most prominent changes in the female's body during pregnancy are increases in blood volume, resting heart rate and cardiac output, resting respiratory rate and oxygen consumption, a decrease in blood pressure (especially in the latter trimester), loosening of hip joints, displacement of abdominal organs, and increased pressure on the inferior vena cava (Table 13-3).

These changes result in an increase in susceptibility to cardiovascular and respiratory emergencies, while at the same time they reduce the patient's ability to compensate for the insult.

Finally, it is also extremely important to realize that you have two patients: the mother and her unborn child. Treatment you administer to the mother must, therefore, serve the twin goals of reversing the mother's emergency as well as ensuring uninterrupted and sufficient oxygenation and circulation to the fetus. While there are numerous factors that can lead to fetal complications, the number one cause of fetal death is maternal death.

Treatment of the Pregnant Cardiac Arrest Patient

Cardiac arrest in a pregnant female, while relatively rare, is possible from medical and traumatic causes. And when it does occur, the resuscitative interventions and medication normally used during an arrest should be administered. This includes electrical therapy, closed chest compressions, and ventilatory management with intubation.

It is also important to take measures that will help reduce the pressure of the gravid uterus on the inferior vena cava to avoid a decrease in venous return to the heart as the weight of the fetus collapses the inferior vena cava between the uterus and the sacrum. The resulting drop in preload will reduce arterial pressure. This "supine hypotensive syndrome" can result in hypotension by itself, or it can worsen any hypotension that may already be present from the initial traumatic or medical insult. To minimize this effect, place the patient on her left side at a 15- to 20-degree angle or tilt the backboard if the patient is immobilized. This will help displace the uterus off the vena cava and improve venous return. Manual displacement is another option, but it is physically tiring and is not any more effective.

TABLE 13–3 | Physical Changes in a Pregnant Woman

- Increase in blood volume by approximately 50%
- Increase in resting heart rate and cardiac output
- Decrease in blood pressure (more pronounced near term)
- Increase in resting respiratory rate
- Overall increase in oxygen consumption
- Loosening of hip joints (leads to increased trauma from falls)
- Displacement of abdominal organs from the gravid uterus
- Increased pressure on the inferior vena cava by the uterus

If the pregnant patient is in cardiac arrest and her fetus is viable, it may become necessary to perform an emergency cesarean section to save the baby. This should be an option only after the following measures have been proven unsuccessful in restoring effective spontaneous circulation in the mother:

▶ Properly performed artificial circulation (CPR)

▶ Displacement of the gravid uterus to the left

▶ Fluid therapy for vascular volume

▶ Medication therapy appropriate to the presenting cardiac rhythm

The decision to perform an emergency cesarean section is one that should not be taken lightly. Numerous additional factors need to be taken into consideration—for example, the factors that precipitated the maternal arrest, availability of personnel capable of performing the procedure, the gestational age of the fetus, and the amount of time since the onset of the maternal arrest. Optimally, the procedure should be performed within 5 minutes of the arrest; however, successful infant survival has been documented after 20 minutes of maternal arrest. In the prehospital management of maternal arrest, the possibility that the baby may survive even if the mother cannot be saved underscores the importance of proper oxygenation, ventilations, compressions, IV therapy, and medication administration.

Specifically, initial management of the pregnant cardiac arrest patient should include the following:

▶ Performance of CPR with the patient rolled to her left at 20 degrees. This may be best accomplished by placing the patient on a backboard and supporting it with pillows or blankets.

▶ Airway management with intubation, ventilation, and maximal oxygenation

▶ Pharmacological support and fluid therapy as appropriate for the patient's cardiac rhythm and physiological condition

▶ Consider the feasibility of emergency cesarean section and/or early notification of the receiving facility that an emergency cesarean may be warranted

In summary, treatment of the pregnant female who suffers cardiac arrest includes appropriate treatment for the mother while ensuring the best opportunity for survival of the fetus should the mother fail to have a return of spontaneous circulation. To this end, proper treatment of the cardiac arrest is essential. The care provider should administer the normal modalities for the arrest, as well as specific interventions discussed above for the pregnant female. Remember, also, that the mother is still the best incubator for the fetus, and all efforts should be extended to reverse the cardiac arrest and return normal circulation.

⊞ LIGHTNING STRIKES

Lightning strikes are the number one cause of deaths from natural environmental phenomena. Hundreds of persons die from lightning strikes every year, while many others sustain injuries, and numerous survivors of lightning strikes have residual effects.

The mortality rate from lightning strikes is about 30%. It is actually an interesting question why more people do *not* die, considering that a lightning strike can deliver over 100 million volts. One reason for the relatively high survival rate is thought to be the "flash-over" effect. The theory is that the energy of a lightning strike is delivered in such a brief instant that most of it "flashes over" the outside of the body. Since a relatively small amount of electricity actually enters the body, there is a relatively good chance for survival.

Despite the "flash-over" theory, some individuals apparently receive a flow of energy through their body that is high enough to disrupt normal cardiac and respiratory activity, or it may be that certain individuals are more susceptible than others to the effects of a lightning strike. In either case, the primary cause of death from a lightning strike is asystole or ventricular fibrillation (which is usually secondary to prolonged apnea).

With a lightning strike, the electrical current flow acts like a massive direct current defibrillation that depolarizes the heart, producing asystole. In numerous instances, following this depolarization, the heart is able to repolarize appropriately and restore normal electrical activity and spontaneous circulation. Unfortunately, however, there is also depression of the brain stem secondary to the lightning strike that causes prolonged periods of apnea. As a result, the patient may develop spontaneous electrical activity of the heart producing blood flow, but then, since the apnea has been shown to persist, the patient deteriorates into ventricular fibrillation or asystole secondary to hypoxia.

Treatment of the Patient in Cardiac Arrest from a Lightning Strike

The management goals for a patient in cardiac arrest following a lightning strike are similar to those for a patient who has experienced a cardiac arrest under more "normal" circumstances. The purpose of your treatment should be to provide aggressive ventilation or oxygenation and perfusion to the heart and brain until cardiac activity is restored and ventilatory efforts again become spontaneous.

Specifically, initial management of the patient in cardiac arrest from a lightning strike should include the following:

▶ Precautionary spinal immobilization
▶ Securing the airway with tracheal intubation (in the presence of facial burns from the strike, early intubation may avoid the problems seen later with laryngeal or pharyngeal edema)
▶ Oxygenation and positive pressure ventilation
▶ Cardiac monitoring, and administration of defibrillation if necessary
▶ IV therapy for medication administration; limit fluid boluses unless necessary
▶ Appropriate stabilization of related injuries secondary to the strike (e.g., fractures, burns)

In a situation where numerous people are injured in the same lightning strike, it behooves the prehospital provider to alter his assessment format to allow those who "look dead" to be treated first. This way, you will be sure to provide ventilation, oxygenation, and artificial circulation to those individuals until a perfusing rhythm and spontaneous respirations return. In the instance where you have a patient displaying only apnea after the strike, the provision of ventilation and oxygenation will help prevent secondary hypoxic cardiac arrest.

⊞ HYPOTHERMIA INDUCED ARREST

Hypothermia in association with respiratory and cardiac arrest deserves special discussion, because the body tends to decrease all metabolic and related activity as the core temperature decreases, and this in turn allows the body to survive longer periods of arrest. This is especially true when hypothermia occurs rapidly. The cardiac arrest event precedes organ ischemia and necrosis and this allows cells of the body to live slightly longer, thereby increasing the likelihood of resuscitation. Although rare in its episodes, it has been documented that under certain circumstances of hypothermia, patients may still have full neurological recovery despite prolonged arrest.

Physiologic changes that accompany hypothermia include:

▶ Decreased metabolic rate, cerebral blood flow, and oxygen requirements

▶ Decreased cardiac output

▶ Decreased respiratory activity

▶ Diminished mental function (confusion)

▶ Progressive hypotension

▶ Flaccid muscles

▶ Eventual unconsciousness and cardiac arrest

In the hypothermic patient, resuscitative measures should be instituted as soon as it is safe to do so, with less attention paid to the length of time in arrest than in other arrest situations. How long can the period of arrest be, and still have neurologic recovery? There is no concrete answer to that question since there are so many variables that play a role in eventual recovery. The length of time submerged or exposed to the cold environment, the exact temperature of the environment, the age of the patient, the general health condition of the victim, presence of associated trauma, and length of time till rewarming is initiated—all factor into the potential for a successful resuscitation.

Basic-Life-Support Treatment

The hypothermic patient may still be in an environment that is dangerous to the provider of initial emergency care. As with all prehospital calls, it is your responsibility to keep yourself and your team safe, as well as eager bystanders who want to help with the rescue. The goal here is to minimize the risk of danger to yourself, your coworkers, and bystanders, as well as to avoid additional harm to the patient.

The first goal of management is to assess and support lost vital functions. Assess vital signs in any hypothermic patient for about 30–45 seconds. This is to assure that you will not miss an extremely bradypneic or bradycardic rhythm. Airway maintenance and rescue breathing or ventilations with a BVM should be initiated as early *as safely possible* when the spontaneous respirations are lost or diminished. Concurrently, full spinal immobilization should be maintained, since there may be an unknown risk that trauma was associated with the emergency.

Chest compressions for the hypothermic patient should be carried out according to normal CPR standards. Another intervention appropriate during the initial management is to remove any wet/cold garments, and to protect the patient from heat loss by shielding the patient from the environment and/or wrapping the patient in dry material.

When hypothermia is present, as confirmed by a temperature recording, rewarming interventions may be indicated. The degree of hypothermia may predispose the patient to the "after-drop" phenomenon. (After-drop is the sudden return of cold, acidic blood to the heart from the cold extremities after the extremities have been rewarmed and the peripheral vessels begin to dilate). However, after-drop can be mitigated by rewarming the patient. Remember, however, that a cold heart is also very susceptible to the irritability caused by rough handling of the patient. During treatment, be cautious and handle the patient gently to avoid precipitating ventricular fibrillation.

Advanced-Life-Support Treatment

Treatment goals for the hypothermic patient in cardiac arrest share the same as those for any other cardiac arrest patient: Early intubation, defibrillation, IV access, and drug therapy as appropriate—however the application of these interventions do come with special criteria. Without having a thermometer capable of assessing core temperature extremes (most "standard" thermometers do not register high nor low enough for environmental emergencies), it may be impossible to determine the exact core temperature, which is key to the interventions recommended for the patient.

Treatment for the hypothermic patient in cardiac arrest is slightly different than for patients in arrest from other causes. As mentioned earlier, many physical manipulations and interventions (e.g., moving the patient, intubating, pacing) have been shown to precipitate ventricular fibrillation in a hypothermic patient who is not yet in full cardiac arrest. While these interventions must never be withheld when needed, it is important to keep this in mind when dealing with hypothermic patients.

The severely hypothermic heart may not be as responsive to cardiac drug and electrical therapy as the normothermic heart. Also, medications may not "work" in hypothermic, acidic environments. Additionally, movement of IV push drugs to the core circulation may be delayed by peripheral vasoconstriction, sludged blood, and diminished perfusion pressures with CPR. The concern is that the drugs will accumulate to toxic levels in the extremities and then be "dumped" on the heart as rewarming begins. Thus the primary treatment for the severely hypothermic patient (core temp < 30°C) is aimed at internal rewarming until the core temperature is brought up to a range where the body will respond to more aggressive therapy. Once this has been achieved, the other interventions and therapies may be carried out. Utilizing this approach will afford the hypothermic cardiac arrest patient the greatest chances for a successful resuscitation.

■ WATER SUBMERSION EMERGENCIES

Cardiac arrest associated with submersion, like hypothermic arrests, also deserves special discussion because of how the precipitating event influences the body's physiology's. Even though a submersion emergency is a distinctly different emergency from hypothermia, it is mentioned because almost all submersion victims have some degree of hypothermia. For this reason, the treatment of the two is very similar. As with hypothermia, the physical appearance of the submersion victim may be deceiving, presenting much like death. Oftentimes, the exact length of time underwater is not known, so attempts at resuscitation should be started immediately unless grossly obvious signs of death are present (such as rigor mortis, dependent lividity, or putrefaction).

In submersion, in addition to hypothermia, other physiological factors increase the likelihood of successful resuscitation with neurological recovery. The "mammalian diving reflex" occurs in any person who dives into cold water (< 68°F). This reflex causes:

▶ Inhibition of breathing
▶ Slowing of heart rate

▶ Vasoconstriction of peripheral vessels

▶ Constant blood flow maintained to heart/brain

▶ About a 50% drop in metabolic activity

In the submersion emergency, resuscitative measures should be instituted as soon as it is safe to do so, with less attention paid to the length of time in arrest than in other arrest situations. How long can the period of arrest be, and still have neurologic recovery? The same variables that play a role in eventual recovery for the hypothermic patient apply to a submersion victim. The length of time submerged, the exact temperature of the water, the age of the patient, the general health condition of the victim, presence of associated trauma, and length of time till rewarming is initiated—all factor into the potential for a successful resuscitation.

Basic-Life-Support Treatment

As with the hypothermic patient, the submersion victim may still be in an environment that is dangerous to the provider of initial emergency care. In a hazardous situation like this, trained and experienced experts must carry out water rescue. It is your responsibility to keep not only yourself and your team safe, but also to keep eager bystanders safe should they want to "jump-in" and help with the rescue. Remember, the goal here is to minimize the risk of danger to yourself, your coworkers, and the bystanders, as well as to avoid additional harm to the patient.

The first goal of management is to assess and support lost vital functions. Airway maintenance and rescue breathing or ventilations with a BVM and oxygen should be initiated as early as safely possible when the spontaneous respirations are lost or diminished. Concurrently, full spinal immobilization should be maintained, since many times there is trauma associated with the emergency. This is especially true with diving emergencies, since the patient may have struck his head while diving into shallow or unknown water. In these instances, immobilization needs to be carried out while the patient is still in the water. Even if trauma isn't confirmed, immobilization is recommended until x-rays rule out any spinal injury.

Chest compressions for the submersion victim should be carried out according to normal CPR standards. Another intervention appropriate during the initial management is to remove any wet garments and to protect the patient from heat loss by shielding the patient from the environment and/or wrapping the patient in dry material.

Advanced-Life-Support Treatment

Treatment goals and interventions for the submersion victim are the same as for any other cardiac arrest patient: Early intubation, defibrillation, IV access, and drug therapy as appropriate. Often, it may be impossible to determine the exact length of submersion. Therefore, the patient should be provided with full advanced cardiac life support on scene and en route to the hospital, where the emergency department physician can decide whether or not to maintain resuscitative efforts. If the resuscitation is successful, the patient should be transported to a health care facility regardless of patient stability.

Treatment for the submersion victim with some degree of hypothermia is also slightly different than for patients in arrest from other causes. As mentioned earlier, many physical manipulations and interventions (e.g., moving the patient, intubating, pacing) have been shown to precipitate ventricular fibrillation in a hypothermic patient who is not yet in full cardiac arrest. While these interventions must never be withheld when needed, it is important to keep this in mind when dealing with hypothermia.

TOXICOLOGIC CARDIAC EMERGENCIES AND ARREST

Due to the proliferation of drug use in our society, both legal and illegal, emergency cardiac care providers need to become aware that certain drugs at a toxic level can interfere not only with CNS activity but can be cardiotoxic as well. For this reason, patients suffering toxic effects from drugs often require specific treatments that may deviate slightly, or significantly, from normal practices.

For example, tricyclic antidepressants (TCAs) are extremely cardiotoxic at high levels. Because it interferes with neurochemical transmitters, a TCA overdose can have profound effects on the heart, ranging from tachydysrhythmias to axis deviations to ventricular irritability. Yet the primary treatment for TCA toxicity is not geared toward treating the dysrhythmia. Rather the specific therapy here is to alkalinize the blood with sodium bicarbonate. This, as you can see, is a major deviation from normal advanced-cardiac-life-support practice.

The problem is the difficulty, or impossibility, of identifying any and all drugs with cardiac side effects. Realistically, it is impossible and unnecessary to try to discuss how each drug will affect the body. Such extensive knowledge is beyond the scope and purpose of this text.

As an alternative, however, the authors want you to consider treating the toxicologic emergency from a "process" point of view. In the process method, approach all toxicologic patients the same way, have certain management goals, and access information centers that will have the information you need to treat the specific overdose.

In the process method, approach the patient with the question "What vital functions have been lost that need support?" and then provide the appropriate care for these functions as your initial stabilization. For example, it does not matter if your patient has overdosed purposely on a narcotic agent, accidentally on an organophosphate agent, or unknowingly on a new anticonvulsant prescription; the patient may be in need of airway maintenance. The provision of airway suctioning, oropharyngeal airway placement, and eventual intubation could all occur without the knowledge of the specific offending agent. The support of lost functions in the prehospital environment is commonly warranted even before the specific agent is discerned. As such, despite the specific type of cardiac emergency, all patients should receive initial stabilization of the ABCs until specific treatments for the toxin have been identified.

Poison Control Centers (PCCs) have been established across the United States and Canada to assist in the treatment of toxicologic emergencies. Officials at the center can assist you in setting priorities and formulating an effective treatment plan. PCC officials can also provide information about any available antidote that may be appropriate for the patient.

Calls to the PCC are typically toll-free, and most are staffed by professionals 24 hours a day to assist health care providers as well as the public. Staffed by experienced professionals, each center is also connected to a network of nationwide consultants who can answer questions about almost any poison. In addition, information on the poison center's computer is updated every 90 days to provide the latest information on treatment options and antidotes.

Be prepared to tell the poison center officials the patient's approximate age and weight. Summarize the patient's condition, including level of responsiveness, level of activity, skin color, vomiting, cardiac activity, and other pertinent physical findings. Any directions from a poison control center should be administered in consultation with the physician receiving your patient in the emergency department.

If the poisoning substance cannot be identified, or the Poison Control Center or medical direction cannot be contacted, the patient in cardiac arrest from a suspected poisoning should be treated symptomatically, based upon presenting rhythm.

CASE STUDY FOLLOW-UP

Assessment

Mrs. Tieche tells you her nephew was walking on the ice to "test" it—making sure it was safe for the kids to play on. She added that when he didn't return to the house, she looked outside and saw the hole in the ice where he had apparently fallen through. "Somehow," she added, "my husband must have pulled him out while I was around front waiting for the ambulance." Estimating, she adds that her nephew must have been under the water for about 15 or 20 minutes.

Even though the patient looks dead, you and the paramedics begin your assessment. Paramedic Lago assesses for a pulse and respirations for a full 30 seconds while Paramedic Davis readies the "quick-look" paddles of the cardiac monitor. To assist in confirming pulselessness, you assess for heart tones as well. As you touch the patient's skin, you note it to be very cold to the touch, with some minor abrasions to the side of his face from falling through the ice.

Treatment

With no signs of life present, and the cardiac monitor displaying an idioventricular rhythm, Paramedic Lago initiates compressions while her partner goes for the immobilization equipment. After ventilations with the BVM, you intubate the patient and resume ventilations with warmed and humidified oxygen, all the time maintaining cervical spine control. Immobilization is completed rapidly, and a tympanic-membrane temperature reveals a temperature of 32°C. CPR is maintained.

You decide to assist the paramedics in the back of the ambulance. Once there, you complete the removal of wet clothing. Since the patient is cold and has poor peripheral veins, the decision is made to initiate an external jugular vein IV. This, you reason, should help speed the drugs to the core circulation, since the jugular vein is physically closer to the core than an arm vein.

The monitor reveals fine ventricular fibrillation, so electrical therapy is applied—without success, as the patient remains in ventricular fibrillation. One mg of epinephrine is administered, and the patient is now en route to the receiving hospital. The onboard oxygen being delivered to the patient is humidified and warmed to assist in internal warming as heating packs are prepared and placed at the groin, axillary, and neck regions. Since the transport time is short, about 10 minutes, there is time to administer only one additional dose of epinephrine along with one dose of amiodarone. Defibrillation is again unsuccessful. Additional medication and electrical therapy are withheld until the core temperature rises.

Upon arrival at the emergency department, the ED staff assess the core temperature to be 33°C. They maintain your rewarming techniques and start to administer warmed IV fluids, as well as initiating additional internal rewarming techniques. After a short period of time, the core temperature has increased, and defibrillation converts the patient into a bradycardic rhythm with a pulse and systolic pressure.

With continued rewarming, the patient's heart rate and systolic blood pressure continues to rise without the assistance of further pharmacological therapy. Care providers are being careful not to aggressively handle the patient. By the time you leave to return home, the patient is physiologically more stable with a core temperature of 36°C. However, the patient has yet to show any signs of neurological recovery.

⊞ SUMMARY

For the majority of cardiac arrests and other cardiac emergencies, treatment is essentially the same. Consideration must be given, however, to those situations where the normal and accepted practices of advanced life support need to be modified to accommodate the patient's specific situation. In this chapter, we have looked at traumatic cardiac arrests, cardiac arrest and pregnancy, and cardiac emergencies associated with lightning strikes, hypothermia, submersions, and toxic drug effects. Emergency cardiac care providers should note carefully the differences in these emergencies with respect to triage, emphasis of treatment, and techniques.

REVIEW QUESTIONS

1. Which of the following traumatic injuries could lead to cardiac arrest?
   a. massive arterial hemorrhage
   b. spinal cord injury
   c. cardiac tamponade
   d. a and c
   e. a, b, and c

2. What treatment must be provided to any cardiac arrest victim from trauma?
   a. spinal immobilization
   b. nasotracheal intubation
   c. IV therapy of D_5W
   d. oxygen at 10 liters per minute

3. What is the proper fluid bolus amount for the trauma victim in need of fluid replacement?
   a. 10 ml/kg
   b. 20 ml/kg
   c. 30 ml/kg
   d. 40 ml/kg

4. Which patient should **not** receive cardiopulmonary resuscitation with advanced life support?
   a. 25-year-old trauma arrest in a PEA rhythm of 60/minute
   b. 63-year-old trauma arrest with full body burns
   c. 51-year-old trauma arrest with hypovolemia
   d. 33-year-old trauma arrest with a tension pneumothorax

5. Which one of these physiological changes in the pregnant female may mask early signs of shock?
   a. gravid uterus
   b. increased pulmonary function
   c. increased metabolic activity and oxygen consumption
   d. increased resting heart rate and cardiac output
   e. c and d

6. The number one cause of fetal death is
   a. trauma to the uterus.
   b. tearing of the placenta.
   c. maternal hypertension.
   d. maternal death.

7. What causes supine hypotensive syndrome in the pregnant female?
   a. pressure on the pulmonary veins
   b. pressure on the descending aorta
   c. pressure on the inferior vena cava
   d. pressure on the iliac arteries and veins

8. The administration of medications used in cardiac arrest should be altered in what way when treating a pregnant female?
   a. Administer half the dose normally used.
   b. Administer the normal dose, but lengthen the repeat times.
   c. Do not administer anything through a central line.
   d. None. Utilize the medications as appropriate for any other arrest.

9. A patient has been struck by lightning while playing golf. What would be the immediate concern regarding treatment?
   a. intubation
   b. positive pressure ventilation
   c. compressions
   d. IV initiation

10. Your lightning victim has been found in ventricular fibrillation. You should immediately
    a. defibrillate at 360 joules.
    b. defibrillate at 300 joules.
    c. defibrillate at 200 joules.
    d. defibrillate at 100 joules.

11. What is the most likely mechanism causing death in the victim struck by lightning?
    a. apnea resulting from depression of the brain stem
    b. persistent ventricular fibrillation that is refractory to drugs
    c. associated trauma from being thrown
    d. extensive burns from the lightning

12. Would it be appropriate to provide spinal immobilization to the cardiac arrest victim who was struck by lightning while providing initial management?
    a. yes
    b. no

13. Which of the following changes is **not** seen in the victim of hypothermia?
    a. slowing heart rate
    b. increasing respiratory rate
    c. redirection of blood flow to heart and brain
    d. drop in metabolic activity

14. What is the **primary** concern when dealing with victims of hypothermia or submersion emergencies?
    a. personal safety during the rescue
    b. early initiation of mouth-to-mouth ventilations
    c. rapid defibrillation
    d. oxygenation

15. Which of the following is true regarding medication administration in the severely hypothermic cardiac arrest patient (core temp < 30°C)?
    a. You should delay administration of drugs until the core temperature rises.
    b. Drugs may not be effective on the hypothermic heart.
    c. Drugs lose their effectiveness when they are chilled by the blood.
    d. Drug dosages should be doubled since they are less effective.

16. All toxicologic cardiac arrests should receive
    a. tracheal intubation.
    b. defibrillation.
    c. specific antidotes for the drug they ingested.
    d. nasogastric tube for gastric evacuation.

17. Poison Control Centers (PCCs) provide
    a. up-to-date treatment plans.
    b. tracking of emerging toxicologic trends.
    c. follow-up to patient treatment.
    d. specific antidotes when necessary.
    e. all of the above

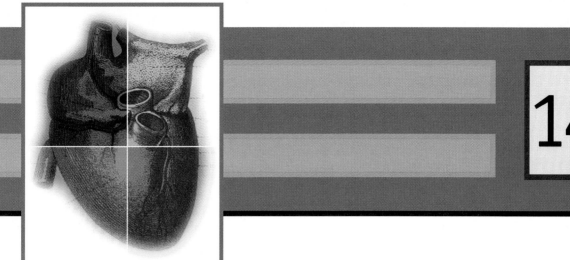

Special Treatment Considerations in the Prehospital Environment

After a cardiac emergency, the patient will be stabilized as best possible in the prehospital environment and then receive continued stabilization by health care providers in the emergency department. Ultimately, the patient will still require definitive care—care that focuses on correcting the underlying problem and restoring the patient, as nearly as possible, to good health. This level of care can best be provided in the coronary care and other intensive care units the patient will inhabit until he is well enough to go home from the hospital. Although they are beyond the normal scope of prehospital advanced cardiac life support education, some of these considerations of definitive care—and other considerations that are not an inherent part of advanced cardiac life support— are briefly introduced in this chapter.

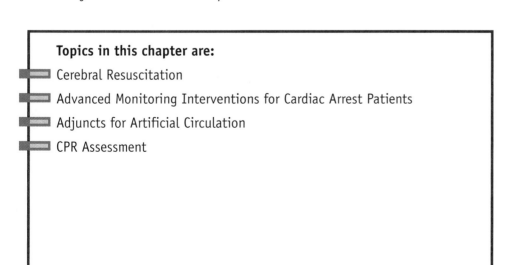

Topics in this chapter are:

- Cerebral Resuscitation
- Advanced Monitoring Interventions for Cardiac Arrest Patients
- Adjuncts for Artificial Circulation
- CPR Assessment

CASE STUDY

Freshly armed with additional knowledge and skills you acquired in a recent advanced cardiac life support lecture during your paramedic program, you have arranged to complete some internship "ride-along" time with your designated ALS service.

The day continues to drag by slowly. After completing 11 hours of your 12-hour shift, you have yet to get even one trip. Finally, about 15 minutes before it's time for you to leave, a call comes in for a "man-down."

When you arrive on scene about 4 minutes later, you see a collapsed man, on his back, with the first responders performing two-person CPR. You think you understood what you learned in your ACLS class, but your heart is pounding anyway as you follow your preceptors Joe and Rich toward the patient.

How would you proceed to assess and care for this patient? This chapter will describe the assessment and necessary treatment of a patient with a cardiac emergency that may require special treatment considerations. Later, we will return to the case and apply the procedures learned.

INTRODUCTION

We begin this chapter by reiterating that the goal of advanced cardiac life support is to temporarily correct (or supplement) altered physiological processes until definitive care can be provided. It is important for you to realize that care rendered in the prehospital and emergency department settings are temporizing measures. Rarely would a patient be cured (let alone discharged) from an emergency department visit after suffering a cardiac arrest. It is not that this level of care is impossible in the ED, but rather that it is reserved for care providers who have the special training and the day-to-day experience and resources to manage patients during that extremely delicate post arrest period.

The obvious example is the typical progression of a cardiac arrest victim through the health care system. First, prehospital advanced life support providers initially resuscitate the patient with early CPR, defibrillation, drug therapy, and airway maintenance while the patient is transported to the emergency department. Secondly, the emergency department staff focuses on continued stabilization with subsequent transport to a coronary care unit. It is in the coronary care unit and step-down units that definitive care takes place.

The following discussion is intended to provide you with an introduction to some of the special treatment considerations that, for the most part, are a part of definitive cardiac care. A full explanation of these concerns is well beyond the scope of this text. The authors recommend that prehospital or intensive/critical care paramedics who need additional information regarding these topics seek the support of the specialty areas of the hospital where these procedures and technologies are more commonplace, and refer to texts devoted specifically to them. (Enlist the help of cardiologists and internal medicine physicians for references.) The authors hope that this approach will encourage you to expand your knowledge of these special areas while keeping the essential purposes of advanced cardiac life support in focus.

CEREBRAL RESUSCITATION

Since the brain is the foundation on which the body must rely, once the heart has been resuscitated it is imperative to restore cerebral blood flow to near normal levels and to correct any concerns of hypoxemia and acidosis. It is a certainty that if the brain is not being properly oxygenated or perfused, it is just a matter of time until cardiac arrest will recur.

After cardiac arrest occurs and cerebral blood flow (CBF) ceases, humans will lose consciousness in about 15 seconds. As the residual levels of glucose and adenosine triphosphate (ATP) are exhausted, the respirations become agonal and the pupils become fixed and dilated. This deterioration of cerebral functioning occurs rapidly, with irreversible damage occurring in roughly 6–10 minutes. (However, be aware that more recent research has indicated some cerebral neurons may be more resistant to ischemia than previously believed.) It is during this period of clinical death that prehospital and in hospital advanced cardiac life support attempts to restore cerebral perfusion by compensating for and/or correcting the effects of cardiac arrest.

The restoration of cerebral perfusion after cardiac arrest is not problem-free. For a period of some hours, in fact, additional brain damage may occur. This "postresuscitation syndrome," as it is called by the American Heart Association, is marked by cerebral blood flow that is still inadequate to meet cerebral demands despite the return of spontaneous cardiac output. While the exact cause of postresuscitation syndrome is yet unknown, it is believed that one influence is the loss of cerebral autoregulation of blood flow. Under normal circumstances, the brain has the ability to autoregulate its blood flow by either vasoconstricting or vasodilating cerebral vessels in order to maintain a constant cerebral blood flow across the variances of systolic pressure. This autoregulation, however, when lost following cardiac arrest (or even following significant head injuries) results in hypoperfusion of the brain with continued cellular ischemia and necrosis. Some hypotheses point to the possibility of reflex vasoconstriction due to abnormal calcium movement, platelet clumping (aggregation), red blood cell deformity, and/or capillary bed edema.

Regardless of the cause of the syndrome, the key for health care providers is to remember that the normal ability of the brain to maintain its perfusion seems to be diminished or lost during a period of time that may last up to 24 hours after a cardiac arrest has been corrected. They must be attuned to certain physiologic considerations and procedures aimed toward ensuring adequate CBF and maximal cerebral outcome for the patient (Figure 14-1).

Cerebral Perfusion Pressures

As mentioned above, under normal circumstances the brain has the ability to autoregulate its own blood flow. So when there are fluctuations in the systolic pressure, the brain will adjust its vascular tone to maintain a constant CBF. However, as a result of the tissue damage and accumulation of acids and metabolites common to cardiac arrest, this ability of autoregulation is temporarily diminished. During the postresuscitation period, the most important extracranial determinant of CBF is systolic blood pressure. For the prehospital care provider, this means that the systolic pressure must be returned to levels that are similar to, or slightly higher than, those observed prior to the cardiac arrest. This should be accomplished by using vasopressors and fluid therapy as appropriate.

Oxygenation

Optimal oxygenation will provide the cells with sufficient oxygen to support their metabolic activity. As a guide, maintaining the PaO_2 above 100 mmHg should

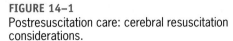

FIGURE 14–1
Postresuscitation care: cerebral resuscitation
considerations.

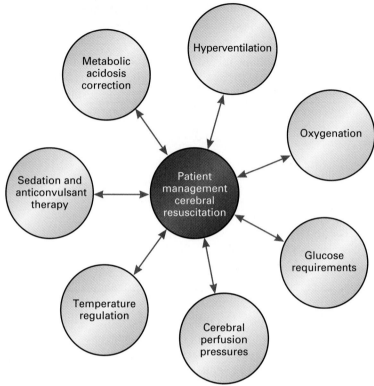

allow for proper oxygenation. Since there may be pulmonary damage as a result of
the arrest that may interfere with oxygen diffusion, positive end-expiratory pressure (PEEP) may be utilized to assure oxygenation across the alveolar wall. The
goal is to maintain a pulse oximetry saturation above 95% with PaO_2 of 100
mmHg.

Hyperventilation

Hyperventilation has been shown to have two main benefits to the post cardiac
arrest patient. First, hyperventilation should help eliminate excessive accumula-
tions of CO_2 (especially after sodium bicarbonate administration) via the lungs,
helping to reverse tissue acidosis that is common during arrest. Secondly, some
research has indicated that, by lowering the $PaCO_2$ through controlled hyperventilation, there is a reflexive constriction of cerebral vessels. The enhanced vasoconstriction, in turn, lowers intracranial pressure (ICP) by decreasing the amount of
blood flow through the brain.

While the concept of vasoconstriction may seem contradictory to improving
cerebral perfusion, in those individuals with high ICP, the vasoconstriction can
actually enhance cerebral perfusion pressure by lowering ICP. (Review the information on intracranial pressure as a factor in cerebral perfusion pressure in
Chapter 12 on strokes.) This effect is only temporary, however. The body's normal
acid-base adjustment systems start to compensate for the drop in $PaCO_2$ and the
effects diminish after about 4 hours. If you are providing mechanical ventilation to
a post arrest victim and simultaneously monitoring end-tidal carbon dioxide levels, one recommendation is to keep the $PetCO_2$ levels between 35–40 mmHg.
There may be clinical reasons to ventilate the patient and maintain a $PetCO_2$ at or
around 25–30 mmHg should evidence of increased intracranial pressure be present

(e.g., evidence of herniation). But as always, rely on medical direction or standing orders if there is a question or concern regarding desired PetCO$_2$ levels.

Metabolic Acidosis Correction

The longer a person is in cardiac arrest, the worse the acidosis becomes. While hyperventilation will help eliminate the carbon dioxide created during the body's buffering of metabolic acidosis, the buffering mechanism can easily become overwhelmed by massive cellular acidosis. In the post arrest patient, the continued acidosis depresses myocardial activity and contributes to eventual death. To help correct this, proper ventilation should be continued with tracheal intubation and an adequate minute ventilation. The administration of sodium bicarbonate should be guided by blood gas analysis and occur secondary to establishment of proper ventilation.

Temperature Regulation

An often-overlooked aspect of patient management, temperature control can be a benefit to post arrest management or become a detriment if left unattended. Research has shown how an increase in core temperature causes an increase in metabolic rate and oxygen demand. As the cerebral metabolic rate increases, it requires an additional flow of oxygenated blood to meet metabolic demands. This increase may be enough to aggravate the already poor balance between supply and demand in a post arrest brain.

Conversely, hypothermia is a widely accepted way to depress cerebral metabolic activity and, consequently, blood-flow requirements. However, in the post arrest scenario, hypothermia also contributes to increased blood viscosity and a drop in cardiac output—both of which are a detriment to cerebral perfusion after cardiac arrest. Researchers cannot agree as to the therapeutic benefits of inducing hypothermia for a post arrest patient. For now, the best guide is to protect the patient from environmental extremes and maintain normothermia.

Glucose Requirements

Glucose levels can have a significant impact on successful cardiac arrest management. Normal levels of blood glucose should be assured by routine monitoring of the blood glucose level (BGL). Excessively high levels and excessively low levels of glucose have both been shown to be detrimental to patient outcomes. Therefore, normal levels should be maintained to allow adequate stores of energy for the body during the repair process following the arrest. It *is not recommended,* however, to routinely administer 50% dextrose as a medication during arrest with the assumption that it "won't do any harm." This practice has been shown to be detrimental to the eventual neurological outcome of the patient. Fifty percent dextrose should only be administered when it is clinically relevant and verifiable that the patient's blood glucose level is low.

Sedation and Anticonvulsant Therapy

An important consideration while managing a patient who has been successfully resuscitated from cardiac arrest is preventing activities that may increase the cerebral metabolic rate. For example, in a comatose patient, a portion of the brain may still respond with heightened metabolic activity in response to external stimuli (for example a sternal rub or suctioning). This causes a localized need for increased perfusion in the face of a diminished supply. The imbalance can then result in a localized deficit and additional damage. It should be a rule, then, to minimize external stimuli to the comatose post arrest patient. Administering sedatives or relaxants may help achieve this end.

Seizure activity, an ever-present danger to the post arrest patient, needs special consideration. A single seizure has the potential of increasing cerebral metabolic activity 300% to 400%. The sudden requirement for increased blood supply and oxygenation will cause a detrimental shift in the balance of supply and demand and worsen neurologic outcomes. While researchers disagree as to the benefit of prophylactic anticonvulsant therapy, all agree that any seizures that occur should be quickly and aggressively terminated. To achieve this, normal anticonvulsant drugs (e.g., benzodiazepines, dilantin, barbiturates) may be employed.

Brain Resuscitation after Cardiopulmonary Arrest

In light of the advancing knowledge about the etiologies that underlie the postresuscitation syndrome, more and more therapeutic modalities are being hypothesized and tested in controlled studies to determine their value. For example, studies are currently being conducted on a newer classification of drugs known as "neuroprotective agents," which are developed to allow brain cells to live longer despite a significant insult or injury that would normally result in progressive cellular death. As yet, however, there are no drugs that can be recommended for routine treatment of post arrest brain damage.

 ADVANCED MONITORING INTERVENTIONS FOR CARDIAC ARREST PATIENTS

The following section is an introduction to invasive monitoring techniques. These techniques are typically not required during the early stages of prehospital advanced cardiac life support, and information about them is considered to be supplemental to the ACLS course for prehospital providers. Should you be assigned to a work area where these more advanced techniques are practiced, you should locate and study an appropriate text on invasive monitoring techniques.

Arterial Cannulation

Arterial cannulation is a process of placing an indwelling catheter into an appropriate artery. Typically, site preferences include the radial artery, femoral artery, axillary artery, or possibly the dorsal pedal artery. It is important to note that there must be evidence of adequate collateral circulation at the chosen site in case the artery should occlude.

Arterial cannulation allows continual and accurate monitoring of arterial pressure. It also allows for sampling of arterial blood without repeated arterial sticks and, to a lesser extent, determination of cardiac output.

Cannulation of the Pulmonary Artery

Cannulation of the pulmonary artery is accomplished by inserting a catheter with a balloon tip into the central circulation until it passes through the right side of the heart and eventually is placed in the pulmonary artery. This placement allows for determination of pulmonary wedge pressures and cardiac output and for sampling of pulmonary arterial blood (which is actually mixed venous blood).

With the data obtained, the care provider can make determinations about left and right ventricular functions, determine mitral valve function, differentiate cardiogenic from noncardiogenic pulmonary edema, and detect the presence of a ruptured intraventricular septum. Additionally, the effectiveness of interventions can be determined, since serial measurements can be performed.

Arterial Puncture

Arterial puncture is the insertion of a needle into an artery to secure an arterial blood specimen. Lab tests are done on the sample to determine such things as arterial gas levels, carbon monoxide levels, or lactate. As noted earlier, if repeated sampling is necessary, placement of an indwelling arterial catheter may be preferred to avoid the discomfort and complications of repeated sticks.

ADJUNCTS FOR ARTIFICIAL CIRCULATION

CPR is now generally considered to be a temporizing measure whose chief benefit is to provide some degree of cardiac output and oxygenation to vital organs until more definitive care (e.g., defibrillation, drugs, intubation) can be provided to the cardiac arrest victim. In essence, CPR delays biological death (irreversible cell death) in the face of clinical death (cessation of heartbeat and respirations). With this goal in mind, proposed new interventions and techniques that make compressions more effective should result in increased blood flow and oxygenation to vital organs and ultimately lead to improvements in cardiac arrest survival in the prehospital environment.

Alternative Techniques to Compressions

Since no newly proposed technique has been shown to consistently improve cardiac arrest survival rates, none has been recommended to replace the standard CPR technique. However, some of these alternative techniques may improve the hemodynamics of compressions.

Interposed abdominal compressions have been shown to improve blood flow, although not consistently in all studies. In this technique, the abdomen is compressed during the relaxation phase of chest compressions. The theory is that this improves blood flow by increasing the aortic diastolic pressure and, as a result, coronary perfusion. This technique requires three people—one to provide ventilations, one to perform chest compressions, and one to perform abdominal compressions—and should be conducted after tracheal intubation is completed. The risks of abdominal injuries, poor ventilation (due to increases in intra-abdominal pressure with compressions), and aspiration, although not reported as significant in the research to date, should still be further considered before interposed abdominal compressions are recommended as a standard.

Of the studies conducted so far, both in the prehospital and in-hospital environments, this technique has been shown to be associated with increased episodes of spontaneous return of circulation. However, it has not yet been demonstrated that this technique, when used in the prehospital setting, has an increase rate of survival benefit when used. So presently, its adoption by the prehospital provider of advanced cardiac life support is not recommended.

High-frequency (or rapid manual rate) CPR is yet another alternative chest-compression technique. In this technique, the standard external compression rates are dramatically increased (>100/min). The theory is that if the heart rate is increased (artificially with the compressions) then cardiac output should improve. (This presumes that the stroke volume, or amount of blood ejected with each compression, stays the same or even improves slightly.) Some laboratory studies, but not all, have shown this to be the case. So while high-frequency CPR shows some potential benefits, additional studies of outcomes for patients in cardiac arrest need to be conducted to determine its efficacy.

Simultaneous ventilation-compression CPR (SVC-CPR) is another new technique that attempts to increase cardiac output. This technique uses the entire thorax as a pump by inflating the lungs (which put pressure on the lateral aspects of the heart), while depressing the sternum (which provides anteroposterior pressure). In hypothesis, this would improve artificial blood flow by providing more complete circumferential pressure to the heart. While promising in theory, studies have not shown improved survivability for cardiac arrest, and therefore this technique has not been recommended as routine.

Mechanical Devices for CPR

A number of mechanical devices have been devised that provide compressions and/or ventilations to the cardiac arrest patient. They are designed to standardize CPR technique, reduce rescuer fatigue, ensure adequacy of compressions, and free up rescuers to attend to other aspects of advanced life support. To date, these devices are intended only for the adult in cardiac arrest.

The cardiac press device has a hinged arm that swings over the patient's thorax and is positioned so the press is over the sternum and adjusted to the proper depth. This permits the device, which is manually operated, to deliver consistent compressions. It is not considered to be a device to replace standard practice CPR; however, it has been recognized as an adjunct to prehospital providers in situations where transport times are prolonged, or when the number of prehospital care personnel are not available.

The automatic resuscitator is a gas-powered device that is programmed to deliver ventilations *and* compressions. While larger and heavier than other mechanical devices, it allows rescuers to attend to other aspects of patient care during arrest management. This is beneficial in those instances when care providers are few.

Another technique that utilizes mechanical equipment for the provision of external compressions is the ACD-CPR (or active compression-decompression CPR). With this technique, a mechanical device, much like a large suction cup, is applied to the anterior chest wall. Following a standard compression of the sternum, the device is manually lifted under the theory that the negative intrathoracic pressure generated will allow better blood flow into the thoracic cavity and heart chambers so that the next subsequent compression yields higher stroke volumes and cardiac output levels. Its use has not been shown effective for prehospital providers, although there is some weak data showing potential benefits to in-hospital arrests.

Vest CPR is an experimental method that compresses the thorax pneumatically with a perithoracic vest. In essence, this device operates under the same hemodynamic principles as simultaneous ventilation-compression CPR. Some preliminary studies have indicated that the vest-CPR device does improve hemodynamic status and that there are some gains in short term survival rates from cardiac arrest. Currently, however, this device is unavailable as FDA approval and device production have not yet occurred. It is anticipated that this device may be used as an adjunct to standard CPR.

A hand-held device, which alternates chest compression and abdominal decompression with chest decompression and abdominal compression is one of the newer mechanical devices under study. Incorporating the theoretical concepts of IAC-CPR and ACD-CPR, this phased approach (known now as PTACD-CPR) has been shown to increase hemodynamic status in both animal and clinical trials. In the absence, however, of clinical outcomes studies and FDA approval, this technique is not yet recommended.

CPR ASSESSMENT

Other than outcome studies (how many patients died vs. how many were successfully resuscitated), there are actually few ways to reliably assess the effectiveness of CPR. In the absence of the ability to evaluate the quality of artificial resuscitation on an ongoing basis, there is minimal opportunity to vary the interventions to meet specific patient needs. Fortunately, there has been additional research in this area, and several options may become viable.

Most commonly, pulses are felt to assess the effectiveness of compressions. It is traditional to assess the carotid pulse for evidence that adequate compressions are being delivered. This, however, has not been shown to be definitively equated with meaningful arterial blood flow. Additionally, since the myocardium is perfused during diastolic relaxation (when the aortic semilunar valves are closed and not occluding the coronary sinuses), the mere presence of a carotid pulse with compression only signifies forward propulsion of blood, and nothing toward the quality of myocardial perfusion or cerebral perfusion.

Femoral pulses felt during compressions are very misleading since you may actually be feeling venous backflow rather than the degree of arterial flow. Remember that the inferior vena cava is devoid of valves and retrograde blood flow may occur from compressions and produce a femoral pulse. For this reason, femoral pulses should be assessed during spontaneous pulse checks only.

Since femoral pulses, when present, tend to be fainter than the carotid pulse location, the carotid site is still the preferred site to check for a spontaneous pulse as well as to check effectiveness of external compressions. Doppler ultrasound may detect spontaneous blood flow that cannot be discerned by palpation of pulse points and may also be useful during the arrest management, especially in patients in pulseless electrical activity.

Respiratory gas measurement via capnometry shows some promise as a reliable test of CPR adequacy. Since expired CO_2 is dependent upon pulmonary perfusion, end tidal CO_2 monitoring has been shown to accurately estimate adequacy of CPR and cardiac output. Experimental models have shown a positive correlation between successful resuscitation from cardiac arrest and higher expired CO_2 levels. Capnometry readings that improve prior to successful resuscitation and may be used to indicate the return of spontaneous circulation. Additionally, end tidal capnography has become more commonplace in the prehospital environment, and could be used as a measure of CPR adequacy.

Despite these promising findings to help improve the delivery and assessment of CPR in arrest situations, continued research is still being conducted to help shape their usefulness and applicability to clinical practice.

CASE STUDY FOLLOW-UP

Having just finished your ACLS course for your EMT-Paramedic program, you are completing your internship phase when a call comes in for a "man down." Arriving on scene, you discover two first responders doing CPR on a supine male.

Assessment

As soon as the ambulance is positioned, you, Joe, and Rich grab the necessary equipment and walk toward the patient. Arriving at the patient's side, you quickly confirm pulselessness while Joe prepares to obtain a "quick look" with the monitor. Rich kneels down beside you and says bystanders report the patient was complaining of chest pain when he suddenly became unresponsive.

Treatment

After doing a "quick-look," Joe says out loud that the patient is in a bradydysrhythmic rhythm. You add, "It must be PEA since there is no palpable pulse." Rich concurs and initiates CPR again while Joe starts hyperventilating the patient with an oropharyngeal airway and BVM. He asks you to prepare a 8.0 mm tracheal tube with the #3 MacIntosh laryngoscope blade and handle.

After about 6 minutes on scene, you are prepared for transport. The patient has been placed on a backboard and has been successfully intubated by Joe. Rich has administered the first epinephrine and atropine down the tracheal tube. Before pulling away from the scene, Joe motions for you to take the BVM and ventilate the patient. He adds that he needs to set up the cardiac press with Rich before he starts driving to the hospital.

You recall that one problem with postresuscitation is the management of cerebral edema. To help minimize this, you remain acutely aware of the end-tidal CO_2 reading on the capnography, to ensure your ventilatory minute ventilation is maintained and chest compressions are ongoing at the appropriate depth. You do so by watching the end tidal CO_2 monitor as it displays the amount of carbon dioxide expired with each ventilation. By this time, the cardiac press is in place, Rich has initiated and IV, and the ambulance is moving with resuscitation continuing en route. You are fascinated to watch the cardiac press administering compressions because you've never seen one in use before.

When you arrive at the hospital, unfortunately, despite all the advanced cardiac life support interventions, the patient is still in arrest. Since the cardiac press is mobile, it is transferred with the patient into the emergency department. It continues to administer compressions as the ED staff takes over treatment of the patient. Joe and Rich then converse with the ED physician, giving him a brief overview of the events. Afterward, Joe and Rich commend you on your performance. Although the arrest was not a "save," you are pleased you had an opportunity to exercise your ACLS skills.

SUMMARY

This chapter has been an introduction to some considerations of definitive cardiac care and several techniques and technologies now being studied that may enhance the chances of restoring the cardiac patient to good health.

Of paramount concern is cerebral resuscitation, taking various measures to compensate for postresuscitation syndrome, the brain's diminished ability to regulate its own cerebral perfusion during a period of 24 hours or so after correction of a cardiac arrest. These measures include oxygenation and hyperventilation, correction of metabolic acidosis, temperature and glucose regulation, and anti-convulsant therapy as needed. Additional special considerations include advanced invasive monitoring interventions such as arterial cannulation, the delivery of external compressions through varied approaches, and other techniques and technologies to improve and measure the effectiveness of CPR compressions.

Research to develop the incorporation of these new devices, technologies, or assessment mechanisms to improve the quality of resuscitation in the prehospital environment is constantly ongoing. It is important to stay abreast of these changes from a provider's perspective, and for medical directors responsible for those providers of prehospital advance cardiac life support to incorporate the newest and most effective strategies into clinical practice to continue the decline in prehospital cardiac arrest death rates.

REVIEW QUESTIONS

1. In relation to cardiac arrest, what does "postresuscitation syndrome" refer to?
   a. the period of time preceding cardiac arrest when the patient is experiencing chest pain
   b. the period of time following the return of spontaneous circulation when the patient exhibits seizures
   c. the period of time following the return of spontaneous circulation when the patient is still hypotensive
   d. the period of time following cardiac arrest when the brain is hypoperfused despite spontaneous circulation

2. What factors can help alleviate the postresuscitation syndrome?
   a. glucose regulation
   b. hyperventilation
   c. temperature regulation
   d. a and b
   e. a, b, and c

3. Seizures are an ever-present danger during the postresuscitation period. They are best managed by
   a. prophylactic administration of an anticonvulsant prior to the onset of a seizure.
   b. administration of a benzodiazepine to terminate the seizures should they occur.
   c. allowing seizures to occur since the medication to stop them is more likely to worsen the postresuscitation syndrome than the seizure itself.
   d. a and b

4. Which advanced monitoring intervention allows for continual monitoring of arterial pressures or sampling of arterial blood?
   a. arterial cannulation
   b. arterial puncture
   c. saphenous line placement
   d. pulmonary artery cannulation

5. By what general principle(s) do the alternative adjuncts for artificial circulation offer an improvement in the performance of CPR for the cardiac arrest patient?
   a. They help reduce rescuer fatigue.
   b. They improve the hemodynamics of compressions.
   c. They are less likely to administer inappropriate compressions.
   d. all the above

6. What is the **currently** approved way to assess the effectiveness of the compressions during CPR?
   a. assessment of the carotid pulse
   b. assessment of the femoral pulse
   c. monitoring end tidal CO_2 readings
   d. monitoring pulse oximetry

7. Drug therapies are currently available that can reverse post-arrest brain damage.
   a. true
   b. false

Review Questions
Answers and Rationales

Chapter 1: Key Concepts of Advanced Cardiac Life Support for Prehospital Care Providers

1. **(a)** In cardiac arrest management, it is necessary to treat the patient as a whole and not just treat the rhythm. The rhythm may be a result of a pre-cardiac-arrest condition that is reversible, such as a tension pneumothorax resulting in pulseless electrical activity. Just treating the PEA rhythm without needle decompression to relieve the pneumothorax will result in a futile resuscitation attempt. However, decompression of the chest may provide immediate results with a favorable outcome. In cases such as ventricular fibrillation and ventricular tachycardia, electrical therapy takes precedence as an initial treatment over medications and tracheal intubation.

2. **(c)** The amount of time that elapses between cardiac arrest and defibrillation is the most critical factor related to patient survival. While the energy level and amount of transthoracic resistance do influence successful defibrillation, time delay to electrical shock is the most significant variable in successful defibrillation.

3. **(c)** Early prevention is not a link in the chain of survival, although it is extremely important in dropping the overall death rate due to cardiovascular disease. To give the adult patient in arrest the best chance of survival, early defibrillation is integral. Early defibrillation is the missing link in the answer.

4. **(d)** The patient must be deemed competent and capable of making a rational decision in order to refuse medical care. Terminal illness or approval from family members, physicians, or hospital administrators does not determine the patient's right or ability to refuse care. If the patient is deemed incompetent or incapable of making a rational decision, the physician relies on advance directives or legal surrogates, if any, in the decision-making process.

5. **(b)** If a question exists regarding a do-not-attempt-resuscitation order, it is necessary to begin full resuscitation to the standard of care that would be provided if no order existed. That is, you treat the patient as if there had never been an order, which means initiating advanced life support until the order is clarified. If the resuscitation is not initiated and the order turns out to be invalid, critical time has elapsed and unsuccessful resuscitation may be directly attributed to your delay in action. Also, emergency care providers must be aware of whether the laws of their state or advance directives can be applied in emergency situations.

Chapter 2: Systematic Approach to Emergency Cardiac Care: The Primary and Secondary Surveys

1. **(c)** You must ensure your own safety first before approaching the patient or scene. Establishing unresponsiveness by shaking and shouting (or talking and touching for a trauma patient) is the first step once you are safely at the patient's side.

2. **(a)** As a health care provider trained in basic and advanced cardiac life support, it is assumed that you have much more training and experience in dealing with medical emergencies. Thus, you need to be decisive and take the most appropriate action based on the presenting situation. It is most appropriate in this situation to establish unresponsiveness, open the airway, and attempt to ventilate, even though you may have a high index of suspicion that the patient is choking. If the patient is choking, it is more important for you, as a health care provider, to attempt to relieve the obstruction than to leave the patient and call for help. You would not begin the foreign body airway obstruction maneuvers until you have confirmed an airway obstruction. Chest compressions would not be performed until the airway is cleared and pulselessness is established.

3. **(b)** Any time you suspect possible spinal trauma, it is necessary to open the airway using a jaw-thrust maneuver while the head and neck are maintained in a neutral in-line position. The head-tilt, chin-lift maneuver will cause hyperextension and manipulation of the cervical spine, possibly aggravating an injury. Keeping the head in a neutral position without performing a jaw thrust will not create an open airway.

4. **(a)** The procedures conducted in the ABCD primary survey are basic skills, including defibrillation. Initiation of an intravenous line, tracheal intubation, and administration of medication are all considered components of the secondary survey.

5. **(c)** The time to defibrillation is the most critical factor influencing the success rate of defibrillation. Delays in defibrillation are paralleled by an increasingly hypoxic and acidotic myocardium which directly decreases the success of defibrillation. Even though airway management, tracheal intubation, and medication administration are critical in resuscitation, initial defibrillation takes precedence.

6. **(a)** When conducting the secondary survey, you should first perform tracheal intubation and assess adequacy of ventilation, then initiate an intravenous line and administer medication, then consider the differential diagnosis.

7. **(c)** Bretylium is not an acceptable drug to administer down the tracheal tube. Drugs used in resuscitation that can be administered down the tracheal tube are lidocaine (Xylocaine), epinephrine, atropine, and naloxone (Narcan). These can be remembered by using the mnemonic LEAN.

8. **(b)** Normal saline is the preferred intravenous solution in the cardiac arrest patient. It is an isotonic volume expander. Any dextrose-containing solutions should be avoided because of potential postarrest neurological sequelae.

9. **(c)** When administering medications by the tracheal route, it is necessary to give 2 to 2.5 times the standard dose diluted to a total of 10 ml with normal saline to assure sufficient and timely absorption, distribution, and action. Tracheal administration of medication is not preferred. An intravenous line must be established as quickly as possible and used as the primary drug

route. Once a patent intravenous line is established, the tracheal route should no longer be used for drug administration.

10. **(b)** The differential diagnosis should be conducted as part of the secondary survey following the initiation of drug therapy. However, there may be times when consideration of a differential diagnosis may occur much earlier to dictate the appropriate patient management. For example, a trauma patient needs more aggressive fluid therapy, which may be initiated earlier in the secondary survey based on the mechanism of injury.

Chapter 3: Airway Management, Ventilation, and Oxygen Therapy

1. **(b)** Sonorous sounds usually indicate a partial airway occlusion at the level of the pharynx. The tongue is commonly the cause of obstruction. Wheezing indicates an increase in airway resistance in the bronchioles. Laryngeal obstruction, from edema or other material, produces stridor or a crowing-type sound. A gurgling sound is heard when secretions, blood, or vomitus is present in the airway.

2. **(c)** Even with an oropharyngeal or nasopharyngeal airway in place, a manual airway maneuver must be maintained. Tracheobronchial suctioning cannot be performed through an oropharyngeal airway. If the airway stimulates a gag reflex upon insertion, because of its hard-plastic construction, it will continue to stimulate the gag reflex when it is in place.

3. **(d)** Stimulation of the sympathetic nervous system may result from tracheal intubation, but it is a complication, not an advantage, of this procedure. Stimulation of the sympathetic nervous system may increase myocardial oxygen demand due to an increase in myocardial workload resulting from tachycardia and an increased contractile force. This may precipitate dysrhythmias and increase intracranial hypertension. Lidocaine, epinephrine, atropine, and naloxone may be given down the tracheal tube; therefore, it may serve as a limited and temporary drug route. Asynchronous ventilation to chest compression may occur with the tracheal tube in place. The major advantage of the tracheal tube is that it protects the airway by isolating it from aspiration of foreign material.

4. **(a)** The curved blade is designed to fit in the vallecula. With an upward and forward lifting motion on the laryngoscope handle, the epiglottis is indirectly lifted, exposing the glottic opening. The straight blade is placed under the epiglottis and is used to directly lift it up to expose the glottic opening.

5. **(c)** In an emergency situation, an 8.0 mm i.d. tracheal tube would be appropriate for both a male and a female. Females usually require a 7.0 to 8.0 mm i.d. tube, whereas males usually take an 8.0 to 8.5 mm i.d. tube.

6. **(a)** When inserting a tracheal tube, the best indicator to use to determine the proper tube depth is to continue until the proximal end of the cuff has passed 1 to 2.5 cm beyond the level of the vocal cords. The centimeter marker is only used as a guide to monitor tube depth once proper placement has occurred, since the depth will vary with each patient. The tip of the tube should sit midway between the level of the carina and larynx.

7. **(b)** With the first ventilation following tube placement, the chest should be inspected for rise and fall while auscultating over the epigastrium for sounds. Auscultation is done in this sequence to prevent unnecessary air

from inflating the stomach while bilateral breath sounds are being assessed with each ventilation. If the tube is in the esophagus while breath sounds are checked, the practitioner may provide several ventilations before then auscultating the epigastrium and realizing that the tube is misplaced. By auscultating over the epigastrium first, you lessen the amount of air insufflation in the stomach and reduce the incidence of possible gastric distention, regurgitation, and aspiration. Condensation in the tube or centimeter marker is not an acceptable method to determine tube placement.

8. **(c)** Patients with blunt trauma to the face have a high incidence of cervical and other spinal injury. Therefore, the head and neck of a patient with facial trauma must be maintained in a neutral in-line position while airway management is being performed, including tracheal intubation. Controlled hyperventilation is indicated in patients with suspected increases in intracranial pressure who exhibit signs of herniation from head injury. Typical cuff volume is 10 ml of air and has no bearing on facial trauma or spinal injury. With the distal end of the cuff at the level of the vocal cords, the tip of the tube will not be positioned midway between the carina and larynx. This will lead to easy dislodgement and misplacement, possibly in the esophagus, upon movement of the patient.

9. **(a)** Secondary confirmation of tracheal tube placement is performed after confirming tube placement using primary techniques including inspection and auscultation. Secondary confirmation is achieved primarily through the use of an end-tidal CO_2 detector and an esophageal detector device.

10. **(c)** The cricothyroid membrane is located inferior to the thyroid cartilage (Adam's apple) and superior to the cricoid cartilage, the large bulky circumferential ring that is the most inferior part of the larynx.

11. **(b)** When providing positive pressure ventilation, a high concentration of oxygen should be attached to the ventilation device as early as possible. If oxygen is not connected to the device or the oxygen concentration delivered is less than 40%, a tidal volume of 10 ml/kg must be delivered with each breath. Once oxygen is connected and an oxygen concentration of 40% or greater is being delivered, the tidal volume delivered is reduced to 6 to 7 ml/kg. The higher oxygen concentration will balance the lower tidal volumes delivered to the patient and will result in less gastric insufflation.

12. **(c)** Because the flow-restricted oxygen-powered ventilation device (FROPVD) provides high rates and volumes of airflow, barotrauma and subsequent pneumothorax may result. The device uses oxygen as its source of power; therefore, 100% oxygen is delivered with each ventilation. Because of the high rate and volume of delivered air, the device is intended for adult patients only. The FROPVD is no longer recommended as a preferred ventilation device.

13. **(a)** The suction should be set at between -80 and -120 mmHg when performing tracheobronchial suctioning to reduce the risk of trauma to the mucosa and other tissue. When performing oropharyngeal suctioning, the pressure should be set at greater than -120 mmHg. The patient should be hyperoxygenated prior to and after any suction procedure. Suction is only applied while withdrawing the catheter; it is never applied while inserting the catheter down the tube. Suction should not be applied for greater than 15 seconds.

14. **(d)** Hypoxemia is the most serious complication associated with tracheobronchial suctioning. When suction is applied, the functional residual volume is removed from the lungs. Along with an interruption in ventilation, both of these lead to serious hypoxemia. Therefore, it is imperative that the patient be hyperoxygenated prior to and after all suction procedures.

15. **(b)** If the liter flow is set at less than 6 lpm, the patient will begin to rebreathe his exhaled gas, resulting in a reduction in FiO_2 and potential increases in carbon dioxide. At 8–10 lpm, the FiO_2 is about 60%. The simple face mask has no reservoir; the nonrebreather mask does. Oxygen masks are not typically well tolerated by pediatric patients.

Chapter 4: Gaining Intravenous Access

1. **(a)** Catheter over the needle is by far the most common IV catheter used for peripheral vein cannulation. Through-the-needle catheters and hollow needles are less commonly used. An intraosseous catheter would be inserted into the medulla of a bone, not a vein.

2. **(c)** Normal saline is the preferred solution to keep the vein open in cardiac arrest. Fluids for resuscitation in cardiac arrest should not contain dextrose. Sterile water should never be used as an IV fluid because of its hypotonicity.

3. **(b)** Delivery of medication to the central circulation is considerably faster when using a central site rather than a peripheral site. The degree of difficulty, however, between the two techniques leaves central cannulation as a less desirable option as it is inherently harder, and yields more complications than peripheral sites. Since peripheral cannulation is an easier skill to master, the peripheral veins are easier to find, and peripheral cannulation can usually be accomplished during CPR, it is the preferred option for achieving vascular access necessary to administer intravenous fluids and drugs in cardiac arrest. Finally, it is important to remember that central cannulation requires interruption of CPR, which is inherently detrimental to the process.

4. **(d)** The antecubital fossa (or the external jugular vein) is preferred because in cardiac arrest peripheral venous circulation is compromised, and it is important to introduce medications as close to the central circulation as possible. The dorsum of the hand and saphenous vein of the leg are peripheral veins, but farther from the central circulation. The subclavian vein is centrally located, but is not a peripheral site.

5. Two strategies for improving delivery of medications to the central circulation in cardiac arrest are: (a) raise the extremity, and (b) follow each medication with a saline flush of 20–50 ml. Although it may seem odd to raise the arm, it actually is just as effective as the saline flush. As such, using both techniques in concert greatly improves absorption and distribution patterns of medications when the patient is in cardiac arrest.

6. One of the greatest concerns deals with the number of venipunctures the patient receives prior to fibrinolytic therapy. The number of IV attempts for a patient who may be a candidate for fibrinolytic therapy should be limited because fibrinolytics act to dissolve clots and will therefore increase the risk of or aggravate bleeding or hematoma formation.

Chapter 5: ECG Monitoring and Dysrhythmia Recognition

1. **(d)** Myocardial tissue is the only muscle tissue that possesses the property of automaticity. Automaticity is the ability of the muscle tissue to contract on its own, without nervous control. All muscle cells in the body depolarize, repolarize, and contract.

2. **(c)** The three specialized types of myocardial cells are pacemaker, conduction, and working cells.

3. **(b)** Pacemaker cells depolarize at regular intervals, causing a depolarization of adjacent muscle tissue. All myocardial tissue contracts when a wave of depolarization reaches it. Repolarization occurs as the ions that flow out of the cell are pumped back in. The delay in conduction between the atria and the ventricles is caused by the AV node.

4. **(a)** The main pacemaker of the healthy heart is the SA node, which depolarizes at a rate of 60–100 times a minute.

5. **(c)** The AV node depolarizes spontaneously at a rate of 40–60 times a minute and functions as a back-up mechanism if the SA node fails to fire.

6. **(c)** Myocardial working cells are responsible for the mechanical contraction of the heart. The pacemaker cells depolarize at regular intervals and cause the regular contraction of the working cells. The conduction cells serve as a conductive pathway to carry the impulse to depolarize from the pacemakers to the working cells.

7. **(c)** The QRS complex is caused by the depolarization of ventricular cells, which results in ventricular contraction. Atrial depolarization and contraction are represented by the P wave. Ventricular repolarization is seen as the T wave. The delay between atrial and ventricular contraction would be represented by the distance between the P wave and the QRS complex.

8. **(a)** A variance of greater than 0.04 seconds between R waves is the definition of irregularity. Automaticity is the ability to contract without nervous control. Ectopy is when beats originate at sites other than the pacemakers of the heart. A dysrhythmia is any disturbance in the normal rhythm of the heart.

9. **(b)** A bundle branch block widens the QRS complex because conduction is delayed on one side of the heart. Hypernatremia has no effect on the QRS complex; hypothermia causes J waves; and an acute myocardial infarction causes ST-segment changes.

10. **(c)** All narrow QRS complexes have followed the normal conduction pathways *below* the level of the AV node and, therefore, must have originated above the ventricles—at the AV node or higher. Impulses generated above the ventricles *may* have wide QRS complexes if they have aberrant conduction. The narrow QRS complex *may* have originated in the SA node and traveled the internodal pathways to the AV node, but it may also have originated at the AV node and not traveled the internodal pathways.

11. **(c)** The maximum normal P-R interval is 0.20 seconds.

12. **(a)** The only "red flag" for sinus tachycardia is a rate above 100 beats per minute.

13. **(b)** The only "red flag" for sinus dysrhythmia is irregularity.

14. **(d)** Atrial fibrillation is the only dysrhythmia that is *irregularly* irregular. Second-degree, Type I heart block and sinus rhythm with PVCs are *regularly* irregular due to beats being dropped from a regular underlying rhythm. Third-degree heart block is often regular.

15. **(f)** b and d—Atrial fibrillation is irregular and has no discernible P waves. The baseline is wavy with fibrillatory (f) waves.

16. **(a)** Atrial fibrillation is not a reentry dysrhythmia. Supraventricular tachycardia, atrial flutter, and ventricular tachycardia are all reentry dysrhythmias.

17. **(d)** Atrial flutter has no P waves but has a sawtooth, or picket fence, baseline caused by flutter (F) waves.

18. **(f)** a and d—Supraventricular tachycardia is a very fast rhythm with no discernible P waves.

19. **(f)** a, c, and d—Ventricular tachycardia is a very fast rhythm with a wide QRS complex and no discernible P waves.

20. **(e)** The only "red flag" in first-degree AV block is a P-R interval greater than 0.20 seconds.

21. **(f)** d and e—Third-degree AV block is identified by lack of a consistent relationship between P waves and the QRS complexes (hence an inconsistent P-R interval).

22. **(c)** Since all PVCs originate within the ventricles, they always have wide QRS complexes. Supraventricular ectopic beats (PACs and PJCs) usually have narrow QRS complexes but can have wide QRS complexes if there is aberrant conduction.

23. **(c)** Most PVCs have a compensatory pause because the SA node does not sense the PVC and continues to fire, unaffected. Most PACs reset the SA node and, therefore, have a noncompensatory pause.

24. **(a)** The term that indicates PVCs occur every third beat is *trigeminy*. *Bigeminy* is PVCs occurring every other beat. *Multifocal* PVCs are those that are morphologically different from each other. *Salvos* are more than one PVC in a row.

25. Answer: ventricular tachycardia.

    Rationale:

Rate	180	⚑
Regularity	Regular	
QRS Complex		
Do all of the QRS complexes look alike?	Yes	
What is the width of the QRS complex?	Wide	⚑
P Waves	No P waves	⚑
Is there a P wave before every QRS complex?	NA	
Is there a QRS after every P wave?	NA	
P-R Interval		
What is the P-R interval?	NA	
Is the P-R interval constant?	NA	

26. Answer: atrial fibrillation

Rationale:

Rate	90
Regularity	Irregular 🏴
QRS Complex	
Do all of the QRS complexes look alike?	Yes
What is the width of the QRS complex?	Narrow
P Waves	No P waves 🏴
Is there a P wave before every QRS complex?	NA
Is there a QRS after every P wave?	NA
P-R Interval	
What is the P-R interval?	NA
Is the P-R interval constant?	NA

27. Answer: normal sinus rhythm

Rationale:

Rate	80
Regularity	Regular
QRS Complex	
Do all of the QRS complexes look alike?	Yes
What is the width of the QRS complex?	Narrow
P Waves	
Is there a P wave before every QRS complex?	Yes
Is there a QRS after every P wave?	Yes
P-R Interval	
What is the P-R interval?	0.16
Is the P-R interval constant?	Yes

28. Answer: ventricular fibrillation

Rationale:

Rate	0 🏴
Regularity	NA
QRS Complex	No QRS complexes 🏴
Do all of the QRS complexes look alike?	NA
What is the width of the QRS complex?	NA
P Waves	No P waves 🏴
Is there a P wave before every QRS complex?	NA
Is there a QRS after every P wave?	NA
P-R Interval	
What is the P-R interval?	NA
Is the P-R interval constant?	NA

29. Answer: supraventricular tachycardia

    Rationale:

Rate	180	⚑
Regularity	Regular	
QRS Complex		
Do all of the QRS complexes look alike?	Yes	
What is the width of the QRS complex?	Narrow	
P Waves	No P waves	⚑
Is there a P wave before every QRS complex?	NA	
Is there a QRS after every P wave?	NA	
P-R Interval		
What is the P-R interval?	NA	
Is the P-R interval constant?	NA	

30. Answer: normal sinus rhythm with PVCs

    Rationale:

Rate	70	
Regularity	Irregular	⚑
QRS Complex		
Do all of the QRS complexes look alike?	No	⚑
What is the width of the QRS complex?	The QRS complexes from the underlying rhythm are narrow. The premature beats are wide.	⚑
P Waves		
Is there a P wave before every QRS complex?	No	⚑
Is there a QRS after every P wave?	Yes	
P-R Interval		
What is the P-R interval?	Not consistent	⚑
Is the P-R interval constant?	NA	⚑

Chapter 6: 12-Lead Electrocardiographic Interpretation

1. **(c)** The 12-lead ECG is best used in the prehospital setting to identify a patient who may be a candidate for reperfusion upon arrival at the ED. A multitude of other conditions or events can be identified on a 12-lead, but most are beyond the scope of prehospital medicine, and none is more significant in improving patient outcome than that of myocardial infarction. Although the definitive diagnosis of an MI is made at the hospital, the acquisition of the 12-lead, clinical symptomatology, and fibrinolytic screening can be easily performed by the paramedic. These actions lead to the positive outcome of decreasing the time between the MI and the reperfusion therapy.

2. **(a)** The left anterior descending artery (LAD) is one of the two major arteries that branches off the left common carotid artery. This blood vessel perfuses the septal and anterior walls. Occlusion of the LAD creates ischemic changes to Leads V_1 through V_4 on the 12-lead. The clinical significance of this is that it commonly causes the development of bundle branch blocks (because

the bundle branches travel through the ventricular septum). Significant changes in stroke volume and cardiac output are associated with occlusion in the proximal LAD or in the left coronary artery (the latter of which is commonly referred to as the "widow maker" infarction).

3. **(a)** Unlike the other walls of the left ventricle, in 90% of the population the inferior wall is perfused by the distal portions of the right coronary artery as it gives rise to the posterior descending artery. Indications of infarction in the inferior leads (Leads II, III, and aVL) point to occlusion of the right coronary artery, which should alert the care provider to obtain right ventricular leads to determine if the right ventricle is also infracting. This is important as it may alter the considerations for pain management with nitrates and dictate the use of fluid rather than vasopressors if the patient develops hypotension.

4. **(c)** The precordial leads are those that view the left ventricle from the frontal plane, and include Leads V_1 through V_6. These leads indicate if the occluded blood vessel is part of the left coronary artery perfusion pattern, and serve as a predictor of the severity of the myocardial infarction.

5. **(b)** Remembering that the mean cardiac vector for a normal axis of $0°$ and $+90°$ helps illustrate that the majority of the electrical impulses are traveling from the right atrial region toward the left ventricular chamber. This causes a large R wave in both Lead I and aVF. If, however, the patient has a large S wave in Lead I and also a large R wave in aVF, this indicates that the mean cardiac vector is traveling toward the right ventricle more than the left. This is called right axis deviation and may be seen in patients with a right bundle branch block, extreme pulmonary hypertension, or right ventricular hypertrophy.

6. **(a)** Left ventricular hypertrophy occurs when the left ventricle enlarges over a period of time due to arterial hypertension or possibly aortic valve stenosis. Although it may be reasoned that enlargement of the left ventricular muscle might be beneficial, it actually causes a decrease in the ventricular lumen size as the thickening myocardium starts to encroach on the size of the ventricle itself. Ultimately this can lead to a drop in stroke volume, diminished cardiac output, and congestive heart failure. The thickening myocardium requires more energy for depolarization purposes and, as such, drags the mean cardiac vector more towards $0°$, or up towards $-90°$. It is diagnosed on a 12-lead by interpreting the amount of voltage seen on specific leads of the 12-lead ECG.

7. **(a)** Early in the progression of ischemia and infarction of the myocardium, the mismatch of blood supply and demand results in repolarization changes to the myocardial cells. Early on, this change results in abnormal ST-segment changes in which the ST segment becomes abnormally depressed. The anatomically contiguous leads that demonstrate this depression correlate to the myocardial wall which is starving for oxygenated blood.

8. **(a)** Although the Q wave of the cardiac cycle is a normal component, an abnormally wide Q wave (>40 milliseconds) indicates that there is the presence of dead (or silent) myocardial tissue which is not capable of propagating an electrical impulse or contracting. Because this "pathologic" Q wave is the result of *dead* tissue, it is impossible to tell exactly when the infarction occurred. As such, the presence of a pathologic Q wave on the 12-lead ECG can only indicate that an infarction *has* occurred, not, however, when it *did* occur.

9. **(b)** The anterior wall of the left ventricle is viewed primarily by the precordial Leads V_3 and V_4. V_1 and V_2 view the septal wall; Leads II, III, and aVF view the inferior wall. The augmented limb leads collectively do not view the same wall of the heart; as such, ischemic findings in the augmented limb leads would be nonsensical. Occasionally, ischemic findings to V_3, V_4, and V_5 is referred to as an anterior wall infarction with lateral extension (owing to the findings in V_5).

10. **(a)** Right bundle branch blocks occur with occlusion to the LAD artery which perfuses the septal wall, and hence the bundle branches themselves. As the septal wall becomes more ischemic, the bundle branches may also begin to fail and result in delayed conduction (hence a bundle branch block). Right bundle branch blocks (widened QRS complexes, evidence of slowed conduction) can be seen in V_1 and V_2 since these leads look specifically at the interventricular septum.

11. **(a)** Potassium is a cation which is extremely important to cellular depolarization, but more importantly, repolarization. As extracellular potassium levels rise (as a result of myocardial infarctions, crush injuries, or errors in medication compliance), a problem with the normal repolarization pattern occurs. Since the T wave is indicative of ventricular repolarization, the T wave may take on a more sharpened and elevated appearance (i.e., peaked T waves).

12. **(b)** Hypothermic myocardial tissue tends to develop a characteristic hump in the cardiac cycle that occurs just after the QRS complex itself. It results in artificial elevation of the J point and is called the J, or Osborn, wave. It is most characteristically seen in Lead II or V_6, but it may be seen in virtually all leads.

Chapter 7: Electrical Therapy: Defibrillation, Cardioversion, and Cardiac Pacing

1. **(c)** Defibrillation (otherwise known as asynchronous cardioversion) is the treatment of choice for a heart in ventricular fibrillation. It is not used in bradycardic rates since these patients mainly need drug therapy to control the rate. Defibrillation is not warranted in asystolic rhythms confirmed in multiple leads. Atrial fibrillation is not life threatening in and of itself, so it is also controlled by drug therapy, and occasionally by synchronized cardioversion.

2. **(c)** Regarding successful cardioversion, the general rule is the earlier it is provided the greater the chance for successful conversion. After that, it is important to take steps necessary to reduce transthoracic resistance. In this instance, timing the countershock with end expiration will reduce the distance from the paddles to the heart, thereby allowing more energy to reach the myocardium. Since the delivery of electrical therapy is time-dependent in the unstable patient, it is often indicated prior to any drugs or other interventions.

3. **(a)** Asynchronous cardioversion is known more commonly as defibrillation. Synchronous cardioversion is the preferred treatment of tachydysrhythmias and starts with lower energy levels of 50–100 joules. Remember also that all forms of cardioversion need to use conductive medium. Lastly, the energy levels must be tailored for pediatric patients when defibrillation is necessary.

4. **(d)** Defibrillation of asystolic hearts is actually damaging, because it can cause a profound increase in vagal tone. Although asystolic arrests are rarely

reversible, the use of electrical therapy in this situation may remove any likelihood of spontaneous initiation of an impulse.

5. **(c)** Monophasic defibrillation is carried out in a step-wise sequence of increasing energy levels. The initial stack of three shocks is administered at 200, 200–300, then 360 joules. The specific energy levels used for biphasic shocks is actually determined by the defibrillation unit based upon several factors beyond the operator's control.

6. **(a)** Automated external defibrillators (AEDs) are indicated for cardiac arrest patients in ventricular fibrillation, regardless of the underlying cause of cardiac arrest. Since defibrillation is time-dependent, it should be applied as early as possible.

7. **(a)** The AED is preprogrammed to administer a stack of three shocks after the analysis mode has determined that VF is still present each time. This differs from the manual defibrillator, which the operator should use to administer only one countershock each time after the initial stack of three. The energy levels are the same for the two types of defibrillators, and studies have shown that the AED is just as effective as the manual defibrillator in terminating VF.

8. **(b)** Synchronized cardioversion delivers the energy during the R wave. This will avoid the T wave and reduce the likelihood of precipitating VF. The energy may be slightly delayed after depressing the buttons, since the synchronizing circuit needs to identify the R wave prior to discharge.

9. **(d)** Because of the synchronizing circuit of the defibrillator, it avoids the T wave and thus reduces the likelihood of causing ventricular fibrillation. Since it also uses a lower amount of energy initially, it can also reduce the chances of direct myocardial damage.

10. **(b)** Identification of the "hemodynamically unstable" patient is imperative to proper management. It is necessary to make the decision to treat the patient with electrical therapy rather than drugs initially. Although other indicators may exist, the main four indicators are chest pain, hypotension, pulmonary edema, and altered orientation. These findings clearly identify the patient who is extremely unstable as a result of the tachycardia, and termination of the rhythm is imperative.

11. **(b)** A risk of synchronized cardioversion is the development of ventricular fibrillation. Should this occur during patient management, you should immediately turn off the synchronizing circuit and charge the machine to 200 joules to deliver an asynchronous countershock. Normal patient management would then occur, depending upon the resultant rhythm.

12. **(a)** True. AED use in pediatric patients has always been avoided, but more recently, may be considered as technology allows AED machines to deliver the small energy levels needed for pediatric defibrillation and the incidence of ventricular fibrillation in pediatric patients is greater than once perceived. Despite this, however, it is integral to remember that pediatric cardiac arrests occur commonly because of respiratory complications, and aggressive ventilation and oxygenation should remain a primary management concern.

13. **(b)** This is a false statement for a number of reasons. Implantation of an automatic implantable cardioverter/defibrillator (AICD) does not preclude possible malfunction due to poor batteries, inaccurate sensing of the rhythm, or exhaustion of the preprogrammed number of countershocks. Therefore, you

should administer electrical therapy, as appropriate, to these patients. Remember to avoid placing your paddle directly over the AICD mechanism.

14. **(a)** External cardiac pacing is the preferred treatment for symptomatic brady-cardias. It is quick, doesn't interfere with other interventions, and is highly effective. It may also be considered for asystole and tachydysrhythmias, but these rhythms typically respond better to drugs first. Therefore, pacing in these individuals is indicated for problems that are refractory to other therapies.

15. **(e)** Not only is it important to assure that the pacer is creating a QRS complex, it is obviously necessary for the QRS complex to create a pulse (hence blood flow). The presence of a blood pressure is not a reliable indicator in the patient who already had a pressure before pacing, and the patient may complain of pain from the electrical impulse whether or not it captures.

Chapter 8: Pharmacological Therapy

1. **(c)** Any patient experiencing any type of cardiovascular emergency should initially receive oxygen to help prevent cellular hypoxia. Additional drug therapy (e.g., atropine, nitroglycerin) will be based upon the specific needs or management regimen of the cardiac abnormality. While a sodium chloride IV infusion is appropriate, it should be the 0.9% concentration, rather than the 0.45%, which is actually hypotonic.

2. **(b)** Atropine is known as a vagolytic (or parasympatholytic) drug. As such, it exerts its action by decreasing the degree of vagal stimulation on the heart by inhibiting the actions of acetylcholine (the neurotransmitter of the parasympathetic nervous system). If vagal tone is blocked, the degree of sympathetic tone present should have a more pronounced effect, causing an increase in the heart rate.

3. **(d)** Epinephrine is known to be a relatively equal stimulator of both beta and alpha sites. During cardiac arrest, however, there is profound vasodilation due to hypoxia and the failure of the vasomotor center. Epinephrine administration in this situation will help restore vascular constriction which will increase the systolic pressure generated with compressions. In turn, this will increase cerebral and coronary perfusion.

4. **(a)** Stimulation of alpha adrenergic receptor sites results in smooth muscle contraction. Since the vasculature is composed of smooth muscle, this results in vasoconstriction. Beta stimulation is either beneficial to the heart by increasing its activity (beta 1 stimulation), or promotes smooth muscle relaxation and peripheral vasodilation (beta 2 stimulation). Dopaminergic stimulation results in renal and mesenteric vasodilation. "Synaptic" is not a type of adrenergic stimulation.

5. **(a)** Atropine is a parasympatholytic drug. It will block the vagal tone and allow the sympathetic nervous system stimulation to have a pronounced effect. Since pupillary dilation is caused by sympathetic stimulation, it is an expected side effect of atropine administration because of the blockade to the parasympathetic nervous system. The other listed drugs do not affect the pupils.

6. **(d)** ACE inhibitors are drugs that prevent the formation of angiotensin II in the blood stream, which is a potent vasoconstrictor. Since angiotensin II is blocked, the SVR is reduced, myocardial workload decreases, oxygen requirements diminish, and the disparity between myocardial blood flow and

demand lessens. Ultimately, these promote an environment in which the infarction size may be limited in its developed size. The inhibition of calcium movement across cellular walls to decrease conduction velocity and contraction strength is characteristic of a group of medications known collectively as "calcium channel blockers".

7. **(d)** In clinical trials, the drug procainamide has seen a wide variety of applications. Although this drug's administration method and side effects commonly preclude it from being a first-line agent for rhythm management, it has been shown effective in patients with PSVT refractory to adenosine, wide complex tachycardia, and V-fib refractory to amiodarone and lidocaine.

8. **(a)** Both verapamil and diltiazem are calcium channel blockers, substances that interfere with calcium ionic movement across cellular membranes. This in turn slows conduction velocity and repolarization times and also diminishes the force of muscle contraction. Typically these drugs are used to slow tachycardic rates or to reduce vascular resistance.

9. **(a)** Since verapamil and diltiazem both interfere with calcium movement during the depolarization of a myocardial cell, they slow conduction and prolong the repolarization phase. This makes them beneficial in paroxysmal supraventricular tachycardia (PSVT) rhythms where rate control will help restore the patient to a more normal cardiovascular status. This drug class would be detrimental for the patient with bradycardia, pulmonary edema, or hypotension; it would only aggravate these conditions due to its vasodilitory and cardiosuppressive effects.

10. **(c)** Procainamide's action is most similar to the action of lidocaine. Although their exact actions are slightly different, they are both useful drugs in the management of ventricular irritability. Adenosine and verapamil are primarily for tachydysrhythmic rates, and atropine will increase myocardial activity by diminishing the degree of vagal tone.

11. **(d)** Adenosine is the preferred drug for patients with symptomatic tachydysrhythmias from Wolff-Parkinson-White (WPW) syndrome. Adenosine has a short half-life and does not increase the conduction velocity in the accessory pathway as verapamil does. It is well documented that a WPW patient who receives calcium channel blockers (verapamil or diltiazem) will most likely experience a deterioration of the dysrhythmia. Morphine is used as an analgesic or vasodilator and is not indicated to control tachydysrhythmic rates. The administration of morphine for an unstable PSVT rhythm would most likely be detrimental.

12. **(d)** Diltiazem is the most dissimilar since it is used to control atrial dysrhythmias or hypertension. Magnesium sulfate, lidocaine, and procainamide are used to control ventricular irritability and have no appreciable effect on controlling atrial dysrhythmias. Additionally, among antidysrhythmics, diltiazem is classified as a drug used for rate control while magnesium, lidocaine, and procainamide are classified as drugs used for rhythm control.

13. **(c)** Since epinephrine is both an alpha and a beta adrenergic receptor site stimulator, it may have applications in a variety of cardiac emergencies. For example, it is beneficial in the cardiac arrest patient since it increases vascular tone by alpha stimulation, which in turn increases perfusion pressures. Additionally, being a beta stimulator as well, it has been used to help correct bradydysrhythmic rates unresponsive to more traditional therapy such as atropine and pacing. This drug would be detrimental in the treatment of

hypertension or ventricular irritability since it would only potentiate the irregularity through sympathetic stimulation. Epinephrine is not used for chest pain.

14. **(d)** Sodium bicarbonate administration is indicated in the cardiac arrest patient only after more appropriate therapy (CPR, intubation, drug therapy, defibrillations, etc.) has failed to generate a response. Since the cardiac arrest patient will eventually develop metabolic acidosis, it is indicated only after 10–20 minutes of arrest management to help buffer the increased hydrogen ions. Hypotension is not affected by sodium bicarbonate. Respiratory acidosis is controlled by increasing alveolar ventilation, and hyperkalemia (not hypokalemia) may be benefited by bicarbonate administration.

15. **(c)** Morphine is a narcotic agent which has the ability to reduce both preload and afterload by promoting vascular relaxation. This may be desirable to reduce intramyocardial wall tension and drop oxygen requirements in ischemic tissue during a myocardial infarction (MI). Dopamine is a sympathomimetic which can increase the blood pressure. Procainamide slows conduction velocity in the ventricles which may lead to hypotension, but not from vasodilation. Nitrous oxide is used primarily for its analgesic properties in certain patients with chest pain.

16. **(c)** Diltiazem is a calcium channel blocker which will slow the heart rate and reduce the force of contraction by hampering calcium movement across the cellular membrane during depolarization and contraction. These effects will depress the pumping action of the heart. Atropine, calcium chloride, and epinephrine will increase the pumping action by either increasing the heart rate by blocking vagal tone (atropine), or increasing the force of contraction by supplying additional calcium ions for muscle activity (calcium chloride), or stimulating beta receptor sites (epinephrine).

17. **(a)** At therapeutic doses, lidocaine (a ventricular antidysrhythmic) will have no depressive effect on the contractility of the myocardium. By contrast, diltiazem, a calcium channel blocker, will depress the activity of the heart by interfering with calcium movement. Propranolol and atenolol are both beta blockers, which inhibit the stimulation of beta 1 receptor sites, which in turn will also depress the activity of the myocardium.

18. **(b)** While all the choices are sympathomimetics with varying degrees of alpha stimulation, norepinephrine is primarily (>90%) an alpha site stimulator. Epinephrine is about a 50-50 stimulator of alpha and beta sites, and dopamine stimulates alpha sites primarily at higher infusion rates.

19. **(d)** By the same rationale as for Question 18, the sympathomimetic drugs (epinephrine, norepinephrine, and dopamine) are all vasoconstrictors. They will achieve this effect in varying degrees.

20. **(b)** Dobutamine, a synthetic sympathomimetic drug, has the ability to stimulate both beta and alpha sites according to a dose-dependent response. The major dissimilarity between dopamine and dobutamine is that dobutamine does not stimulate dopaminergic sites; however, dobutamine, like dopamine, does increase renal output by increasing renal perfusion. Atropine is a parasympatholytic drug, isoproterenol is a sympathomimetic drug with primarily beta effects; and metoprolol is a beta blocker.

21. **(d)** Esmolol is a drug that is in the "beta-blocking" category of agents. With this mechanism of action, the net effect of inhibiting beta 1 stimulation is diminishment of cardiac workload and cardiac output.

22. **(a)** Esmolol decreases the sympathetic tone received by the heart. As such, this can help to control stable angina in the patient prone to chest pain from coronary artery disease. If used in hypotension or bradycardia, it would only worsen the patient's clinical status as cardiac output would drop further as a result of the drug administration.

23. **(c)** Digitalis is a drug that slows conduction velocity through the AV node. Although this may interfere with cardiac output, it does not change vascular tone at therapeutic doses. The other drugs mentioned all promote vasodilation, which will diminish preload and systemic vascular resistance.

24. **(d)** Beta blockers decrease, not increase, blood pressure. They also decrease heart contractility and rate, so (a) and (c) are true. As a result, (b) is also true, since a myocardium not working as hard will require less oxygen.

25. **(d)** The problem in congestive heart failure (CHF) arises from a myocardium that cannot efficiently eject its given blood volume. As a result, increased venous hydrostatic pressure results in fluid back-up into the lungs and periphery. Administration of a drug that will increase venous capacitance (nitroglycerin or morphine) will reduce the preload. As a result, the volume of blood delivered to the left ventricle may be more manageable. Additionally, administering a diuretic such as furosemide (Lasix) will help remove excess fluid, also reducing preload. However, verapamil administration will decrease myocardial contractile force by slowing calcium movement, thus making the heart less effective and the CHF more severe.

26. **(b)** The initial dose of verapamil is 2.5 mg IVP. Oxygen is administered at rates from 1 to 15 lpm; the initial IV dose for adenosine is 6 mg, for diltiazem is 0.25 mg/kg.

27. **(b)** Oxygen is always the first drug administered to a patient with cardiovascular instability. To ensure oxygenation, use a nonrebreather mask until blood gases dictate otherwise.

28. **(a)** The standard repeat dose for epinephrine is 1 mg. Higher doses should be considered if several attempts at the traditional dose fail.

29. **(d)** The maximum dose of atropine, when administered for unstable bradycardia, is 0.04 mg/kg. This is not the maximum dose for epinephrine, isoproterenol, or dopamine, although all of these drugs may, at times, be used in the treatment of bradycardia. (See the bradycardia algorithm in Chapter 10.)

30. **(a)** Initially, lidocaine can be administered at a 1–1.5 mg/kg IV bolus. Amiodarone is given at 300 mg IVP for patients in V-fib, and procainamide and magnesium sulfate for the same problem is given at at 20–30 mg/min and 1–2 grams IVP, respectively.

31. **(c)** The initial dose of sodium bicarbonate is 1 milliequivalent per kilogram (1mEq/kg). Epinephrine and atropine can be administered at 1 mg.

32. **(c)** When repeated during ventricular fibrillation, the proper dose of amiodarone is 150 mg IVP.

33. **(b)** The initial bolus for adenosine is 6 mg rapid IVP. Verapamil is 2.5–5 mg IVP, and diltiazem is 0.25 mg/kg.

34. **(d)** None of the given drugs is administered at 10 mg initial bolus for PSVT. Verapamil is 2.5–5 mg; adenosine is 6 mg; and diltiazem is 0.25 mg/kg.

35. **(b)** 1 to 2 grams of magnesium sulfate should be diluted into the D_5W to achieve a therapeutic dose and concentration of the drug.

36. **(a)** Sodium bicarbonate is administered according to its unit of measure, milliequivalents per kilogram (mEq/kg). Lidocaine and diltiazem are given according to the patient's weight in kilograms.

37. **(a)** The initial dose of sodium bicarbonate is 1 mEq/kg.

38. **(d)** Morphine should be administered in 1–3-mg increments IV push, repeated at 5-minute intervals until the desired effect is achieved.

39. **(c)** The initial bolus should be at 8–16 mg/kg of a 10% solution. Responses (a) and (b) would be insufficient.

40. **(b)** The dose range for epinephrine in refractory bradycardia is 2–10 μg/min. The traditional dose of epinephrine is 1 mg, and the the dose range for dopamine is 2–20 μg/kg per minute.

41. **(a)** The effects of dopamine are dose dependent. Lower doses of dopamine (2–5 μg/kg/min) allow for renal dopaminergic stimulation. Moderate doses (5–10 μg/kg/min) cause primarily cardiac beta effects, while high doses (10–20 μg/kg/min) cause alpha vasopressor responses.

42. **(d)** As mentioned in the rationale for question 41, dopamine is dose dependent. As such, in order to promote the alpha effects of dopamine, a higher infusion rate needs to be achieved. Generally speaking, infusion rates of 10–20 micrograms per kilogram per minute promote vasoconstrictive properties.

43. **(c)** The maximum dose of dopamine is 20 μg/kg/min. Both epinephrine and isoproterenol infusion maximums are at 10 μg/min.

44. **(a)** The proper initial dose of amiodarone for ventricular fibrillation is 300 mg given IVP.

45. **(c)** Procainamide is administered at 20–30 mg/min as a loading infusion. After suppression of the dysrhythmia is achieved, a maintenance infusion of procainamide can be started at 1–2 mg/min.

46. **(b)** The proper sublingual dose of nitroglycerin is either 0.3 mg or 0.4 mg, repeated three times. As such, the maximum allowance would either be 0.9 mg or 1.2 mg respectively.

47. **(b)** When administering lidocaine via constant infusion for continued suppression of ventricular ectopy, an appropriate starting dose would be 2 mg/min.

48. **(d)** Vasopressin is a newer drug used in cardiac arrest patients in ventricular fibrillation. It can be administered as an alternative to the first dose of epinephrine since its mechanism of action is the promotion of vasoconstriction. As with epinephrine, this vasoconstriction helps to improve coronary and cerebral blood flow during external cardiac compressions. In the future, vasopressin may also be used for other cardiac arrest rhythms, but clinical trials for this purpose must first demonstrate its applicability to these other situations.

49. **(a)** Furosemide is commonly given at 1 mg/kg for the initial loading dose. As such, in a 55 kg patient, this would be a total of 55 mg of the drug.

50. **(c)** Fibrinolytics work by dissolving newly formed clots within the vasculature. As such, when the embolic clot formation occurs in the heart (MI) or brain (stroke), this type of drug may prove beneficial in restoring blood to the distal capillary beds from the site of occlusion.

Chapter 9: Acute Coronary Syndromes

1. **(a)** Increased afterload with diminished preload would most effectively decrease cardiac output. In this situation, while the heart is receiving less blood to pump, it must also pump against a higher pressure. Therefore, the stroke volume will be lower with a subsequent diminishment in the overall cardiac output. An increased heart rate with unchanged stroke volume would increase cardiac output. A decreased heart rate with increased stroke volume, or increased heart rate with decreased stroke volume will both amount to a cardiac output with no notable increase or decrease.

2. **(b)** The acute MI patient who presents with systemic hypotension and clear lung sounds is most likely suffering an infarction of the right ventricle. A right ventricular MI causes blood to back up in the periphery of the body and not the lungs. Consequently, you would note jugular vein distention (JVD), pedal edema, and clear lung sounds. In light of the systemic hypotension, a left ventricular infarction would most likely manifest itself with adventitious lung sounds as the hydrostatic pressure inside the pulmonary capillaries increases.

3. **(c)** Anything that serves to decrease the heart's workload will also decrease its demand for oxygen. So a decrease in the pressure which the heart must pump against (afterload) will effectively decrease the workload and oxygen demand. An increase in afterload, increase in preload, and increase in contractility all serve to increase the workload of the heart and ultimately raise its demand for oxygen.

4. **(d)** Administration of oxygen works to reverse ischemia and improve function to ischemic tissues of the heart. While the delivery of oxygen can help reverse the damage to some injured cells, it will most likely not restore normal activity in all injured cells. Oxygen administration will not increase the workload of the heart but decrease it as the heart does not have to work as hard to deliver adequate quantities of oxygen to the body and itself.

5. **(a)** The patient suffering the greatest damage will be the patient with an occlusion of the left coronary artery. The higher the occlusion, the greater the number of cardiac cells effectively deprived of oxygenated blood. The left descending and left circumflex coronary arteries are inferior to, and fed by, the left coronary artery. The subclavian artery is not part of the coronary artery system.

6. **(c)** Aberrant conduction of electricity through ischemic and injured tissues is the correct choice. Electrical instability that produces dysrhythmias is the most common cause of death in the acute MI. A myocardial wall rupture can occur but is rare in comparison to electrical dysrhythmias. Infarcted tissue does not conduct electricity at all. Aneurysms can lead to myocardial wall weakening and rupture but, like the ruptures themselves, are relatively rare.

7. **(b)** Of the choices given, the indication that most supports an evaluation of acute myocardial infarction would be the presence of ST elevation in two contiguous leads. Remember, an acute MI can occur in the absence of chest pain, and chest pain can have a non-cardiac cause. Hypotension can have many causes other than MI.

8. **(d)** The provider must suspect an anterior wall MI. The ST elevation in Leads V_3 and V_4 and the shortness of breath, even without chest pain, would seemingly indicate myocardial ischemia occurring in the anterior wall. COPD

should be placed low on the diagnostic list because the ST elevation noted indicates myocardial ischemia. The location of the ST elevation in Leads V_3 and V_4 does not indicate right coronary artery occlusion (this would show up in Leads II, III, and aVF). Remember that myocardial infarctions can occur without the symptom of chest pain.

9. **(a)** While the other choices would lead the practitioner to suspect an MI, the serum enzyme changes and the development of pathologic Q waves confirms an acute MI.

10. **(c)** Based upon the presented information, it would appear that the patient is suffering from a right ventricular wall MI. In the presence of such an infarct, oxygen and aggressive fluid therapy should be initiated in an attempt to stretch the right ventricular wall for a greater contractile response (Starling's Law). This will hopefully increase cardiac output and decrease the chance of severe hypotension and reduced coronary artery perfusion. While the administration of oxygen is correct, it does not represent the best (most complete) choice of the listed items. Nitroglycerin and morphine produce vasodilation. Vasodilation should be strictly avoided, in that this will decrease the amount of fluid returning to the right sided pump and further worsen the situation. Also, beta blockers would serve to decrease the cardiac output by decreasing the heart rate and contractility and should therefore not be employed.

11. **(a)** Even though fibrinolytic therapy dissolves the obstructing clot, the rough atherosclerotic surface upon which the clot formed is still intact. Upon this surface, platelets can collect and form another thrombus. Therefore, the administration of heparin with its anticoagulatory effects would prove beneficial in preventing reformation and in keeping this artery open and patent. Heparin does nothing to lower the preload or decrease the myocardial workload. Also, heparin is an anticoagulant and exerts no action that serves to prevent hemorrhage elsewhere in the body.

12. **(d)** In the presence of an acute MI, warning dysrhythmias such as PVCs usually occur in relation to an underlying abnormality. Therefore, correcting this abnormality will most likely abolish the dysrhythmia. To accomplish this, the provider must give interventions such as oxygen, nitroglycerin, morphine, etc., as a first shot at correcting abnormalities such as hypoxemia or a high state of circulating catecholamines. If these interventions do not abolish the rhythm, only then should specific pharmacological therapy such as lidocaine be initiated.

13. **(a)** Because this patient has a low pulse oximeter reading, a high concentration of oxygen administered by a nonrebreather is prudent. Never withhold oxygen from a patient who needs it! Even in the setting of COPD, a patient with a myocardial infarction needs supplemental oxygen. In the short term emergent setting, the respiratory drive will most likely not be affected.

14. **(b)** Nitroglycerin causes vasodilation, which can effectively decrease the blood pressure along with coronary artery perfusion. If cardiac arrest ensues secondary to the administration of nitroglycerin, relative hypovolemia is most likely the culprit. Therefore, fluid should be administered to bring the coronary perfusion back up to an acceptable level. While placing the patient supine with the legs elevated is a good technique to return blood to the heart, defibrillation should not occur in the presence of PEA. Dopamine may be indicated to raise the blood pressure, but not until fluid therapy is well underway to correct the underlying problem of hypovolemia. CPR is appropriate

but would be ineffective as the sole therapy since it would do nothing to correct the underlying problem.

15. **(b)** The female patient with the transmural MI and stroke 11 months ago would be the most eligible for fibrinolytic therapy. A stroke in general is only a relative contraindication for the administration of fibrinolytic therapy. Only when the stroke has occurred within the last 6 months is fibrinolytic therapy absolutely contraindicated. A diastolic pressure of greater than 110 mmHg, head trauma, and pregnancy are all absolute contraindications to the use of fibrinolytic therapy.

16. **(d)** Ventricular fibrillation occurs with the highest incidence within the first hour of infarction. The remaining dysrhythmias do occur, but with a lower incidence.

17. **(d)** In the cardiogenic shock patient, aggressive airway control via intubation should be attempted, followed by oxygen, dopamine, and norepinephrine if needed.

18. **(b)** Oxygen is the most important drug in the management of the acute MI, because the infarcting heart is oxygen-starved. Oxygen is the drug that is administered first and is indicated in any type of myocardial infarction. While the other medications all play an active role in the treatment of the acute MI, none of them is as universally indicated as is oxygen.

19. **(a)** This patient appears to be in pulmonary edema. Oxygen is always the initial drug of choice for any cardiovascular emergency. As discussed, oxygen can help alleviate chest pain and assist in preventing further infarct that may well worsen the pulmonary edema. While the remaining choices all have application in pulmonary edema, they are not initial interventions, as oxygen is.

Chapter 10: Prehospital Algorithms and Emergency Cardiac Care Protocols

1. **(c)** The most common initial presenting rhythm in the cardiac arrest patient is ventricular fibrillation. Due to the hypoxia and acidosis, the ventricular fibrillation, which is the most viable rhythm for the cardiac arrest patient, will deteriorate within minutes to asystole. Thus, with response times greater than a few minutes, the rhythm will commonly present as asystole.

2. **(a)** Amiodarone cannot be administered down the tracheal tube. Lidocaine, epinephrine, atropine, and naloxone are all acceptable drugs that can be administered tracheally.

3. **(a)** Vasopressin can be used as an alternative vasopressor agent in ventricular fibrillation. The dose is 40 units, and it is administered only once. If the patient remains in cardiac arrest, epinephrine is administered 10 minutes following the vasopressin.

4. **(b)** Administration of sodium bicarbonate is not recommended in a patient suspected to be in hypoxic lactic acidosis. The treatment of choice in this case is intubation and aggressive alveolar ventilation with supplemental oxygen.

5. **(a)** Immediately upon identifying ventricular fibrillation on the monitor, your priority is to defibrillate. Defibrillation terminates ventricular fibrillation. Medications, tracheal intubation, chest compressions, and ventilation are all adjuncts to defibrillation and are contributing factors to how successful the defibrillation might be.

6. **(b)** Upon identification of asystole on the monitor, it is necessary to check another lead to ensure that the patient is still not in ventricular fibrillation. Ventricular fibrillation waves may be more prominent in one lead and very fine in another. Defibrillating the asystolic patient can unnecessarily lead to and increase in parasympathetic tone and worsen the resuscitation efforts. Chest decompression should be considered in a patient in pulseless electrical activity who is suspected of having a tension pneumothorax. Asystole is not a primary indication for sodium bicarbonate administration.

7. **(c)** The treatment of choice to terminate ventricular fibrillation is defibrillation. Defibrillation should not be delayed for any other interventions. You start at the energy level that was last effective in terminating the rhythm, which was 360 joules or the biphasic equivalent in this case. A lidocaine or amiodarone bolus and infusion along with tracheal intubation will follow the defibrillation.

8. **(a)** Amiodarone is administered at 300 mg IV and repeated in 3 to 5 minutes at 150 mg.

9. **(b)** Immediately following the administration of a medication while treating the patient in ventricular fibrillation, you should perform CPR for 30 to 60 seconds, then defibrillate at 360 joules or the biphasic equivalent. The sequence is drug–shock. The drug is thought to reach the core circulation after a 1 to 2 minute period; however, defibrillation should not be delayed for that period of time.

10. **(d)** Possible etiologies of pulseless electrical activity include hypovolemia, hypoxemia, hypoventilation, cardiac tamponade, tension pneumothorax, pericardial tamponade, hypothermia, massive pulmonary embolism, drug overdose, hyperkalemia, acidosis, and massive myocardial infarction.

11. **(b)** Needle thoracentesis or needle decompression is the treatment of choice for the patient in pulseless electrical activity (PEA) secondary to a tension pneumothorax. Administration of medications, fluids, or transcutaneous pacing will not correct the etiology of the PEA.

12. **(c)** The total maximum cumulative dose of atropine in asystole is 0.04 mg/kg. Therefore, the total cumulative dose for a 70 kg patient would be 2.8 mg. A total maximum cumulative dose for the symptomatic bradycardic patient is 0.03 mg/kg.

13. **(a)** Provided the patient is not exhibiting any signs of having (nor is suspected of having) fluid overload, a fluid bolus of 250–500 ml of normal saline is recommended. If the fluid bolus does not reverse the hypotension, or the patient is potentially fluid-overloaded, the administration of dopamine, norepinephrine, and other inotropic and vasopressor agents would be considered a first choice intervention.

14. **(b)** Unless the patient is hypotensive or exhibiting signs and symptoms of hemodynamic instability, leave the rhythm untreated. Supraventricular tachycardias are commonly a result of high amounts of circulating catecholamines following resuscitation.

15. **(c)** Transcutaneous pacing is the intervention of choice in the third-degree heart block patient. Administration of lidocaine can abolish the ventricular rhythm and lead to ventricular asystole and subsequent cardiac arrest. Atropine has little effect on the ventricle; thus it is of no real value in the third-degree block. An epinephrine infusion would follow unsuccessful transcutaneous pacing and dopamine infusion.

16. **(c)** If the external pacer fails to capture, it is necessary to proceed to other pharmacologic interventions. (You will have administered atropine before attempting the pacing.) The next drug of choice is a dopamine infusion beginning at 5 μg/kg/minute and titrating it to the heart rate and blood pressure. If the dopamine fails to work, initiate an epinephrine infusion at 2 to 10 μg/minute.

17. **(b)** The initial treatment of choice for a stable supraventricular tachycardia (SVT) patient is vagal maneuvers. If these fail to convert the rhythm, then adenosine should be administered. If still no conversion occurs, consider the administration of digoxin, beta blockers, diltiazem, and synchronized cardioversion.

18. **(a)** This patient obviously deteriorated from a stable SVT to an unstable SVT. The treatment of choice for the unstable SVT patient is synchronized cardioversion. You can consider sedation prior to cardioverting.

19. **(c)** Management of torsades de pointes (polymorphic ventricular tachycardia) is the administration of magnesium sulfate at 1 to 2 grams IV. Isoproterenol can be used to overdrive the ventricular rate in an attempt to abolish the dysrhythmia. Ventricular antidysrhythmic agents are not a standard treatment for torsades de pointes.

20. **(c)** Amiodarone 150 mg bolus over 10 minutes or at 15 mg/minute is the drug of choice in the monomorphic wide complex tachycardia patient who is presenting with signs or symptoms of congestive heart failure or left ventricular failure.

Chapter 11: Prehospital Cardiac Emergency Scenarios: Application Exercises

1. **(a)** The first step on any scene is to ensure scene safety. If the scene is not safe, you must either make it safe or retreat until the appropriate resources can make it safe.

2. **(d)** The best, easiest, safest, and fastest method of opening the airway in the non-trauma patient is the head-tilt, chin-lift. An oropharyngeal airway and tracheal tube are used to manage the airway after the initial techniques are employed. The chin lift without head tilt is generally used to open the airway in trauma patients.

3. **(c)** The first defibrillatory shock must be delivered within 90 seconds of the arrival of an AED.

4. **(d)** Immediately upon determining unresponsiveness, you must manually open the airway, assess the respiratory status, and check for a pulse.

5. **(b)** You should immediately confirm tube placement by auscultating the chest and epigastrium after inflation of the tracheal tube cuff. Also inspect the chest rise and fall. Pulse oximetry is an unreliable indication of proper tube placement in the patient in cardiac arrest due to the extremely low perfusion state. After confirmation of tube placement, secure the tube and insert a bite block.

6. **(c)** It takes 30–60 seconds for a medication to reach the central circulation during CPR. You should follow any medication administration by a fluid bolus and elevation of the extremity.

7. **(d)** Bretylium is no longer indicated in the treatment of ventricular fibrillation.

8. **(a)** Epinephrine is given in any case of cardiac arrest to increase myocardial and cerebral blood flow during CPR. Amiodarone is indicated for ventricular fibrillation and pulseless ventricular tachycardia. Atropine is indicated for bradycardia and/or asystolic rhythms. Sodium bicarbonate is indicated for the specific treatment of hyperkalemia, or profound metabolic acidosis.

9. **(d)** Cardiac tamponade is a complication of chest trauma. The main signs are distended neck veins, muffled heart tones, bilaterally equal lung sounds, hypotension, and decreased QRS amplitude.

10. **(b)** Asystole typically represents the endpoint of resuscitation efforts. The survival rate of patients in asystole is very low. Continued resuscitation of patients in asystole who do not respond to epinephrine and pacing is considered futile. High dose epinephrine, sodium bicarbonate, and fluid resuscitation are not indicated in the routine management of asystolic patients unless you suspect specific etiologies.

11. **(b)** The initial supplemental oxygen therapy for the suspected acute coronary syndrome patient is guided by the pulse oximetry reading and the physical signs and symptoms of the patient. Remember, it is important to treat the patient. Thus, look for clinical evidence of hypoxia in your patient.

12. **(a)** Magnesium sulfate at 1 to 2 grams is the drug of choice for polymorphic wide complex tachycardia with a prolonged QT interval while in a sinus rhythm.

13. **(c)** The external pacer should be set at 80 beats per minute and the output gradually increased until mechanical capture is accomplished.

14. **(d)** Unstable wide complex tachycardia should be treated with synchronized cardioversion. If a delay to cardioversion is evident, a trial of adenosine can be administered at 6 mg and repeated at 12 mg. However, if the defibrillator is immediately available, synchronized cardioversion must be performed as the first line of treatment.

15. **(b)** Paroxysmal supraventricular tachycardia should be treated with synchronized cardioversion if the patient is unstable or if pharmacologic intervention is not effective.

Chapter 12: Acute Stroke

1. **(d)** An acute ischemic stroke is caused by an interruption in cerebral blood flow that will result in necrosis of tissues distal to the site of interruption. A TIA is a temporary occlusion of a cerebral vessel caused usually by an embolus which the body dissolves, which is why the effects resolve within 24 hours. Finally, a massive acute stroke is capable of causing cardiac arrest, especially if it involves or encroaches on the brain stem.

2. **(a)** A TIA is sometimes referred to as a "warning stroke," because many victims of a TIA will eventually experience an actual acute ischemic stroke. Identifying a TIA is important so additional diagnostic tests can be performed to assess the likelihood of an acute ischemic stroke.

3. **(a)** True. An acute stroke or TIA can potentially occur in any portion of the brain or stem that receives blood flow. The presenting signs and symptoms will vary according to the area affected.

4. **(d)** On the Glasgow Coma Scale, 2 points would be awarded for eye opening to pain; 5 points for localizing the noxious stimulus and moving it away; and 2 points for incomprehensible sounds. The total would be 9.

5. **(a)** Reduction of ICP is an important component of acute stroke management. Without it, ICP may continue to rise and cause additional complications, including death. Controlled hyperventilation at 20 to 24 ventilations/minute has been shown to initially reduce ICP by promoting cerebral vasoconstriction by eliminating excessive carbon dioxide. IV therapy and anticonvulsants have no action that will decrease ICP. Trendelenburg position may actually be harmful since it will inhibit venous drainage from the brain.

6. **(b)** An abrupt onset of a severe headache is most typical etiology of a hemorrhagic stroke. An occlusive stroke, thrombotic or embolic, may present with a headache; however, the onset is usually not as abrupt and the intensity not as severe. The patient typically complains of a "pistol shot" headache or "the worst headache in my life."

7. **(c)** Cheyne-Stokes respirations usually occur when bilateral cerebral hemisphere damage has occurred due to a large hemorrhagic stroke. Central neurogenic hyperventilation results from early herniation or damage to the pons or lower midbrain. Apneustic breathing occurs from lower pontine lesions seen in basilar artery occlusion. Biot's breathing occurs when the medulla is compressed.

8. **(a)** The doll's eye maneuver provides an indication of the integrity of the brainstem. An indication of an intact brainstem is when the eyes remain focused upward when the head is turned; the eyes do not move in the direction of the turned head.

9. **(b)** Fibrinolytics typically must be administered within 3 hours following the onset of signs and symptoms of an acute ischemic stroke.

10. **(c)** Aggressive hypertension management should be considered in the hemorrhagic patient when the blood pressure exceeds 220 mmHg systolic and 120 mmHg diastolic. The hypertension in an embolic and thrombotic stroke typically decreases within a couple of hours after the onset. Reducing the blood pressure in an occlusive stroke may subsequently reduce the cerebral perfusion pressure.

Chapter 13: Special Resuscitation Situations

1. **(e)** A massive hemorrhage can precipitate cardiac arrest from a loss of circulating volume; this in turn reduces perfusion pressures necessary for organ (including the brain and heart) function. Spinal cord injury above C-5 can affect the phrenic nerve which provides innervation of the diaphragm. This paralysis causes hypoxia which can lead to arrest. Tamponade causes a mechanical pressure on the heart which inhibits diastolic filling. Since the heart can only pump as much as it receives, this reduction can also cause arrest. All of these mentioned injures are also common causes of PEA.

2. **(a)** Spinal immobilization is mandatory for any trauma patient until x-rays prove otherwise. Intubation is also necessary but may be achieved orotracheally (which is the preferred method in the arrested patient). IV therapy should be with a volume expander (normal saline or Ringer's lactate), and oxygen therapy should be maximized at 15 liters per minute.

3. **(b)** 20 ml/kg is the proper bolus amount for fluid replacement. This can be repeated as appropriate; just ensure you do not accidentally cause fluid overload or pulmonary edema.

4. **(b)** It is important to recognize patients for whom full resuscitative measures would be futile in order to avoid an unwarranted waste of health care resources. In arrest patients with full body burns, resuscitation is almost always futile. The other listed causes of arrest may be reversible with appropriate treatment.

5. **(d)** While there are many changes in the pregnant female's body, the cardiovascular changes are most likely to interfere with shock recognition. Early signs of shock include tachypnea and tachycardia, and these may go unrecognized since those findings would be expected in the pregnant female. The care provider has to rely heavily on the mechanism of injury to guide initial treatment.

6. **(d)** While all the conditions listed can potentially cause arrest, maternal cardiac arrest is the number one cause of fetal death. Thus, treatment should be aggressive in restoring and maintaining the mother's cardiovascular hemodynamics. Remember that two lives are at risk.

7. **(c)** While lying supine, the gravid uterus puts excessive pressure on the inferior vena cava. Since this can markedly drop cardiac preload, hypotension ensues. Treatment includes displacement of the uterus to the left by rolling the patient to the left 15–20 degrees.

8. **(d)** The treatment of a maternal cardiac arrest will follow the same algorithms and drug dosages as the non-pregnant cardiac arrest. This includes the provision of electrical therapy when appropriate.

9. **(b)** Often, immediately after a lightning strike, the patient is found to be apneic and asystolic. However, the heart recovers more quickly and may restore cardiac activity in the absence of spontaneous respirations. For these patients, then, positive pressure ventilation (with or without intubation) is imperative. The patient will have a better chance of survival if the blood stays oxygenated while the heart stabilizes itself. Failing to do so will lead to a hypoxic arrest.

10. **(c)** The provision of electrical therapy in the victims of a lightning strike is the same as in the normal arrest. The initial defibrillation will start out at 200 joules and progress by steps to 360 joules as a maximum.

11. **(a)** All of the injuries listed are possible as a result of a lightning strike. But respiratory arrest from brain stem depression is the most likely cause of death. Persistent ventricular fibrillation is most likely to be a result of the hypoxia that results from apnea. Trauma and burns are also possible from the strike but usually do not cause as extensive damage as once thought.

12. **(a)** Yes. Since the electricity of a lightning strike can cause violent muscular contractions and the explosive expansion of air can cause the patient to be thrown, spinal immobilization is a good preventative measure until x-rays can rule out associated fractures or spinal injury.

13. **(b)** As a response to hypothermia, the body will begin to slow down its cardiac, respiratory, and metabolic activity. Peripheral vasoconstriction occurs to preserve body heat and to assist in redirecting blood to vital organs.

14. **(a)** As in any patient care situation, the primary concern is your personal safety. An injured health care provider is of no use to the patient and becomes a burden to the other care providers by being added to the injured/sick list. In

any rescue or patient contact, only proceed if you are adequately prepared and equipped to help—without falling victim to the same problem as the patient.

15. **(a)** Because the hypothermic patient has sluggish perfusion to the extremities, movement of IV drugs to the core circulation may be delayed and they may accumulate to toxic levels in the extremities before being "dumped" on the heart as rewarming begins. For this reason, it is recommended that drug administration be delayed until internal rewarming increases the core temperature above 30 degrees C. Because the heart is less responsive to the medications when cold, with a core temp < 30 degrees C, the standard repeat times for the medications should be lengthened. Although a hypothermic heart is less responsive to drugs, the drugs do not become "ineffective." They should not be doubled, since increasing the dosage does not make them "more effective."

16. **(a)** Any patient in cardiac arrest should be intubated with an tracheal tube to secure and control the airway. There is no specific contraindication to intubation for the cardiac arrest patient. Defibrillation, antidote treatment, and NG tube placement are not used on *all* toxicologic arrest patients since those treatments are administered only when appropriate. For example, if the arrested patient is never in V-fib, defibrillation should not be performed.

17. **(e)** Poison Control Centers are a valuable asset to the management of any poisoning or overdose. They have a constantly updated databank which holds the current treatment plans and specific antidotes when appropriate. They also provide tracking of current trends and perform follow-up on patients during recovery. They are accessible in every large community 24 hours a day, usually by a toll free number.

Chapter 14: Special Treatment Considerations in the Prehospital Environment

1. **(d)** The postresuscitation period following cardiac arrest refers to the state of cerebral hypoperfusion that occurs despite the return of spontaneous cardiac output. Regardless of the varied causes, attention needs to be directed to those factors that help limit the postresuscitation syndrome initially and, consequently, influence survivability. The prefix post-, meaning "afterward," is your clue that this is not a syndrome that precedes cardiac arrest; it is not related to chest pain. The syndrome occurs whether or not the patient is otherwise hypotensive. Although it may precipitate seizures, this syndrome is not characterized by seizures.

2. **(e)** Answers a, b, and c are all correct. The goal in limiting the effects of the postresuscitation syndrome is to improve cerebral blood flow and to maintain a balance between the brain's demand for oxygenated blood and the available supply. The necessary steps include glucose regulation to avoid the detrimental effects of hyperglycemia; hyperventilation to help reduce cerebral edema after the arrest and improve oxygenation of the brain cells; and temperature regulation to prevent either hyperthermia (which increases metabolic activity) or hypothermia (which reduces metabolic demand but increases blood viscosity).

3. **(b)** Should a seizure occur during the fragile postresuscitation period, it needs to be terminated, since it can greatly increase cerebral blood flow demands due to the increased metabolic activity. In this instance, seizures are best treated by administering diazepam (Valium) or barbiturates. However, since seizures are not a common occurrence during this phase, automatic prophylactic therapy is not warranted. Lastly, a decision to withhold anticonvulsant medication because of possible ill effects is also not warranted since the seizure is capable of precipitating a cardiac arrest.

4. **(a)** Arterial cannulation is the method of choice when repeated assessments are needed from arterial blood. Arterial puncture is simply the process of passing a needle into the artery to obtain just one sampling. The disadvantage to this is the necessity of making repeated sticks for further sampling. The saphenous vessel is a vein and cannot be used to monitor arterial pressure. If intravascular access is warranted, initiation of an IV through a peripheral vessel is preferred. Finally, pulmonary artery cannulation is actually performed to assess deoxygenated venous blood.

5. **(d)** Adjuncts for artificial circulation assist in the improvement of cardiac output and core perfusion during cardiac arrest, provided the adjuncts are used correctly. The net effects in using one of these devices are the elimination of rescuer fatigue (which also means more personnel available for other tasks) and the reduction in inappropriate compressions due to rescuer error. In conjunction, these considerations stand to improve the hemodynamics of the cardiac output during compressions.

6. **(a)** The safest and most reliable method of assessing the adequacy of compressions now recommended for clinical practice is palpating the carotid pulse. The femoral pulse should be avoided since you may actually feel venous backflow caused by increased intrathoracic pressure from the chest compressions, rather than arterial flow. Monitoring end tidal CO_2 readings shows promise as a means of assessing CPR effectiveness, but research on its usefulness in clinical practice is still being conducted. And lastly, pulse oximetry is usually not an option for a person in cardiac arrest since the perfusion pressures generated during CPR are not great enough to perfuse the distal capillary beds of the extremities.

7. **(b)** False. In light of the increasing understanding of the causes and effects of cardiac arrest and postresuscitation syndrome, more and more therapeutic modalities to improve patient outcome are being tested. So far, technologies and methods have been developed to help improve brain perfusion and prevent some of the ill effects of postresuscitation syndrome. Unfortunately, however, no drug has yet been identified as capable of reversing postresuscitation brain damage.

INDEX

W

Y